Whole Health Shiatsu

Whole Health Shiatsu

Health and Vitality for Everyone

By Shizuko Yamamoto

and

Patrick McCarty

Foreword by Benjamin Spock, M.D.

Japan Publications., Inc.

Note to the reader: Those with health problems are advised to seek the guidance of a qualified medical or psychological professional in addition to qualified macrobiotic teacher before implementing any of the dietary or other approaches presented in this book. It is essential that any reader who has any reason to suspect serious illness seek appropriate medical, nutritional or psychological advice promptly. Neither this nor any other related book should be used as a substitute for qualified care or treatment.

Published by JAPAN PUBLICATIONS, INC., Tokyo and New York

Distributors:
UNITED STATES: *Kodansha America, Inc., through Farrar, Straus & Giroux, 19 Union Square West, New York, N.Y. 10003.* CANADA: *Fitzhenry & Whiteside Ltd., 91 Granton Drive, Richmond Hill, Ontario, L4B 2N5.* BRITISH ISLES AND EUROPEAN CONTINENT: *Premier Book Marketing Ltd., 1 Gower Street, London WC1E 6HA.* AUSTRALIA AND NEW ZEALAND: *Bookwise International, 54 Crittenden Road, Findon, South Australia 5023.* THE FAR EAST AND JAPAN: *Japan Publications Trading Co., Ltd., 1–2–1, Sarugaku-cho, Chiyoda-ku, Tokyo 101.*

First Edition: June 1993

ISBN 0–87040–874–7
LCCC No. 91–076144

Printed in U.S.A.

Foreword

I have to confess that I slid into macrobiotics and shiatsu, in the beginning, without any intention—or even awareness—of what they might mean for me. That is unlike me; all the earlier turns in my life—to become a children's physician, to devote my career particularly to the everyday emotional aspects of child management, to go from pediatric practice to medical school teaching, to branch out into political activism when I realized that the major unsolved problems of childhood (day care, good schools and health care for all, housing, nuclear disarmament, to avoid a holocaust, and to save money for desperate civilian needs)—all these shifts had come from deliberate analysis and planning.

Then a good friend in a neighboring town, suffering from a serious disease, asked my wife Mary to save a date two months hence for an appointment with her health advisor who would be coming from out of town. When the date approached, Mary could not remember just what the therapy or activity was. I guessed it was massage because both Mary and the friend are great enthusiasts.

We were introduced to Dr. Marc Van Cauwenberghe a macrobiotic counselor who is also a doctor of medicine trained in Belgium. He asked for a brief summary of my health history, which included a heart arrhythmia being treated with a pacemaker and digitalis, a mercifully brief stroke for which I was on coumarin, a "blood thinner." I had had a miserable previous year with half a dozen attacks of bronchitis that required antibiotics, and a chronic prostatitis that got me up five times a night and left me sleepy all day. Dr. Van Cauwenberghe noticed that my fingertips were unusually pink and asked how much fluid I consumed. Aerially I answered, "Two or three large iced teas at lunch and the same at dinner." He said my circulation was overloaded with fluid and that iced drinks and caffeine were unwise, too.

I was impressed with the concept of overloaded capillaries and Mary with the interpretation of her muscle aches. We decided to go along with the macrobiotic diets prescribed, basically whole grains, beans, leafy vegetables and seaweeds. No meat (except for occasional white fish), no eggs, no potatoes, no dairy foods. That last item was by far the most painful derivation for me, for I loved butter on my vegetables, half-and-half on my cooked cereal, Brie or saga cheese on my crackers, creamy soups.

The first couple of weeks we felt sorry for ourselves and apologetic to our stomachs. I might have quit, but Mary never compromises on health. Next came tolerance of the diet. Then a positive though moderate enjoyment. But what impressed us and bound us most was the loss of weight—fifteen pounds for Mary and thirty pounds for me along with a good appetite. That proved to the skeptical Western-trained physician in me that something very real and significant was going on, whatever the explanation. My nocturnal trips to the bathroom diminished a lot; I was much more wide awake in the daytime. Most welcome was the abrupt and complete absence of respiratory infections from early September until July. By the way, my fifty-year-old wart has shrunk almost to nothing, as was casually predicted. Most impressive of all to the Western-trained physician was reading *Recalled by Life* by Anthony J. Sattilaro, M.D. and *Recovery* by

Elaine Nussbaum which describe how two people close to death from advanced cancer were able to halt their cancers and then recover robust health with macrobiotics.

Mary was the first to receive barefoot shiatsu massage, from Shizuko Yamamoto the originator of the technique and Patrick McCarty her associate, because her primary problem was a chronically lame upper arm, and because she has always loved and benefited from massage. I had always shied away from it because of my New England uneasiness about self-indulgence and I had had no limb or back pain for many years. But Mary wanted to practice shiatsu on me and I gradually came to accept it—even enjoy it—on this family basis.

So I was thereby prepared to appreciate and enjoy and benefit from the expert shiatsu of Shizuko Yamamoto when she offered it. I was amazed by her strength and delighted with her considerateness. Another occasion when I received whole health shiatsu therapy was when we were staying in the same house with Shizuko and Patrick and they offered me shiatsu mainly because my bad cold was hanging on and I now seemed to have overcome my resistance to receiving treatment thanks to Mary. Patrick added three days of acupuncture and my bronchitis responded dramatically to the two-pronged therapy.

As for my giving shiatsu to Mary Morgan, my 110 pound, 5 foot 2 inch wife, it took me longer to get up the courage. I was afraid of crushing her with my 190 pounds, but she gradually reassured me.

You may have been puzzled—or irritated—by my references to the skepticism of the Western physician. It is not just that the methods of macrobiotics, and shiatsu, and the implication that they can prevent, arrest, or even reverse such dread diseases as cancer and coronary heart disease, in at least some cases, sounds impossible to the Western physician on first acquaintance. Even harder to believe are the macrobiotic explanations of how diseases originate and how they can be cured. There is no obvious connection between anatomy as taught in our medical schools and the "channels" between well defined areas on the surface of the body and the internal organs, which are utilized in shiatsu massage. And macrobiotic leaders point out the marked philosophical contrast between Western physiology and medicine which seems obsessed with dividing, sub-dividing, and analyzing the processes of the body, and Eastern medicine, Chinese and Japanese, which strongly leans toward broad generalizations such as the contrast or balance between yin and yang (expansion versus contraction) which is at the center of the explanations of macrobiotics.

So I am pointing out that most Western physicians have an enormous wall of skepticism to surmount in order to accept macrobiotic and shiatsu concepts. The fact that gradually increasing numbers are succeeding is to me a good sign. The increasing numbers will make it easier, even compulsory for Western physicians to open their minds and to study macrobiotic concepts. If Western medicine and macrobiotics both have validity (and it is hard to see how they could not) the interconnections should become apparent —for the benefit of humanity.

Benjamin Spock, M.D.

Preface

Working with a living master in the traditional healing arts has exposed me to life in ways that I never could have imagined. This is not to say that I may not have discovered much of what I have learned on my own and in other ways, but it has thrown me into the lion's den of life and I have had to scramble, constantly readjusting my position to discover the simplest and quickest solutions to life's way.

From my first introduction to Shizuko Yamamoto in a class with over one hundred students; to observing hundreds of her private counseling sessions; to arranging our classes in the United States and Europe; and our coauthoring books on natural healing and shiatsu, I have learned so much. But that is not the end of it. This exposure has made me uncomfortable. It is not often that you get to work with a master. I feel that I am in a unique position. I have had years of work and discussions with one of world's leading experts in shiatsu. I have had the opportunity to ask Shizuko every question that has ever entered my brain about shiatsu, diet, healing, and health. After having an intimate glimpse of the suffering that so many people experience, and seeing the living proof that indeed there are simple, practical, effective solutions, I am left with a responsibility. My participation in the preparation of this book is a partial fulfillment of that responsibility. To help Shizuko record some of her life's study is a wonderful task. Now students are able to share her secrets.

I remember experiencing a particular feeling more than once while observing Shizuko's private treatment sessions. People in the most desperate conditions come to see her hoping that her advice and treatment will benefit them. On a number of occasions patients labelled "terminal" or "incurable" would suffer through a treatment session. I would sit as an observer taking notes and occasionally assist in one way or another with the treatment. On these intense occasions when the patient was so desperately ill and every treatment technique would bring from them a scream, sigh, or murmur, sweat would bead up on my forehead and roll from my underarms as the electricity in the air was so overwhelming that you would have to be made of stone not to be able to feel the intensity. Pain, anxiety, and fear, emotions the patient may have harbored for years were brought to the surface and exposed. When the treatment session ended and we all could breathe again, the patient would always exhale a sigh of relief as new found life began to flow in their veins. It was obvious that the renewal process had begun. They were lighter and freer. An intense experience had just occurred and without speaking we all knew that it was healing and powerful.

If it is possible to sum up the unique quality that Shizuko Yamamoto possesses that makes this style of shiatsu so valuable, it would have to be the word *simplicity*. Her direct approach to understanding the source of problems and to solutions is refreshing in the complexity of modern living. In a nutshell, Shizuko teaches that the causes of our problems come from not following the way of nature. Of course the solution is to remedy this error.

We in the Western world have created a valley that has separated science and art. We normally view science as superior and tend toward literal interpretations, while in the East, art and its less distinct, intangible, metaphorical views predominate. Jacob Bronowski, mathematician, physicist, and scientist, has said in *The Ascent of Man,* "A popular cliché in philosophy says that science is pure analysis or reductionism, like taking the rainbow to pieces, and art is pure synthesis, putting the rainbow together. This is not so. All imagination begins by analyzing nature." This is so true in *Whole Health Shiatsu.*

In a practical way *Whole Health Shiatsu* gives everyday people and professionals alike the tools to make adjustments to the imbalances that we have created. One tool that has never been included in the shiatsu world before Shizuko Yamamoto's influence has been diet. Her dietary approach adds a dimension to shiatsu that can only be described as phenomenal. With this added tool in the practitioner's bag of tricks, problems that until now have not responded to shiatsu can be affected in a positive way.

This book has been put together to help you understand both the surface and the depths of shiatsu. Understanding your purpose for giving shiatsu treatments as well as understanding diagnosis and techniques make for a well-rounded approach. This is our intention.

For convenience I have taken a literary liberty. Throughout the book I have written in the singular, first person, "I" form. Even though there are two authors we felt that information given from one person would be less distracting and perhaps less confusing.

Because of the seriousness of illness and the usual heaviness surrounding the healing and medical world, we have attempted to lighten the load. You will note the cartoon-like illustrations found in the book. When you begin to study the complexity of tongue diagnosis and look to the accompanying illustration you will be reminded that life actually is joyful and even a bit playful. These illustrations may remind you not to take everything too seriously, especially yourself and your work.

In Chapter 3 of this book we use many Oriental medical words in a capitalized form. The reason for this is so that you do not confuse our use and meaning of the words with common usage. For example the word *spleen* refers to the internal organ located beneath the left rib cage that deals with the immune system. Spleen with a capital *S* refers to the traditional extensive meaning that includes all the functions that Oriental medicine has given to it such as controlling women's menstrual cycles, keeping the blood flow within the confines of blood vessels, serving as the principal digestive organ, and so forth. Whenever you come across capitalized words the meaning goes a bit deeper than is used in daily language.

After studying this book you the reader and student should catch a glimpse of what it is like to be an apprentice of a learned teacher. We hope you find the information presented in *Whole Health Shiatsu* challenging, practical, and useful.

Patrick McCarty
January 1992

Acknowledgments

The people who influenced the writing and completion of this book both directly and indirectly are many. We want to acknowledge our gratitude for the many thousands of people that we have seen in the treatment sessions we have given. Without these patients who have come to us there would be no material nor experience to write about. A special thanks must go to those who allowed us to print their case histories. Their positive lifestyle changes are representative of many who have experienced the power of Whole Health Shiatsu. Thanks to: Elaine Nussbaum, Rosemary Stark, Sarah and Richard Deslauriers, Sophie Regenstein, Lou-Ella Merin, Miriam Hausman, Maggie Dukakis, Lilo Mandel, and Frances Alexander.

Taking the photographs for this book was an immense undertaking. Beginning in southern California with Guy Webster, to New York with Jeff Niki, and back to northern California with Mark Oliver, we sought out the best photographers to help display our technique. Thanks to the expertise of these three professionals the spirit and dimension we had hoped for was indeed captured on film.

Their photographic genius was made a bit easier to display with the cooperation of the many models who worked with us on this project. We would like to thank each of them for the quality of their work and for making our ideas live and breathe. Thanks to: Natalie Wolfe, Tracy Shields, David Hevey, Allison Fiske, Joyce Ostin, Charity Carlin, and Delphine Robertson.

Without a doubt the illustrations in this book will not be overlooked by the reader. Their lightness and humor add a welcomed dimension. Thanks to Dan Fletcher, professional cartoonist of London, for creating such a happy tone.

Thanks also to Meredith McCarty, Karen Bandy, and Laurie Richardson (Arupa) for attending to the many details that facilitated this project.

Mr. Yoshiro Fujiwara of Japan Publications, Inc. was encouraging and helpful in several decision-making details. For your help, thank you very much.

And finally a heartfelt thanks to the people who are the future. Thank you to the growing number of serious teachers of Whole Health Shiatsu who dedicate their time and energy to sharing the information they have learned in order to lighten the burden of others on this planet. In the United States: Edward Spencer, Kerry Loeb, Dale Belvin, Clyde Motosue, Michael Anthony Joutras, Jan Ste. Germaine, Susan Krieger, Joya Sexton, Reneé Kelley. And in Europe: Frans Copers, Gerard Heynan, Simon Brown, Helga Krimphove, Patrick Heckelmann, Rochelle Hood, Janice Jaeger, Michel Bik, Adelbert Nelissen, Danielle Serres, Jaime Bort Anducas, and Aurea Sierra.

Contents

Chapter *1*

The Power of
Whole Health Shiatsu

Clutching her husband's arm as she slowly walked into my office, Elaine Nussbaum did not have more than a glimmer of hope left in her. This was the first time we met in March of 1983. For years she had been suffering with oppressive pain and the complications of uterine cancer that had spread to her spine and lungs. Complications of her illness had depressed her immune system. This affected her kidneys and created an uncomfortable urgency to urinate. She did not look nor feel very well. After checking her vital signs with traditional techniques I applied my style of shiatsu and recommended a variety of foods to be included in her daily diet that included some special dishes and preparations. She had been taking strong chemotherapy at the time without much success. Her body was almost completely debilitated and wracked with pain. Fortunately a major change occurred in this woman. It was not easy for Elaine. She worked and suffered trying to apply the new information she was learning. Because of Elaine's faith in her natural healing abilities and her strength of will she recovered. Against all odds she survived and healed herself. Observing precise age-old techniques that included simple but correct application of my way of life, dietary and shiatsu suggestions, she transformed her body and her life. Now some years later her healing is complete. Her story is unique. I wish I could say that all who attempt to understand and apply this method will be successful. But the truth is life is complicated. However, Elaine's story encourages us never to lose hope and to continue to try. These days she continues to transform herself by helping others who are suffering. She now serves people who, like her former self, live without hope. Her remarkable story is reported in her book, *Recovery: From Cancer to Health through Macrobiotics* (Japan Pablication Inc., 1986). Elaine Nussbaum's story is a magnificent example of the power of Whole Health Shiatsu.

While this remarkable story of recovery is unique the methods used are not. These techniques have ancient and simple beginnings. It started many centuries ago when humans attempted to help their friends and neighbors. This humane activity developed throughout recorded history to become our healing systems. Prompted by the human spirit of invention and compassion, this unending search to maintain health and longevity advanced. Many types of healing evolved, each with the basic aim of alleviating suffering. Even before humans moved out of caves, tribal society recognized healing techniques as a valuable service.

While the aim of alleviating suffering is the primary goal of every healing system, the means by which this is accomplished vary greatly. There exists a diverse view of the cause of illness. Our primitive ancestral cave dwellers had particularly earthy, frequently superstitious reasons for the cause of ill health and disease. When a tribal member fell ill it was because he had angered a god or demon. The cause of a foot infection may very well be the wrath of the angered deity. An extreme example of this superstitious belief system concerned the birth of a new baby. The conception, development, and subsequent delivery of a newborn child was often an unexpected event, delivered to a woman for no apparent reason. As society developed from a nomadic hunter/gatherer existence to an agrarian one many things changed. Since the tribe could supply their food needs without having to move about, society developed stable activities such as advanced agriculture, architecture, a written language, and a different medicine. The foundations for modern ideas and techniques in the healing realm come from ancient civilizations. In the West it was Greece and Rome. And in the East it was China, India, and Persia. These foundations are the basis of the present scientific, non-superstitious methods.

For many people science, an often dry, humorless activity, has become the religion of today. Strictly speaking the word *science* means "a systematized knowledge derived from observation, study, and experimentation." The methods of science are laboratory and field research and the double-blind experiment. The double-blind technique is a method of evaluating the effects of a drug or course of treatment in which neither the subjects nor the researchers know who specifically is receiving the drug or treatment under study. Such information can then be expected to give similar results when administered elsewhere.

This method functions well when the methods of treatment are the administration of medications and to a lesser degree surgery. It is relatively easy to disguise the contents of a pill, and most patients are usually unconscious and therefore less then attentive during surgery. So the patient can easily be fooled into believing they received treatment when in fact they received a placebo or surgically cut open but no actual internal surgery done. What happens when the method of treatment is something other than medication or surgery? Is the double-blind experiment valid then? When research investigates areas outside drug therapy the limitations of a method become obvious. What if the effects of diet and lifestyle are to be looked into? Can foods be disguised and the consumers convinced they are eating the same thing when one group eats hamburger and another oatmeal? Obviously it would be very difficult. What happens in the case of shiatsu, breathing techniques, or acupuncture? Can the patient discern if he or she is being treated or not? Those who have received acupuncture will attest that there always is a sensation while receiving treatment. Under these circumstances it is impossible to construct a double-blind study. It simply cannot be done. Does that fact invalidate their effectiveness?

With the double-blind scientific method an amusing catch-22 situation arises for modern medicine whose stated purpose is to discover truth and to separate fact from fiction. A few years ago after a lecture discussing the use of acupuncture in incurable eye disease, the lecture and slide presentation reported the results of years of research and treatment by Dr. Renald Ching of Hong Kong. Dr. Ching, a Western trained ophthalmologist, began using acupuncture in his medical practice because of the failure of drug therapies to affect retinitis pigmentosa, a degenerative eye disease. His results demonstrate that the disease can be controlled by his therapy. Normally the disease will continue to degenerate until blindness occurs. While not reversed, with Dr. Ching's therapy, the progress of the disease slowed or stopped stabilizing vision at this point.

A mother in the audience asked a local ophthalmologist if he would use Dr. Ching's therapy on her son. There is no known effective treatment. His response was negative.

He could not use the treatment without the results of a double-blind study. When asked if a double-blind experiment was possible with such a treatment method he responded he felt it would be impossible. Like many scientists he was stuck. No experiment could be set up, no testing could be done, therefore he could never accept the treatment although over 2,000 patients' case histories had successfully proved its effectiveness. While shiatsu and acupuncture are medically sound and accepted methods of treatment for over one-quarter of the world's population, the United States considers them experimental. It is an experiment that has been going on for over two and a half thousand years!

Medical research is coming around with the investigation of epidemiological studies. This investigative method measures the prevalence and occurrence of disease and looks into causes of epidemics. It also investigates all the elements contributing to the occurrence or non-occurrence of a disease in a population. The relationship between a diet high in fat and the occurrence of breast cancer in women comes from an epidemiological investigation. The Framingham Heart Study is also an example. This long-term study traced individuals for many years. It proved that dietary fat, exercise, smoking, and other lifestyle aspects played a major role in the occurrence of heart and vessel blockage and therefore heart disease. Another example is Cornell University's work in China in 1990. It is an epidemiological study of grand proportions. After recording the eating habits of over 6,500 Chinese people regarding dietary calories, carbohydrate, fat, and protein contents, initial findings indicate that diet can positively affect cholesterol levels, calcium absorption, reduction of the risk of developing certain kinds of cancers, and help to maintain normal body weight. High cholesterol levels, osteoporosis, heart disease, diabetes, also breast and colon cancers are major problems in the United States and Western Europe while still rare in China. This study points at factors that influence their spread.

While twentieth century medicine lays its foundation on Greek and Roman models such as the work of our friend Hippocrates, the Father of Medicine (460–377 B.C.) and others, there are many fundamentals of these ancient methods that have been excluded in the modern version. The single most important idea, is the idea of the ultimate cause of illness, and human beings' place in the universe. Greek, Roman, Persian, and Oriental medical thought felt that man was not separate from nature. Therefore the occasional occurrence of illness is a natural phenomenon. Less viewed as a curse and more as an inconvenience, it was a reminder that individual or societal behavior and lifestyle needed to be adjusted to correct the condition that was creating the original sickness. While many terms used to describe the older traditional causes of illness such as heat, cold, wind, dampness, and dryness are not medically descriptive to modern scientists and honestly does not make much sense to them, this does not diminish the accuracy such terms convey within their medical model.

Having stood the test of time, many principles and practices from these former civilizations survive today. They have been incorporated into many traditional healing models such as Western herbology and traditional Oriental medicine. These consist of herbs, acupuncture, shiatsu, massage, meditation, visualization and so forth. Also modern holistic healing models combine the rare occasion of patient participation in the healing process—a novel idea.

One modern method based on ancient beginnings stands out in a unique way. It stands out because it reconnects humans with their natural healing power. It gives individuals the information and technique necessary to reestablish equilibrium. It uses the combination of sound dietary practices and a healing touch method. I call this remarkable combination *Macrobiotic* or *Whole Health Shiatsu*. Inherent in this system is the knowledge that individuals are both the creators and healers of their problems. When understood this fact generates a tremendous amount of energy. When applied systematically, this power is a strong healing force. This system is generally easy to understand and even easier to apply.

Whole Health healing includes many unique curative techniques. Among them "shiatsu" or finger pressure relies on traditional medical knowledge still in use today in Japan, Asia, and many Third World countries. This natural approach understands that external environmental elements (such as wind, cold, moisture, heat, dryness, bacteria, virus, yeast, and other microbes) and internal emotional factors (including anger, anxiety, pensiveness, sorrow, pleasure, fear, and terror) cause disease. Exposure of a weary, run-down, or weak person to the previously mentioned physical or emotional elements creates sickness. Simultaneously with external and internal factors, lifestyle also must be included as a cause of disease. Lifestyle, the way you spend your time day after day, has a tremendous effect on health, and subsequently on the possibility of developing illness.

Whole Health Shiatsu treatment focuses not only on eliminating harmful toxins but also on strengthening vitality and the body's resistance to disease. Modern medical treatment, on the other hand, mainly adopts palliative localized treatment. The modern system administers medications that treat the head for headache or that treat the feet for aching feet. This method is accurate only if the source of headaches or aching feet is the specific area in question. If the cause is outside the treated area the treatment will be ineffective or partially effective and may even harm the body by creating new problems with chemical side effects.

Whole Health healing seeks wholeness by applying a whole body treatment because the body is one, interrelated entity. Restoring the body's balance eliminates the cause of headaches or of aching feet. It also restores a sense of humor. This radical or holistic treatment uses not only physical technique, but also diet, breathing, and exercise in therapy. Macrobiotic Whole Health Shiatsu is a powerful approach to health that has stood the test of time. Elaine Nussbaum understood this unique view and applied it in her life. She can smile and testify what a powerful combination natural remedies can be. The understanding and systematic application of this approach is the purpose of this book.

Revolutionary Health Care

Everyone is always in such a great hurry to rid themselves of their illnesses and physical problems. Because of this compulsive hurry and anxiety they may put themselves at the mercy of a doctor or health-care professional whom they have had the fortune or in many cases, the misfortune, to visit. When pain and illness affects them often there is no easy solution to their problem. The patient would like but cannot receive a guarantee of a cure from the physician. If after a series of treatments are attempted and fail, the patient's sense of confidence erodes as he or she begins to understand that medical information and the treatment arsenal is limited by the education and experience of the treater. There are no absolutes in a changing world. Even if the patient knew where to look for other answers, the current medical approach is geared for the alleviation of symptoms rather than fundamental changes. In the unhappy event that treatment does not give the result that you had hoped for, you, the health-care consumer, must live with the results.

Dissatisfaction stems from this reality forcing increasing numbers of people to look seriously for a different approach. With the failure of modern methods to control most cancers coupled with the alarming increase of AIDS and other immune diseases, people are looking for prevention measures, rather than temporary remedies. Many are fed up with the recurring routine of tests, medication, and surgery, only to find their initial problem remains unchanged.

Over the years this type of person has come to visit me as well as other macrobiotic and holistic health care practitioners. They have confided in us and shared their disappointment and frustrations. They have expressed that they have distrust of the current medical establishment. They feel that the current system has nothing to offer them. They have often wondered if there would ever be a solution for them.

The natural state of humanity is to be healthy. It is mainly up to us if we are healthy or sick, happy or sad. We are responsible. No one can cure you. People tend to depend on the doctor too much. They do not realize they can cure themselves. The manner in which we live, especially the way we eat and drink, creates our physical body and mental and emotional states. If we become sick, to a large degree, it is our own fault. The only effective way to achieve a cure is through our will. If the will is in accordance with nature many things are possible. For most people this attitude is both liberating and revolutionary.

With observation we can see there is a definite and distinct order in nature. Nature's power guides all things. When we do not follow nature's order we can become sick. We are often reminded of nature's order by the presence of sickness. Sickness can be our teacher. From a traditional point of view the specific name of an illness is not so important. Physical ailments such as headache, gallbladder pain; emotional states such as anger, depression, irritability; and mental conditions such as paranoia, lack of concentration, and forgetfulness; are all various states of dis-equilibrium or dis-ease. Theorically there is no disease that is incurable, if we are able to change the way we think, eat, and live. Of course, this is easier said than done.

While it may appear that the success or failure of achieving meaningful change is unique for each person, there is a formula. What changes your life is the ability to make decisions. Once a decision is made you must then take consistent action. Here are my four keys which, if followed, will increase your chances of success.

1. Know your outcome. What do you want to accomplish? You must know what you want to achieve it.
2. Get yourself to take action by deciding to do so. Only you can decide to change yourself. So do it!
3. Notice what you are getting from your actions. Are you getting what you want from your action? Are you going in the right direction?
4. If what you are doing is not working, change your approach.

Each individual must depend on their inner strength and commitment to succeed and achieve their goal of sound health and contentment. The following is my personal story. It is an account of my change to a better, healthier way of living. It is a journey that began many years ago.

At one time I was seriously ill. It was when I was in my twenties in Tokyo. My doctors felt that I was very close to having leukemia. I also had vision and eye troubles. I suffered over ten operations trying to correct my eye problem. Even more than the eye troubles generally I just did not feel well. I was in and out of hospitals for three years. After my hospital traumas I stayed at home, almost hiding out for more than eight years. Because of these experiences I lost trust in Western medicine. From my education and upbringing I grew up with a deep sense of trust and confidence in Western ways. After my prolonged experience, I completely lost trust in this approach. Therefore I began looking for some alternative. I was committed to change and I knew what kind of outcome I was looking for. I wanted to be healthy.

While I was living at home with my parents I was introduced to shiatsu (Japanese style of finger-pressure massage). There was an older women, a shiatsu practitioner, who came to the house once a week to give my parents shiatsu treatments. She was an honest and sympathetic person. However at that time I hated the idea of the classical Oriental healing arts. My educational background had trained me to reject such unscientific and primitive nonsense. The problem was that because of my eye trouble and its effect on my neck and shoulder I had a great deal of stiffness and pain. I was deeply uncomfortable and complained to my mother. Finally I relented to my mother's request that I take one of Mrs. Fukumorita's shiatsu treatments. It felt so good! She was a nice person so I could talk to her about what I was going through. From this initial experience I began my study of the Oriental healing arts.

The first step began with my reading a book on Yoga that was given to me by my aunt. This led me to attend Yoga classes. After taking these classes I immediately changed my way of life. I began with my diet. I started by cooking brown rice. I completely stopped eating animal foods, such as meat, chicken, and pork as well as sugar. Not eating sugar was very difficult for me, as I have since discovered is the case for almost everyone. I cooked brown rice, a variety of local vegetables, and sea vegetables. Everyday I would go out and walk a lot. I would do exercises and I began to meditate. In the morning I would open all the windows to let in the fresh air and perform deep breathing exercises for sometime. I practically changed my life overnight. Within one month I felt different. I felt much better.

From there I began to help out and teach at a Yoga training center. I saw many people guiding them with the Yoga exercises that I had learned. The Yoga style that I know has more movement than regular Hatha Yoga. It also includes individual corrective exercises. As I worked with more and more people I could see that each had variations of the same problems. The symptoms appeared to be different. But really the problems were the same. No one knew how to breathe or to move correctly. Each person improved using correct breathing and movement exercises. It was proven to me that if you make simple lifestyle adjustments you can get results. Sometimes students would need some extra help. They would do the Yoga techniques the best they could by themselves but their healing progressed slowly. At such times I would help them with shiatsu. I had taken beginning studies at the Namikoshi and Nishizawa schools of shiatsu. These shiatsu styles relied on the use of the practitioner's hands to do the treatment. While working at the Yoga *dôjô* (training hall) one of my fellow teachers showed me how to use the foot during a partner exercise. After trying it during a shiatsu session I realized that using the feet was easier than using only the hands. I treated my friends with my feet and gradually developed a barefoot shiatsu style that included this foot technique. I never learned about using the feet in a class or school. It naturally evolved.

I continued my search of alternative healing methods with the study of *seitai*. Seitai is a system of guided self-corrective exercises. This study was accomplished with Hideo Noguchi. His techniques are very effective.

I began to incorporate martial art principles into my style after my study of Aikido. Aikido was founded by Morihei Ueshiba and is considered a unique martial art. Through this study not only was I exposed to technical skills but also to universal principles of how nature functions. Realities such as the illusion of conflict and the unification of opposite forces deepened my understanding about the nature of reality. This further helped to develop my shiatsu style. I found the corrective exercises of Yoga particularly useful so I combined them with shiatsu treatment. The two together achieved a much greater response than either one alone.

Fundamentally my initial search in Japan led me to the understanding that the foundation of the macrobiotic diet coupled with corrective exercises and shiatsu had tremendous power to cause change within an individual and the alleviation of suffering. For me this was a revelation. Especially considering my original outlook seeing natural healing techniques as foolish and a waste of time.

For the next ten years I applied myself to understanding traditional healing methods. While I was pursuing my studies of the healing arts in Japan I developed a holistic beauty school. People would come and be introduced to macrobiotic foods, healthful cooking, Yoga, and exercise as well as beauty tips such as facial treatments and cosmetics. The school was developing nicely when my teacher, George Ohsawa suggested that I could be more useful working in America to spread macrobiotics.

I carefully considered Ohsawa's point of view and decided that he was correct. I would go to America. My purpose for coming to America was, following Ohsawa's wishes, to help promote macrobiotic activities. At that time I did not have any plans to do shiatsu treatments. After I arrived in New York there was some legal trouble regarding macrobiotics. Consequently there were not many activities going on. Because of this I decided to work with Gloria Swanson, a famous film star, helping her with macrobiotic cooking. From Gloria Swanson's job I got another job working in a macrobiotic restaurant. While working in the restaurant some employees would complain about stiff neck and shoulders so I would quickly work on them for a few minutes and apparently they felt better because soon I was being asked to do many treatments. The employees would come to me and they told their friends who also would come for treatments. The fact that I was giving shiatsu spread by word of mouth. It was soon after that I began to earn a living from shiatsu.

My treatment style had developed to include both the skills that I had learned from schools in Japan that primarily used the fingers and hands, plus the foot technique from my time at the Yoga center. These two styles along with the technical additions that I invented while working on the people of New York and the use of the macrobiotic diet became the "Barefoot Shiatsu" style.

New Yorkers are hard working people who tend to eat large amounts of beef, pastrami, hot dogs, eggs, and other animal source foods. This excessive consumption of animal protein together with their stressful mental work and lack of physical exercise produces exceptionally stiff, tight bodies. I developed a technique that is specifically directed toward addressing such inflexible conditions.

Technique wise from the beginning I would put a great deal of energy into giving a treatment. As time has progressed and I have seen tens of thousands of patients, the technique has become simpler and simpler. I have always taught this holistic style of treatment that includes diet, breathing, and corrective exercise with shiatsu. Before there were any macrobiotic training schools many young people would gather at Michio and Aveline Kushi's house in Boston and I would spend time sharing my experience with them. We did this many times. I was always treating patients and teaching students what I had learned. Later as interest grew large seminars were developed to share shiatsu with the public. Now many years later this information is being taught around the United States and in Europe. Shiatsu continues to grow and is sought after by many people.

Though I had many physical and emotional troubles, they were all healed. After I made the profound change to macrobiotic living principles my problems were cured. With these changes I developed more of a positive outlook. It has become easier for me to look on the bright side. When I was sick everything appeared negative to me. As my body healed itself I was able to do more work. I became involved in many interesting activities. I was able to forget my personal troubles. I soon began to feel good about things again.

After forty years of living in Tokyo with my parents and friends, life gave me an opportunity to start over. It started with my practice of Yoga and macrobiotics. It has continued with my move to the United States. This process initiated my new life. Before that time I had hardships with my illnesses but I never really had to work hard nor to depend on myself. To break away from my old ways and start a new life really felt good to me.

I feel that human beings who are in really good condition, those who are healthy in body and mind, will naturally have a positive outlook. Even if the environment is difficult and there are many hardships we can have a positive outlook. When your body and mind become weak everything looks bad, even if you are in a great environment. Everything is in a moving balance in nature. As we all belong to nature we are not supposed to have many troubles. If we are healthy, we are able to cope and adjust to the challenges that inevitably affect us all. We have to follow nature's order to survive. When we violate nature's order trouble is sure to come. Most people however, never realize we are part of nature. My experience has proven the truth of this to me. To fundamentally change for the better we must learn from nature. We have no choice. If you do not have the will to change, your life is finished. You will not die right away but you will never change and your physical and emotional miseries will remain. Is this the life you were born to experience? If we as human beings cannot understand the simple message that we belong to nature we will be incapable of curing physical or emotional troubles. Nature created us. We cannot control nature. The key here is "how to discover what is nature's order." As humans, we have lost this sense. We must be able to feel it.

If we can practice self-reflection, meditation, and even honest talking to ourselves, we will discover that we are part of nature. Nature is in us.

Much of the illness that exists today can be traced back to lifestyle. The number one cause of death is heart and vessel disease. This illness is practically 100 percent avoidable with dietary modifications. Although all scientific evidence points out this fact it has not been acted on by either the medical nor lay communities. I suggest that common sense action be taken immediately. This stance appears to be revolutionary. It may be revolutionary as it meets the current needs of a serious problem in an innovative, untried manner. It is my desire that individuals within society take it upon themselves to make appropriate changes. To take a stance individually and act upon it with logic and reason, particularly when it is outside the norm, takes courage. If society is to continue without extreme financial and emotional burdens, significant change must occur. The numbers of people afflicted with serious illnesses are ever increasing. A fundamental and rapid change to preventive health care and holistic techniques is essential to turn around human kind's race toward degeneration. The solution is simple and it can be done. In one of his poems American poet Robert Frost said, "I took the road less traveled and that has made all the difference."

Developing a New Style

Every technical skill evolves over a long period of time. It is tempered by time and experience and honed by trial and error. The development of the Whole Health or Macrobiotic style of Shiatsu is no different. As my story in the previous section describes, my style of shiatsu developed slowly over many years, evolving and changing as life's circumstances changed.

The most important underlying principle of Whole Health Shiatsu is that everyone has the power to heal themselves. This power comes as standard equipment with each human being. However, we can abuse, lose, or enhance this ability. It all depends on how we live our lives.

This style of shiatsu developed to include both the skills that had been learned from formal training in Japan that primarily used the fingers and hands, and an intuitive foot technique. Additionally, beyond the formal training and martial arts exposure, intuition and common sense blend into the technique to make it what it is today. Its principal beauty is that it has a large sense of caring for others, of course, in a very practical way.

- *Principles of Whole Health Macrobiotic Shiatsu*
  1. Health is the natural condition of human beings.
  2. Illness and unhappiness are unnatural conditions.
  3. Health or sickness is not an accident or something without explanation.
  4. Sickness arises from how we live because of our own actions and thoughts.
  5. Food is one of the more important factors in determining sickness.
  6. We should eat foods that grow in our environment.
  7. The strong will naturally help the weak.

8. People will naturally help themselves.
9. Through interaction with others, you naturally develop beyond your limitations of body, mind, and spirit.
10. Purpose of treatment is to stimulate people to go beyond their previous limitations.

Whole Health Shiatsu Technique

Technique wise from the beginning a great deal of physical energy was put into giving a treatment. As time has progressed and tens of thousands of patients have been treated, the technique has become simpler and simpler. Less physical effort is used today, yet the power and effect remains. This holistic style of treatment has always taught the importance of diet, breathing, and corrective exercise with shiatsu. In short, it has always included lifestyle adjustments. One major addition I have included in my style is breathing. Throughout the entire shiatsu session the receiver is continually being asked to open the mouth and lightly breathe out. There is special emphasis on the exhalation. This heightens the relaxation effect of the treatment while at the same time facilitating a more penetrating pressure without pain. It opens the body and flushes out toxins in the tissues and internal organs.

Whole Health Shiatsu was developed by working on rather large, very stiff individuals. When people say that New York is a hard city, you better believe it! As for the future development of Whole Health Shiatsu, it depends on the giver of the treatment. Each giver will naturally develop his or her own style. As long as the principles of Whole Health Shiatsu are followed, the technical style used is of secondary importance. Here are some important things to think about:

1. What can the giver learn from the treatment?
2. What can the receiver learn from the treatment?
3. Without food you cannot live.
4. Receiving treatment does not guarantee success.
5. Techniques should be developed for the benefit of the receiver.
6. Future style development is stimulated by meaningful life encounters.

What Is Whole Health Shiatsu?

In a very practical way every shiatsu session is in reality a lifestyle education session. Sometimes the communication between giver and receiver is verbal but always it is tactile, that is, there is always communication through touch. But what exactly are we communicating? Without a penetrating understanding of Whole Health Shiatsu your work may become a relaxing way to pass time. While relaxing times are often beneficial, is that the main purpose of your session? To deeply understand this complex question let us investigate what Whole Health Macrobiotic Shiatsu is.

Shiatsu is a time-tested healing and balancing technique that uses touch and pressure. However, shiatsu is not only pushing magical points located on the surface of the body. It is a holistic treatment for both giver and receiver. The practitioner's body is the tool that is used. While based on Chinese medical massage, its primary development took place in Japan. It is from Japan that we get the name *shiatsu* meaning literally finger pressure. It has been used as an effective technique to help others who are unwell or suffering from a variety of complaints. Usually shiatsu practitioners never discuss anything other than the most obvious with the receiver. Aspects of the patient's way of life, such as the need for better breathing and exercises, and so forth, are sometimes discussed, but essentially practitioners of shiatsu rarely address the cause of the illness they are treating. One of the fundamental shortcomings with this standard approach is the absence of corrective information concerning diet and lifestyle. The reason the receiver developed trouble is never addressed.

Major Difference in Focus

Whole Health Shiatsu	Other Shiatsu Styles
Preventive health care	Relaxation
Total treatment	Area of concern
Involvement of receiver	Detachment of receiver
Practitioner uses whole body	Practitioner uses mainly hands

In the past, macrobiotic lifestyle and dietary information and the application of shiatsu treatment were usually presented separately. There were few qualified practitioners trained in both arts to adequately apply these health giving practices.

Each aspect, macrobiotic dietetics and shiatsu, are effective, but alone they sometimes are not enough to bring about a total and fundamental change within an individual. Many peoples' defensive and healing power is weak. They are unable to help themselves. Their condition demands they receive help and support from others. In short they need a powerful treatment.

Natural Power

Nature's forces are everywhere. This power is absorbed by healthy people. This same energy flows through the practitioner's body. This energy nourishes and electrifies the receiver's nervous system. It stimulates the correction of imbalances. Former inadequate living habits are corrected by Whole Health Shiatsu. The practitioner is teaching the receiver's body how to correct itself.

There are many books describing shiatsu and other massage techniques. These approaches have the same basic purpose, which is to correct physical imbalance, and I would like to add, to serve and help others. They can all be considered various forms to promote healing. The study and use of these books can be worthwhile. Particularly if they serve as a stepping stone to develop further and evolve the theory and practice of shiatsu.

Shiatsu is based on nature as well as human instinct. The foundation of the finger-pressure system originates in traditional Oriental medical practices. Primarily this comes from traditional Oriental massage with many amendments from the Japanese experience. Nowadays this process has continued with the variety of shiatsu styles that exist. The Whole Health style (also known as Barefoot and Macrobiotic Shiatsu) continues along in this evolutionary development. It is steeped in sound traditional principles yet its application is contemporary. Because of the changing nature of human life, our style of treatment must continually change and evolve so that it too remains an effective and therefore useful tool.

Shiatsu deals with the physical body in a practical way. The body is made from cells, blood, food, air, exercise, and so forth. Therefore we have to think about the total picture. Shiatsu acts like a spark or catalyst to the human body. It stimulates the receiver to realize that they must do what is necessary to maintain and balance their health. Treatment stimulation makes energy flow well within existing channels or energy pathways. The combination of treatment and way of life suggestions form the basis of total care.

We humans are group or social animals. We gain a great deal of happiness when there is harmonious interaction between individuals, family members, friends, and in society as a whole. Families make up society. Every living person came from parents. Each of us owes gratitude for those who have come before us such as our grandparents and parents and, we have the responsibility to care for those who come after us. There is a harmony, a vibration that exists with each relationship.

When a mother pats her crying baby she is demonstrating a distinct form of healing power. The mother's gentle touch is another type of harmony or vibration. Every human has healing power within them. Because our nervous systems are constructed similarly we can expect that every human has some degree of healing power. If this were not true, the first time you cut yourself you would bleed to death. But the fact is for most cuts, without any effort on your part, the body stops the bleeding and the wound heals. Months later there is no sign of the cut, scratch, or scrape. This is natural healing. This power comes from our creator. It comes from nature.

Vibration and Consciousness

Humans have about the same vibrations compared to other animals because our body systems are similar. The combination of digestive organ function mixed with breathing, elimination, immune, reproductive, and nervous system functions work together to produce our individual vibration. Individual differences come about from heredity, environmental influences, and education. What makes for the flavor difference between Canadian, American, and Mexican carrots? What produces the difference between the grapes that become California, French, or Italian wines? The taste difference is because of environment.

Consciousness is a vibration. It is the totality of one's thoughts, feelings, and impressions. With practice the mind can concentrate and focus. These thoughts can be directed and put to use. It is consciousness that sets the direction for shiatsu treatment. The nervous system through an unconscious mechanism directs the body of the giver in the treatment. Because your nervous system and the nervous system of the receiver are similar, the practitioner's fingers and hands as well as the feet are directed in treatment application. These invisible, intuitive commands lead the practitioner to do a correct treatment. Simultaneously, the practitioner perceives the receiver's body consciousness and directs his consciousness to correct imbalances in the receiver. This process occurs at a subtle level.

Antagonistic-Complementary Relationship in Shiatsu

Whole Health Shiatsu is based on the universal principle of antagonism-complementarity. This is demonstrated in the treatment style. While one location on the body is being pushed, another is pulled. The practitioner sometimes appears antagonistic to the receiver for example when he or she guides the receiver to stretch more than they would otherwise like. A complementary action occurs when both giver and receiver inhale and exhale together throughout the treatment. This dynamic interaction mirrors natural motion. For a bird to fly the wings must move both up (the direction they want to go) and down. It is this opposition that creates flight. Using the principle of antagonism-complementarity allows us to successfully treat many difficult cases.

A New Kind of Shiatsu

As the natural flow of a river continues onward from the mountain to the sea so too goes the natural evolution of the healing arts—forever onward. Whole Health Shiatsu corresponds to this natural phenomena. Over the years it has continued to evolve and change. This fact of change plus two very important others make this style a new kind of shiatsu.

The general effectiveness of all styles of shiatsu is being documented and becoming common place. What differentiates Whole Health Shiatsu from other forms of shiatsu? The first of two points is the thrust of Whole Health Shiatsu toward preventive care. Prior and during treatment there is often a long and thoughtful study of all aspects of a patient's condition, physical and mental, ancestral, and even environmental. The idea of an instant cure, such as that promised with drug therapy, is seductive. Often times many illnesses or debilitations are the result of deep-rooted problems and without concise, accurate and sometimes long-term attention by both patient and practitioner, the problem will simply manifest itself again and again, in different forms and in different parts of the body.

Normally in Japan, shiatsu therapy is given to relax the receiver. Because it has been known to lower blood pressure and relax tense muscle in the neck and back, shiatsu is used principally as a de-stressor. Very few practitioners talk to their clients about posture, diet, breathing patterns, and so forth. While I consider this a minor form of preventive therapy, it does not go deep enough.

Preventive medicine should involve two basic approaches. The patient must cultivate proper personal habits of health and hygiene, and the practitioner must detect illnesses to which the patient is prone and treat his vulnerable condition before disease strikes. The first approach includes such measures as proper diet, plenty of exercise, proper breathing, regulated sex life, and other daily preventive routines. We call these the *fundamentals of health*. Changes in season and weather must be met by appropriate adjustments in diet and other routines so that the optimum relative balance of energies within and without the body is maintained. This personal daily approach to preventive care is especially effective in preventing chronic and degenerative diseases from developing. It also raises one's general level of health, vitality, and resistance to infectious diseases.

The second part of the preventive approach depends on the skills of the shiatsu practitioner. The various forms of diagnosis used in Whole Health Shiatsu can detect existing troubles and/or give valuable information about impending troubles that may develop if not attended to. Observation of a patient's skin color, tongue, texture of hair, tone of voice, abdominal condition, bowel and urinary habits, and many other telltale signs give an accurate picture of where the patient has been and perhaps more importantly, where he or she is going. These signs reflect a patient's vulnerability to certain forms of disease long before they strike. If the conditions that make the body vulnerable are corrected early enough, disease is prevented. It is the combined efforts of the skilled practitioner and the diligence of the patient that determines if prevention will be successful.

The other major addition that Whole Health Macrobiotic Shiatsu includes is total treatment. The arsenal of tools used is not limited to acupressure, massage, or body-work. It is from understanding the underlying reasons for ill-health, such as the patient's breathing patterns, emotional changes, dietary preferences, and so on, that we get our direction concerning what must be adjusted in the patient's lifestyle. Besides treating the patient with shiatsu, we must look into the *fundamentals of health* and make appropriate adjustments in these areas also. Therefore a patient's shortsightedness in his or her life outlook is oftentimes pointed out. When inappropriate breathing patterns are noted, appropriate exercises are suggested. Physical movement such as Yoga and walking, dietary recommendations, pointers on relationships, sex, and sleeping patterns are some of the counselling given to the receiver of Whole Health Shiatsu. Any area that is weak is fortified with suggestion and homework. All aspects of an individual's life are treated. This is what we mean by total treatment. This total approach affects the cause of disease by rectifying the energy imbalances and tonifying the weak organs that permit disease to develop. It also adjusts the living patterns that promote the disease in the first place.

The concepts of change, preventive care, and total treatment, traditional in Oriental medicine, are recognized as integral and important elements in Whole Health Shiatsu.

Shiatsu throughout History

Since the beginning of time people have used various styles of touch to try to soothe and heal family and friends. While scholars feel that massage originated in China it is certain that each country throughout the world has developed and passed down their methods for treating the body with the hands. Ancient writings of Egypt, Persia, Greece, Rome, and Oriental countries mention the positive effects from the use of massage.

We instinctively rub, press, pat, or in some way touch when we ache, feel pain, or just do not feel right. Intuitively we are applying self-treatment to try to create a more balanced state. Everyone is qualified to help themselves and with a little effort, are able to help others too. The simple understanding that humans are equipped to heal themselves, and that we can also help others, is the underlying foundation of shiatsu. If we live according to natural laws we really should not have many troubles. Unfortunately we do not consistently live that way and humankind has had to devise ways to deal with the suffering that we create for ourselves. Ultimately to regain wholeness we must change our way of living. There are many tools that we can use in this process. Shiatsu is one of them.

Today, shiatsu, acupuncture, and moxibustion are becoming more prevalent all over the world. Scientists and medical practitioners from both East and West are conducting research and publishing books on shiatsu, while an increasing number of people are seeking shiatsu treatment.

The origin of the Japanese word *shiatsu* is not certain. Over the centuries, information that makes up the shiatsu techniques was gathered through trial and error. The healing techniques that are fundamental to shiatsu probably originated in ancient China, and later came to Japan. Shiatsu is a synthesis of Judo principles, Dô-In (self-massage), and ancient massage. It is an evolving process derived from the unique experience of healers. The first syllable in shiatsu, *shi,* means fingers and the second, *atsu,* indicates pressure. Therefore, shiatsu means "to apply pressure on the body with the fingers." Recently in the West, it has become known as acupressure.

It is only recently that the Japanese government became interested in and recognized shiatsu as a complementary medical practice. In 1955, the Japanese parliament adopted a bill on revised *Amma* treatment (ancient Oriental massage). Thus, for the first time in Japan, shiatsu was given official endorsement. Along with Amma and massage, which had already received recognition, shiatsu was thereafter legally and officially taught in schools. To understand shiatsu, we can compare it with two other healing techniques that involve the touch of a practitioner's hands. These two forms are Amma and massage (of Western origin). Let us examine the theory, practical application, and historical background of these techniques.

Amma (ancient Oriental massage) originated in ancient China and later was introduced to Japan. The first syllable in Amma, *am,* denotes pressure and non-pressure, and the second, *ma,* means rubbing. Amma is a technique of pressing and rubbing the body. During the early part of the Nara period (A.D. 710–784), Amma was recognized by the official medical authorities. Sometime later it lost popularity and in the Edo period (1603–1868), it was revived once again. In 1793, a comprehensive handbook on Amma was completed. It was one component of the Oriental healing arts. Its working principles are based on theories of meridians (channels of energy) and pressure points.

As far back as the fourth or fifth century B.C., written records indicate that Hippocrates, the father of modern Western medicine, advocated massage and exercises for a variety of problems. His prescriptions were used on patients as well as athletes. In Rome, Plutarch records that Julius Caesar had himself pinched all over to cure body pains. It is thought that Julius Caesar suffered from epileptic seizures. Massage undoubtedly helped him cope with his affliction. In the ensuing years, records prove that interest still remained, but in small degree. As the Renaissance flourished in France during the latter half of the sixteenth century, massage was revived. It continued to grow especially in the early nineteenth century in Sweden. Only in the late 1880s was it introduced to Japan, during the middle of the Meiji period. Although the word *massage* is French, it is derived from Arabic, Greek, and/or Hebrew and denotes "rubbing, kneading, touching, and so on." In today's medical world, massage is used as a complementary treatment in widely ranging applications for general health maintenance.

Amma, deeply embedded in the Oriental approach, and "massage," of Western origin, took different courses in their conceptual development. Each evolved by modifying its weaknesses and exploring its strengths. However, there is a strong tendency to consider the two methods as having the same type of applications. Since both Amma and massage have been fully assimilated into Japanese practice, they are administered together rather than independent of each other. In the hands of highly experienced and intuitive practitioners, distinguishing Amma from massage techniques becomes especially difficult.

In the Edo period, the majority of Amma practitioners were blind, and they gave treatments in their patients' homes. By the time Western massage was introduced in the late 1880s, there existed many vocational schools of Amma for the blind all over Japan. Both Amma and massage were taught mostly to this group. Just as the performance of certain Japanese musical instruments was dominated by blind players and therefore, because of their visual limitation did not develop to a high degree, so the development of Amma technique stopped and it became a mere tool for comfort and relaxation.

Unlike Amma, shiatsu was further refined in its working principles and applications. In the beginning of the Taisho period (1920s), shiatsu practitioners adopted some bodywork popular in America (such as chiropractic, occupational therapy, and so on). Tokujirô Namikoshi and the late Shizuto Masunaga are but a few examples of excellent practitioners who continued their research. As a result, today, shiatsu represents Oriental "bodywork." Amma and massage also fall into this category.

In analyzing these three healing techniques, it is clear that all are based on the laws of dynamics. This is a study of motion and reaction produced by external forces. There is a physical law that states that when there is a force exerted on one object there is an equal and opposite force or reaction on a first object by the second. Likewise, when stimulation is applied to the body either as pressing, rubbing, or kneading, the body accordingly produces some internal changes. Detecting these internal reactions, an experienced practitioner then applies other stimulation, which is based on one's intuitive reactions to the internal changes in one's patient. Thus, a practitioner of these techniques applies dynamic stimulation to the patient. All three massage methods promote the circulation of body fluids and regulate the functions of the organs. Physiological reactions to this dynamic stimulation follow the same basic route. In the case of shiatsu, the application of energy force is at one point applied, for example, with the thumb. The pressure is administered rhythmically in varying degrees, so that the recipient feels the compound results of varying applications of pressure. The direct administration of pressure in shiatsu is simpler and more linear than in the other two techniques.

Neither a thorough physical checkup by a doctor of Western medicine, nor a complete laboratory analysis, can adequately diagnose and cure symptoms caused by nervous and mental disorders and the imbalance of the autonomic nervous system. Shiatsu, with other forms of massage, is a system that has developed from centuries of experience, and has proven effective in curing many symptoms. Among these symptoms are headaches, dizziness, ringing in the ears, eyestrain, general fatigue, stiff neck and shoulders, lower backache, constipation, numbness of limbs, chills, flushes, insomnia, and lack of appetite. Shiatsu and related techniques have also proven effective for curing chronic and painful conditions such as high blood pressure, rheumatism, and general neuralgia.

Shiatsu practitioners have long been considered authorities on treating minor diseases in Japan. In general, the Japanese public favors shiatsu treatment and, for many years, these practitioners have played a major role in health maintenance. The previously mentioned forms of massage and shiatsu are wonderful tools for the betterment of health. With the fact that life is forever changing, even these techniques must continue to evolve.

The practice of eating large amounts of animal food has created bodies that are very tight and rigid. To effectively deal with this hard, stiff situation an appropriate shiatsu technique naturally evolved. The Whole Health Shiatsu style (also called Macrobiotic and Barefoot Shiatsu) developed as a response to the Western condition. It is a technique that deals with the common problems that many westerners have. When someone is tight, they need a vigorous style of treatment to loosen them up. Anything less than this will be ineffective and often a waste of time. Do not forget, however, that the aim of treatment is to create balance within the individual. We are always attentive to the needs of the receiver.

This style of shiatsu coordinates the breathing of the giver and the receiver as an important part of the treatment. Breathing together creates a lot of energy that is used in the correcting process. A vigorous style, which includes not only pressing with the hands and thumbs but the use of the giver's whole body, helps to loosen up the stiffness that so many people have. Stretching is also an important element of this style. In the diagnosis segment of a shiatsu session the senses of touch, vision, and smell are used. By understanding the imbalances that are present, accurate way of life recommendations can be made. Recommendations that include diet, breathing and movement exercises, and way of thinking are combined with the shiatsu treatment. In this way the individual can be guided toward wholeness. These methods are used because they are effective. After so many years of treating people I have realized that this style of shiatsu, which deals with the aspects of everyday living, promotes the fastest recovery from illness and suffering. It is also good for the one who gives the treatment.

In sharing shiatsu, you are participating in the healing arts at a high level. The act of treating someone provides a powerful means of personal growth for the practitioner in a similar way that the practice of the martial arts allows an adept's spiritual nature to develop. The essence of shiatsu is love, which is infinitely available. It is no wonder that after a shiatsu session both giver and receiver are smiling.

Distant Cousins—Shiatsu and Acupuncture

Of the many Oriental healing arts shiatsu and acupuncture descend from the same lineage. Like two brothers from the same parents they share origins. Yet, they have distinct personalities and each thinks about life uniquely. Most teachers group the two arts together for convenience. For the public already burdened with details why add to the mental load? This point of view is reasonable. But it is a simplification, a matter of convenience. It is like saying that your brother or sister and you are the same just because you share a similar family name. While such a statement lets us begin to meet the family, we remain ignorant of individual siblings.

What is your favorite musical style? Do you prefer classical, jazz, country and western, rhythm and blues, or rock and roll? Each style creates sound, rhythm, harmony, and melody in addition to pleasure it brings to the listener's ear. Many styles exist. Each has its own personality. Classical music has a distinct tone, feeling, pitch. So does jazz, country, and rock and roll. To appreciate shiatsu and acupuncture let us compare them to music. Acupuncture is similar to the classical style. It has a long history, is grand, powerful, stable, formal, and heady stuff. Like classical music, acupuncture must follow a score, a system. It is fixed and needs lots of training and study. You do not just pick up some needles and go to work. Shiatsu, on the other hand, is more free flowing, less precise. If you are sensitive it is not necessary to follow a score or format. You do not need much formal training and study. If you have the ear or touch you can play right away.

Shiatsu and acupuncture each have their fans. There is even a small group that appreciates and practices both. These arts share the objective of creating harmony and balance. How each accomplishes this goal is unique. I feel it is important not to mix up the two. Here are some distinctions. Historically shiatsu precedes acupuncture so I will discuss it first.

1. Primary focus is developing an intuitive, nurturing approach, with a feminine, Taoist disposition.
2. Shiatsu uses no tools. The practitioner's body is the tool. The practitioner feels free because there is no worry about losing and replacing the tools of the trade. Because there are no tools, there is no expense.
3. Primary concern for treatment is the transformation of the individual. This is ob served in the receiver's consciousness, behavior, and condition of the muscles, bones, and internal organs.
4. Treatment does not foster dependence. Through interaction with the giver, the receiver is encouraged to make adjustments and continue on without external help.
5. The giver of the treatment gets an effect. The practitioner, who uses his or her body to perform the treatment, receives the benefits of physical exercise. There is give-and-take during the session which is satisfying to both parties.

On the other side of the coin acupuncture is highly skilled and must be practiced carefully. Careless use of needles may severely injure the patient. The attitude of acupuncture is closer to modern medicine, with its doctor-patient relationship. Acupuncture treatment involves insertion of very thin stainless steel needles into vital energy points along the meridians or pathways of energy. Acu-points (*tsubo*) are located at hundreds of locations on the skin on the surface of the body. Stimulation of the acu-point is achieved by rotating the needles until a tight, twisting sensation is felt on the needle. It is a perceptible feeling similar to a tugging sensation. When this occurs the practitioner has "caught energy (*decqi* in Chinese)." Every acu-point has specific therapeutic effects on the related organ, specific effects on the body areas covered by the meridian, and a general effect on the body's vital energy throughout the meridian system. Acupuncture is useful in regulating internal dysfunction as well as external painful symptoms in bones, muscles, joints, and skin.

1. Primary focus is adhering to natural laws and technique, with a masculine, Confucian inclination.
2. Acupuncture uses tools. Before metallurgy was invented, stones and shells were used. Without needles, stones or tortoise shell there is no treatment.

3. Primary concern for treatment is the alleviation of symptoms. This is observed by an adjustment of energy within the organs. Harmony between energy pathways and the internal organs is paramount for successful treatment.
4. The patient is dependent on the practitioner for treatment. The technique is so highly skilled only qualified professionals should use it.
5. The practitioner of the treatment does not get much physical stimulation. Usually the giver does get plenty of mental stimulation. At day's end the wise acupuncturist will do some exercises to balance body and mind.

Distinctions between Shiatsu and Acupuncture

Category	Shiatsu	Acupuncture
Movement:	Free flowing	Systematic
Focus:	Intuitive	Adheres to laws
Theoretical Inclination:	Taoist	Confucian
Quality:	Feminine	Masculine
Tools:	Practitioner's body	Needles
Treatment Goal:	Balance—by becoming whole	Balance—by alleviating symptoms
Interacts with Treater:	Yes	No
Encourages		
Independence:	Yes—immediately	Yes—after treatment series
Physically Strengthens		
Receiver:	Yes	Sometimes
Treater:	Yes	No

While differences exist shiatsu and acupuncture share common history too. You should know some of the great history of traditional Chinese medicine—the source of both shiatsu and acupuncture. It is fascinating.

Long ago the combination of myth and fact was blended to produce the longest recorded medical system in existence. Historians date the foundations of Oriental medicine back at least 5,000 years. The early beginnings are attributed to the legendary emperor, Shen Nong (3494 B.C.), who is said to have introduced agriculture to his people and to have become fascinated and intrigued by the apparent medicinal properties of various plants. He tested thousands of plants to discover their effects.

Not having written records the medical information gathered was passed on by word of mouth. This left much room for individual interpretation that led to much superstition and symbolism. Nonetheless, the accurate and what we could call the scientific portion has survived. The Chinese are a practical people and the fact that the volume of information, with all its lore and symbolism, has continued to flourish and survive to this day testifies to its validity as a time honored truth.

Medicine, as with all parts of Chinese society, was entangled in the cultural philosophy and religious spirit. Far from being just a form of medical treatment, medicine was, and still is, firmly planted at the core of a philosophy that encompasses the well-being of the body and the soul. It includes a code of spiritual and social behavior and even an attempt to define the very meaning of life.

Over the centuries Chinese emperors and philosophers developed the concept that man's role in the universe was to understand nature's knowledge of her opposing principles. They developed this concept of opposing natural forces into a code by which man could come to terms with the mystery of life and define his role with that mystery. These opposing principles are seen as the opposing and yet complementary *yin* and *yang* forces of nature, of all matter, of all action and thought, and of all movement. The universe is seen as the result of the interplay of yin and yang forces, of the strong and the passive, the positive and negative.

Further change occurred with the thinking of two of China's greatest philosophers. Confucius (551–479 B.C.) applied the concepts of the interplay of natural change to societal and personal behavior. He formulated a code of rules and ethics that began with the premise that there is a right order and harmony to the universe, based upon a delicate balance of yin and yang forces. Because of these forces, humankind must act morally. He taught that man must exert a force in the eternal cycle of good and evil, by cultivating the virtues of benevolence, justice, propriety, wisdom, and sincerity.

Lao Tsu is considered the father of Taoism. Taking the Confucian teaching of universal order, Lao Tsu taught that man himself can only achieve personal harmony by surrendering to natural order and pursuing a course of inaction. Lao Tsu's message is that striving and interference is unnecessary as things resolve themselves without effort. Taoism essentially deals with the theory of a cosmic law and structure and man's place within that structure. The Tao became the way, or path. Along that path two basic forces struggled in their never-ending embrace—the active yang, and the receptive yin. Their correlation and balance determine the universal order. This includes man himself. Man as the universe on a small scale, contains within himself the same cycle of yin and yang.

From these influences the foundations of natural healing was born. Thousands of years later this ancient information has combined with modern discoveries to produce techniques that encourage total health and vitality for everyone.

George Ohsawa and the Modern Macrobiotic Movement

At first glance, macrobiotics appears to be a new holistic health system. However, the word *macrobiotics* was used many centuries ago to describe people who were healthy and lived a long time. We can say that macrobiotics is the art of living a long and happy life according to the principles of nature. The essence of macrobiotics has existed for thousands of years. More recently, around the turn of the century, these natural principles were revitalized and reintroduced by George Ohsawa (1893–1966). Borrowing its ancient name, this traditional information is again called *macrobiotics*.

The word *macrobiotic* was used by Georges Ohsawa. It is based on the Greek *makro*, which means great, large, or big, and *bios* which means life. Together they form a concept of living a great life of health and longevity. Ohsawa gathered much of his information from Sagen Ishizuka (1850–1910), a medical doctor who investigated and revived the traditional folk medicine of Japan. Ishizuka based much of his treatment on the use of unrefined whole grains, especially brown rice, and a variety of vegetables, notably *daikon* radish. His success and fame was well known around Tokyo. George Ohsawa never met Ishizuka yet his teaching stimulated young Ohsawa to further develop the connection between diet and health.

Because of Ohsawa's tireless work and promotion the dietary, health, and behavior connection has grown far and wide. In his teachings Ohsawa included the idea that individual's and society's actions were based on nutritional foundations. In other words, food is a foundation in creating individual peace and health as well as global peace. In this direction he met with many world leaders discussing this connection.

I worked with Ohsawa closely. Some of my stories may give you some insight into the character of the "father of macrobiotics." I met Ohsawa when he was already over seventy years of age. He usually wore a Japanese *kimono* and was always very busy giving lectures. He was sometimes very cynical but his heart was always warm. We would call him "Papa." People from all over the world sent him things like cheese from France or dark sugar in blocks from the northern part of Japan. Ohsawa took meals together with his students and he would cut the normally forbidden foods and gave one piece to each of us and say, "Let's share poison together."

He really loved to clean. He questioned me once if I liked to clean corners, and asked me to clean the areas that everyone else overlooked when cleaning. He never asked people to do what he would not do himself. Every morning he cleaned the stairs at his apartment. The stairwell was five stories high yet each day he cleaned the steps by hand from top to bottom. He personally never used the stairs—he had an elevator!

Although generally considered an innovative and free thinking individual in some ways he was a very traditional man. He was very much like my father who also was very traditional. But unlike my father George Ohsawa had a depth of insight and more experience. He was very active physically, spiritually, and mentally. He was such an unusual man. It is not often when you meet such a person. In fact, it is extremely rare.

When George Ohsawa died he was alone with his wife Lima Ohsawa. A friend called me and I came right away. His body was reclining and on his face was a brilliance. It appeared so clean looking. We tried to resuscitate him, to bring him back to life but we could not do anything. He was dead. His spirit had already departed.

In Japan when someone dies, you keep vigil over him all night. Though I was the youngest student I felt I should do it. Candles were lighted and I stayed with him throughout the night. Silently I sat, feeling his presence in a room where his normally active body now remained motionless. I will never forget that experience. George Ohsawa died in April of 1966. He was seventy-three years old.

I really felt he was always pushing us. I never considered to come to the United States myself. In 1965 he came back from teaching in the United States and called me and said. "You go to the United States and help macrobiotics in America." I said, "I can't, I have a job." After time passed I finally told him "I would go." I did not think about doing it. I just said "O.K." Of course my parents were against my decision. At that time it was very difficult for a Japanese woman to go abroad alone. I was able to make the trip when Michio Kushi and my father sponsored me. In February 1966 before I left Japan bound for the U.S., my mother also died. I proceeded with my plans anyway and came to America. One year later my father died in November of 1967. That was a very hard year for me, so many deaths. When I received the news of his death there was nothing I could do. I could not go back to Japan to attend his funeral service because I did not have any money.

Since then I saw and met many nice people both in the United States and in Europe. Ohsawa said that you could make as many friends as you wish. He felt with many friends we could spread macrobiotics all over the world.

The philosophical foundations of macrobiotics originate from many sources. Much of current macrobiotic teaching comes from the writings of Ohsawa. Ohsawa was an avid reader, thinker, and idea processor. He could read and write in Japanese, French, and English. He usually read three to five books each day. In addition to gathering dietetic and potassium-sodium relationship information from his teacher Sagen Ishizuka, Ohsawa studied classical Japanese and other Oriental writings. He sought to understand the physical and spiritual causes of suffering. He felt this could be achieved through the study of nature and nature's antagonisms.

Ohsawa discovered the earliest study of duality and yin and yang in ancient classics. It was a time before the noted Chinese sages Confucius and Lao Tsu lived. It is thought that an ancient emperor, Fu Hi, is the originator of the concepts of yin and yang that he developed into the book *I Ching* or *Book of Changes*. In another ancient Chinese classic, *The Yellow Emperor's Classic of Internal Medicine* or *Nei Jing*, there is a dialogue between the emperor and his chief physicians. During these conversations the concepts of yin and yang are further developed. This occurred by at least 500 B.C. Some scholars say even before this date.

From these and other traditional sources such as Indian, native American, and so forth, the philosophical and spiritual foundations have developed. Essentially this process continues. Each level of teacher passing on an essence to the students and these students passing that essence to their students.

Ohsawa left a volume of teaching much of which continues to be pertinent today. He simplified complex ideas. Generally most concepts were reduced to seven principles. Among his favorites were the "Seven Conditions of Health," "The Seven Stages of Sickness," and "The Seven Levels of Judgment."

- *The Seven Conditions of Health*
1. Never exhausted
2. Good appetite
3. Good sleep
4. Good memory
5. Appreciative
6. Selflessness
7. Abides in justice

- *The Seven Stages of Sickness*
1. Fatigue
2. Pain
3. Infectious disease
4. Autonomic nervous system dysfunction
5. Cell and organ diseases
6. Psychological disorders
7. Spiritual disorders

- *The Seven Levels of Judgment*
1. Physical judgment, which is blind, mechanical, responding automatically to external stimuli

2. Sensory or aesthetic judgment, responding to sensory stimulation and classifying according to pleasant, beautiful or ugly

3. Sentimental or emotional judgment, responding to emotion and classifying according to love or hate, like or dislike

4. Intellectual judgment, responding to ideas and concepts and judging them true or untrue

5. Social judgment, responding to patterns of social behavior and organization and judging them beneficial or harmful to society

6. Ideological judgment, responding to ideologies (social, political, economic, philosophical, and so forth) and classifying them as just or unjust, valid or invalid

7. Supreme judgment, which responds to everything with absolute and universal love and compassion that sees harmony in all antagonisms

Ohsawa's Students

Following George Ohsawa have been many of his students who have enlarged the body of information and experience of macrobiotics. In addition to my work on the east coast of the United States is Michio and Aveline Kushi. Situated on the west coast of the United States are Herman and Cornellia Aihara, Noboru Muramoto, Jacques and Yvette De Langre, and Cecile Levin. Each has added their unique flavor to the stew of macrobiotics. But this is not the end of the modern macrobiotic movement. It is only the beginning. The minds of North and South American, European, African, and Asian students continue to investigate and expand upon this thing we call *macrobiotics*.

Health and Illness Today

In the United States we spend more money per capita on health care than any other industrialized nation, yet we rank lower in life expectancy than sixteen other countries, including Japan, Switzerland, Canada, Greece, Great Britain, and Italy! Today you stand a one in two chance of dying of heart disease, and a one in three chance of dying of cancer. One out of every ten dollars spent in America is spent on health care, yet 4,000 people die each day from these diseases alone.

Life expectancy in 1900 was 47.3 years. In the last century, death came early. Mothers and small children were the first to go, and men who made it to adulthood were still likely to get knocked off from infectious disease before the end of middle age. People feared tuberculosis then as they fear cancer today, and as some fear AIDS. Infections that might develop from surgery or accidents could easily prove fatal. Every industrialized nation has passed through this transition. The first phase was reduction in infectious infant and maternal mortality. By 1900 tuberculosis had declined by about 70 percent since 1850.

In the 1920s life expectancy climbed to the late 50 years, high enough to put many people at risk for the chronic killers. By 1930, heart disease had become the leading cause of death, followed closely by cancer. "Half the gain in life expectancy this century had occurred by 1920, and medicine had nothing to do with it," says Dr. Jacob A.

Brody, dean of the school of public health at the University of Illinois at Chicago. In fact, antibiotics were not widely available until the late 1940s. In the early twentieth century, drugs were of questionable value, he says, "There was a famous saying by Oliver Wendell Holmes that if they threw all the drugs in the ocean, it would be better for people and worse for the fishes."

Social interventions, rather than biomedical ones deserve credit for the life extension. Availability of adequate nutrition, of clean water free of sewage, of sufficient housing to prevent crowding and exposure to the elements, and the institution of rudimentary sanitation practices.

By 1986 life expectancy had reached 74.8 for both sexes, 71.3 for men. For the individual the risk of most cancer or arthritis was no greater for the 65 years old in 1960 than it had been in 1920. For coronary artery disease and lung cancer, the age-specific risk of death actually rose and then later declined. There are some exceptions to these trends. One such group, the Seventh Day adventists, live nearly a decade longer than other residents. From viewing lifestyle factors it appears exercise made the greatest contribution to their life expectancy, adding nearly five years among men: vegetarianism added more than 3.5 years; and obesity subtracted two years.

The average 70 to 74 years old, who has a life expectancy of 13.6 years more years, can expect to be disabled for more than five of those years. The most feared condition affecting senior citizens is Alzheimer's disease. It has been called the disease of the twenty-first century. The 2.5 million victims cost 45 billion dollars a year, nearly 10 percent of which is spent annually on all health care. The average person over 65 years old uses 4,000 dollars worth of health care a year compared with 1,100 dollars worth for someone under 65 years old.

The idea that our modern diet is a major triumph for humanity stands in direct conflict with the health of those who are eating it. Affluent countries like the United States suffer a host of medical conditions that marginally affect the rest of the world. A partial list of the most common illnesses of civilization follows: arthritis, atherosclerosis, heart attacks, strokes, high blood pressure, obesity, diabetes, hypoglycemia, gout, kidney stones, osteoporosis, multiple sclerosis, psoriasis, gallbladder disease, allergies, tooth decay, hemorrhoids, colitis, chronic diarrhea, diverticulitis, and a variety of cancers such as breast, colon, prostate, ovary, kidney, uterine, testicle, pancreas, and lymphoma. The people living in underdeveloped countries suffer mostly from illnesses caused by starvation and poor sanitation. These two basic health problems have been largely resolved by modern technology.

Think about how the technologically advanced health care system that has developed in the United States affects your health care. A major player, the drug industry, makes up a huge component of the medical system and has been an aggressive business since the early days of its existence. It spends hundreds of millions of dollars each year on trying to persuade doctors and layman of the benefits of their products. As a society we encourage researchers to look for drugs as the solution, rather than changing our lifestyle and preventing the problem in the first place. We read about the new genetic breakthroughs and drugs that are going to change our lives, yet as a nation we are becoming flabbier, fatter, and less healthy day after day!

Some treatment methods that are in vogue give cause for consideration. The current opinion of the best treatment method becomes the standard used. Methods outside the accepted standard invite trouble. This conformity breeds a sluggishness to innovation. For example, the death rate for breast cancer has not changed during the past seventy-five years. From 150,000 to 175,000 women are diagnosed with breast cancer each year in the United States. It is estimated that one out of nine women will develop breast cancer. None of the diverse treatment protocols such as surgery, radiation, and chemotherapy have produced any significant advantage in terms of survival time. As length of life cannot be increased by present day breast cancer surgical therapies a simple lumpectomy (lump removal) is as effective as a radical mastectomy (breast amputation). Yet in the United States more than 100,000 women annually, on the advice of their doctors, accept mastectomy. Dr. William Kelley, stated in *Business Week*, 22 September 1986, "Often while making a biopsy, the malignant tumor is cut across, which tends to spread or accelerate the growth. Needle biopsies can accomplish the same tragic results…. Of the nearly 1 million Americans diagnosed with cancer each year, only half will be alive in five years. Surgery, radiation, and highly toxic drugs all tend to fail for a stunningly simple reason: a tumor the size of your thumb has 1 billion malignant cells in it. Even if a treatment gets 99.99 percent of them, a million remain to take root all over again."

The United States General Accounting Office (GAO) released a study of how the survival of breast cancer patients has changed since the introduction of adjuvant chemotherapy. The February 1989 GAO report entitled "Breast Cancer—Patients Survival," focused on premenopausal, node-positive, Stage II breast cancer patients because this group was acknowledged to benefit most from chemotherapy. Despite a threefold increase in the use of chemotherapy since 1975 (23 to 69 percent), there has been no detectable increase in survival for the patients who should have benefitted most from the advent of this therapy. Dr. Alan Levin of the University of California stated: "Most cancer patients in this country die of chemotherapy…. Women with breast cancer are likely to die faster with chemotherapy than without it."

Radiation severely damages bodily systems, and various studies have shown that it offers no survival advantage. Radiation therapy following breast surgery may actually increase death rates, according to a study reported in *The Lancet* (British Medical Journal). Other studies suggest that women who receive no treatment whatsoever survive longer than those who receive any method of treatment.

Are we winning the war on cancer? The most common cancers, cancers of the lungs, colon, breast, prostate, pancreas, and ovary, together account for most cancer deaths. The death rate from these cancers has either stayed the same, or increased during the past fifty years. Every thirty seconds another American is diagnosed as having cancer. In November 1985, Dr. John Cairns of the Harvard School of Public Health, writing in *Scientific American*, found no significant gains against the primary cancers since the 1950s. He estimated that only 2 to 3 percent of the nearly half-million Americans afflicted with cancer every year were being saved by chemotherapy. Virtually all chemotherapy drugs are toxic. Many of them have devastating side effects and weaken the immune system. Many of them are carcinogenic. Typical cancer patients spend 25,000 dollars in their treatments. Every minute, another American dies of cancer. That is 1,440 deaths daily.

American women fear and suffer from osteoporosis (softening of the bones). The standard treatment for this debilitating illness is estrogen therapy. Hormone pills do stop bone loss, but they increase the risk of developing uterine cancer by fourteen times.

Statistics demonstrate that women in countries (such as Asia and Africa) that do not consume high amounts of protein and dairy products do not have osteoporosis.

Many people believe that when the inevitable heart attack occurs (remember one in two have a chance of dying of heart disease) they will submit to coronary artery bypass surgery. A lifetime of eating meat, eggs, cheese, and other fats damages the arteries causing a hardening that diminishes blood flow. At a critical stage blockage occurs and the heart is deprived of oxygen causing a heart attack. Coronary heart disease accounts for over 700,000 deaths annually in the United States. At an average cost of 25,000 dollars over 200,000 people receive bypass surgery each year. That is 5 billion dollars per year. What are we buying for 5 billion dollars? The five-year survival rate for by-pass surgery patients and those who only used diet is essentially the same (90 percent). Until recently very few patients were educated about the cause of the hardening in the first place. Nor were they instructed in preventive measures to increase their survival. The primary factors in developing hardening of the arteries are, first, dietary habits, which we can control, and second, heredity, which we can do nothing about. Secondary factors, which are also very important and need our attention, include smoking, obesity, high blood pressure, physical inactivity, and emotional stress.

The study of human populations has enabled reasonable estimates to be made of the proportion of cancers in the population that result from food. As was reported in the *San Francisco Chronicle* about 40 percent of fatal cancers in American men can be attributed to food factors, and about 60 percent in women. Dietary change would produce a 90 percent reduction in deaths from cancer of the stomach and large intestine, a 50 percent reduction from cancer of the uterus, the gallbladder, the pancreas, and the breast, a 20 percent reduction from cancer of the bladder, the cervix, the mouth and the esophagus; and a 10 percent reduction in deaths from cancer arising at other sites.

The financial burden heaped on the physical and emotional destruction caused by the AIDS epidemic is staggering. Governmental agencies predict that treatment and care costs may bankrupt social and medical services. AIDS is the leading cause of death for men between the ages of 35 and 44.

Environmental pollution escalates worldwide. Air and water quality is in a deplorable state. Exceptionally high rates of childhood leukemia exists in several towns of California's San Joaquin valley, the source of most of the fresh produce of the United States. Water from the areas where illness is highest contain high levels of toxic chemicals. The same chemicals that are used as fertilizers, herbicides, and pesticides. Officially, in many places the water is declared contaminated and undrinkable. One official for the Environmental Protection Agency of the U.S. government stated on public television that he would not drink the water. A similar situation has occurred in Massachusetts and to one degree or another this process is occurring nation wide.

The infrastructure of many of America's major cities such as New York and Boston, are deteriorating. Roads, bridges, sewage, public water works are falling apart faster than cities can afford to replace them. Crime makes walking on the street dangerous. Parents are frightened to allow children outside to play in New York because of the violence and insanity. It is the children who suffer as they appear to be under house arrest. In Los Angeles children are confined indoors because of the unhealthy air quality. It appears that many stalwarts of American civilization are tumbling. Is there hope for the future? Can anything be done?

Fig. 1 Scene of Toxic Material and Drugs in the Ocean with Dead Fish

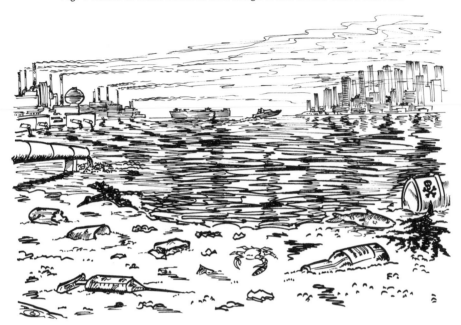

What could possibly destroy such a powerful force—our modern civilization? The answer is simple. Mankind, each of us, is destroying the things we hold so dear. Yet the majority of destruction is not done consciously. Rather deterioration continues from ignorance and inaction. If only man could see the obvious and change his direction, how can we change our direction? The fact is each individual decision shapes the direction of our destiny. Everyday decisions about what you eat, which products you buy, how you use your body, what thoughts you think on a consistent basis. These decisions lead to *actions*, setting a *cause* in motion, creating an *effect* that builds on the day before, moving you in a mental and physical *direction*. And every direction has an ultimate *destiny*.

In a practical sense every individual's consciousness is the source of trouble. Our way of thinking mainly stems from over-reliance on other people, the government, and the medical profession to name a few sources. A big question we need to ask is where does our way of thinking come from? While every answer will be incomplete there are several sources that greatly influence us. Of primary importance is how we were reared by our parents. How parents live serves as a model for us. The things they valued or disliked are observed by us as youngsters and without doubt has made some influence on us. How we were treated by them educates us in relationships, love, marriage, and how to deal with other people. Outside the family other sources also exist. These include the physical environment such as living in the city or countryside. If you were reared in a small town your world-view will be different from someone reared in Chicago or Europe. The type of education you received lays a foundation for how you think. If the educational system you attended (or you may not have attended formal schools) was public or privately run, or if your schools were in a free society or a socialist society, your outlook and way of thinking may have certain distinctions. Your daily life including your workplace, number of children, satisfaction level, ability to travel or not, molds your thoughts. The individual must reeducate himself to change his consciousness. Because we live in society we have to help each other. Investigating the *fundamentals of health* provides a focus for change. With all the world's problems that exist, the realms where solutions can be found are not infinite. They are limited. They are manageable. As human beings we must take responsibility for the world we are creating. If we look into the time periods that make up our day to day life we can discover the sources of our problems and therefore the solutions. One question remains, "Do we have the strength to investigate?"

Chapter 2

Daily Living

Fundamentals of Health

Longevity has always been the most prized and respected achievement among Oriental as well as other world peoples. The ideal longevity picture, however, does not envision years spent in wheelchairs and old-age clinics. Nor does it include enduring sexual impotence, the inability to digest food properly, irritating nervous disorders, senility, and other common realities of old age. A human being deserves to live out their years with dignity, health, and vitality, remaining fully active and alert to the end. Is there a method to ensure longevity? Or at least is there a way to live the present moment in reasonably good fashion while laying a foundation for golden quality years?

Although most of us at one time feel that abundant energy and good health should be our birthright, we soon discover that this is rarely true. Being in good health and maintaining that state takes constant attention and diligent work. We can all think of someone close to us who suffers from some chronic or serious illness. We may wonder, is it possible to prevent these problems?

How long do you expect to live? Remember life expectancy is an average of 74.8 years in the United States. Unfortunately many people never think about such a practical question. If you do think about it the logic of planning how to survive becomes obvious.

Genetic inheritance, education, and job activities throughout life build not only one's character, but also one's body. Food, drink, emotions, stress, and what we think add to the body chemistry and make us who we are. We are a combination of our family genes and environment.

In addition to our family heritage and growth environment, the things that we do throughout the day are extremely important in helping to shape our wellness picture. These day-to-day activities can be considered our fundamentals of health. These aspects of living are the cornerstones upon which our health and vitality rests. If we care for the foundation, all which is built upon it will withstand the storms of life. It is the little everyday things in life that are important and have the possibility of bringing the greatest happiness.

In seeking to solve the many problems that affect us we habitually use the same methods and techniques which have created the problem in the first place. For example when someone has chronic back pain they tend to hold themselves in a misaligned way thereby adding to the continuation of their misery. They may use special back support devices or other direct methods which affect only the back. When this approach does not bring about the expected relief back surgery is recommended and usually accepted. The sufferer has a condition and wants a direct solution for their specific problem. However without considering the cause of the back condition, the direct solution may miss the mark and be unsuccessful at changing the condition. There are preexisting habits that promote our troubles.

Our aim is to discover a method of dealing with the problem of habit and change. From the previous example we discover that our assumption of directly trying to change the back's condition by using support devices or surgery may be ineffective. We may realize that this assumption is illusory and that a fundamental change of habit can only be achieved by considering the organism as a whole. Our changes successfully come only by indirect means. Instead of going directly for our end goal (the relief of back pain), we have to first discover and inhibit the habitual response. In order to ensure that the habitual response remains inhibited we have to practice the projection of conscious direction. In other words we have to be attentive to those things that we do day-to-day.

Imbalance in these day-to-day components is the source of chronic and acute problems. In an opposite way, correct adjustment in these areas can lead to solutions. You may want to carefully observe how you think, breathe, eat, move, sleep, and maintain relationships, for these are the six fundamentals of health. Within these realms lie success or failure in your physical health and emotional happiness. To better understand the significance of these fundamentals let us look at each one and discover how it relates to your overall health picture.

Fig. 2 Circle with Six Fundamentals Displayed

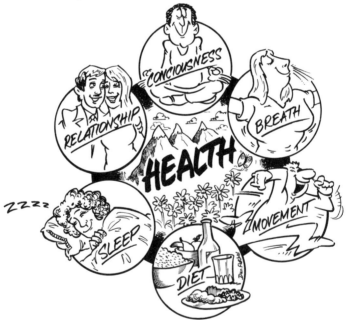

Thinking

The brain is the origin of the central nervous system that rests inside the skull. It is the body's most important organ because it acts as the central computer or corporate headquarters that processes information and gives direction to the other parts of the body. Perceptions, observations, and decisions that lead to action process through the brain.

Each personal decision from rolling out of bed in the morning to deciding if you should marry, is a small electrical charge circulating through the brain's trillions of cells.

The autonomic nervous system, that portion of the nervous system over which there is no voluntary or conscious control, begins at the back of the eyes and travels down the spine to the tailbone. It communicates with all the internal organs, blood vessels, glands (producers of hormones and body secretions), and the skin. Autonomic nervous system dysfunction creates most of the chronic degenerative illness that we witness today. Maintaining balance within the autonomic nervous and central nervous systems is the principal purpose of studying and applying the fundamentals of health.

It is my belief that each individual's blood quality influences their thoughts and thinking patterns; organ function and structure; and hormone production and distribution. Also, blood quality is dependent on the fundamentals of health. To what degree you follow nature's order determines your health level.

Let us begin our investigation with the most important of the fundamentals—how we think. Thinking reflects our beliefs, judgments, prejudices, as well as positive and negative experiences. How we think lays the foundation for how we feel about life. Human nature is full of riddles and contradictions. For every person on the face of the planet there is a unique view of life. No two people think alike. Thinking rules the world. Even possession of the same thinking machinery does not guarantee uniformity or sameness of thought.

All thoughts and body functions are processed by the brain. It serves as the central control office. Located in the head, which is the uppermost or most yin part of the body, the brain function coordinates all physical movement, thinking, and emotions. All body parts are affected by its condition. Likewise, the condition of the body has an effect on the brain. We know that nourishment from food creates blood. The quality of our blood influences the quality of our thinking. The brain and body are inseparable, but it is the brain that determines the direction of the rest of the body.

Messages from the brain to the body and from the body to the brain pass through the neck. It is the neck that acts as the connection. It is important that the neck is flexible, relaxed, and in proper condition.

Our sense organs can be considered receptors of stimuli from the external environment. They transmit the messages they receive to the brain and to the meridian system within the body. The brain's function is to sort, store, and send the messages it receives. Oriental medicine states that every part of the body communicates with other parts through the meridian system. Because of this connection, emotions produced in the brain in response to various stimuli, can be responsible for disturbing the function of any part of the body. The emotions of anger, fear, worry, excitability, depression, anxiety, joy, and so forth have definite effects on the rest of the body. The example of the worried person who develops stomach ulcers is all too plain. If an imbalance of yin and yang exists in either the brain and/or body, a problem will develop. Excessive emotion takes its toll on the body.

The physical brain influences thinking and judgment. The ancient memory of our heritage, as well as the current, immediate learned memory is influenced by the condition and the quality of the brain. Our will, sense of direction, and happiness are the total of the functions of the body, mind, and spirit. If our thinking is to be truly clear and accurate, we cannot overlook the brain. One humorous example of a clear mind is an anonymous quotation that says, "The average girl would rather have beauty than brains because she knows that the average man can see much better than he can think."

Modern thinking has many shortcomings. People's conversations fill with attitudes expressing low self-esteem. The streets of New York are filled with individuals who display irresponsible behavior and manners, while simultaneously shouting loudly that no one cares for them. From the thousands of people who come to see me I have noticed negative thinking patterns that I feel are worth mentioning. These are the most common thoughts that preoccupy and possess us. They warp and destroy the first of the six fundamentals of health—thinking.

1. *Dependence*. Most humans are over-dependent. They are dependent on their doctor, teachers, parents, accountants, and whoever else they listen to. Without the ability to think for ourselves, life cannot be elevated beyond a level of slavery.
2. *Fear*. People are afraid of the uncertainty of what they do not know as well as the certainty of what they do. Many people think all pain is bad and fear the sensations and soul searching that accompany healing. They are afraid of being uncomfortable as the body and emotions adjust. This fear stops progress and they become stuck, experiencing discomfort and pain—the very conditions they feared.
3. *Unrealistic Expectations*. Everyone wants to change fast. Yesterday is too late. They want to throw all their problems out the window and be done with them immediately. They forget that we belong to nature and must follow nature's timetable.
4. *Separation*. Humans are not separate from nature. Many people believing otherwise want to avoid the reality of their lives. They would like to pretend they are separate from their surroundings and circumstances. This separation creates schizophrenia and paranoia. The beauty of separation, of course, is that you feel no accountability or responsibility for what you do. This gives the illusion of freedom but, it only brings pain.
5. *Short-term Orientation*. Infants, children, elderly, and seriously sick people are indulged, to a small degree, in their need for immediate satisfaction of their demands. But as mature healthy adults we should learn that sometimes we postpone immediate pleasure for an assumed greater pleasure in the future. Many people whom I counsel are interested only in the relief of their symptoms. They are not interested in understanding the mechanism of how the problem arose in the first place nor are they interested in curative methods that are dependent on doing something now for effects in the future. They do not understand the total process of healing nor do they understand how life works. For others the idea of prevention lacks meaning. Why change when you are feeling fine? This is short-term thinking. Its shortsightedness will be discovered in the long-term.
6. *Depression*. At some point many people feel life is too big for them. This way of thinking is dangerous because once settled into the mind and emotions all external stimuli are accepted and screened by a depressed brain. The depressed brain uses all stimuli to support the validity of its depression. In other words a hole is dug and it can only get deeper.

What is correct thinking? There is no correct thinking. Yet, there is a correct relationship you can have with your thoughts. If you feel comfortable with thoughts that enter your mind, probably your thinking process goes smoothly. When disturbing or challenging thoughts enter, the thinker influenced by nature searches for their complementary message or silver lining. When we are healthy we are fearless and tireless, filled with contentment, energy, and optimism.

If this is not so, I have a few suggestions. I have found the following process useful in dealing with physical, mental, or emotional challenges. This takes the form of a conversation where you can talk honestly to yourself. This creates an opportunity to listen. My first declaration to myself is the realization that "my condition is not right." When I confirm this is true I continue, " I must do something about it." Notice I did not say, "Why is this happening to me," or "If only I had… " (you fill the blank). Often doing something means stopping what you were doing in the first place. This means doing nothing. After I realize that I am the responsible one who must act, I think, "However I respond, it must be a natural solution." As the examination process continues I remind myself that "no matter how long the solution takes I won't become impatient nor get upset." Through this process we have the opportunity to investigate the factors that allow us to make solid decisions without regret. This is a natural movement of thinking. This may lead you to discussions with professional counselors, doctors, friends, or it may lead you to change your diet, quit smoking, change your job, or move to a deserted island. The point is, our thinking process should be our ally. The content of our thoughts and belief system is our life.

How do you use your brain? What do you think about? There are hidden, almost unconscious behaviors that tip the scales between frustration and fulfillment, pleasure and pain. These unseen influences are: perception of time and personal priorities. Beliefs that we carry with us. When these two areas are better understood we will have clarity about the pressures of time.

The perception of time is a critical, yet an often overlooked issue in most people's lives. Ordinarily people do not think of themselves as past-, present-, or future- oriented. Psychologists know that one's view of the past, present, or future is an unseen determinant of one's relationship to time. Studies have shown that 57 percent chose a balance between present and future, 33 percent were more future-oriented, 9 percent were present-focused, and 1 percent preferred to live in the past. Those with future orientations considered themselves "planners"; individuals with present orientations lived in the moment and, by choice, avoided planning or thinking ahead.

The type of job you choose relates to your relationship with time and how you use time. Not unexpectedly, managers, teachers, and other white-collar types were more future-oriented with semiskilled individuals more present-centered.

Understanding Your Thinking

Time perspective has a direct bearing on one's perception of the need for time management. Your time orientation exerts either a push toward success or a pull toward complacency. A future-oriented individual in a managerial position understands goals, deadlines, and the need to squeeze a lot into very little time. Someone with a present or past perspective placed in a managerial position, no matter how many time-management classes he or she takes, may never grasp the complexities of getting organized.

This imbalance between what is expected and what your tendency is, creates frustration. This is a very good reason you may dislike your job or marriage.

Time Perception as Thought

There is yet another unseen area that influences how your life is organized. Psychologists refer to this component as a "priority base." Most of us tend to have one important base, or focus, around which our decisions are made. If work is the priority and perceived as more important than home, then decisions will benefit office first, and leftover time will be reserved for home. Everyone has a target, priority base, or frame of reference around which thinking and decisions are formulated. Research has shown the four main priority bases are: home; work; home/work combination; and social/extra curricula.

Individuals who are home-based think and organize in a way that maximizes their time at home with their family. They do not do less work than their colleagues; still, if there is an opportunity to manage a group of activities to give them time at home, they will do so. These people tend to be married and place a high value on time spent with family. Many are self-employed or in jobs that allow them to work from their homes. Compared to the other three groups, these "home bodies" tend to be happier and more satisfied.

Individuals who organize their time around work obviously spend much time in that environment. Work is clearly the center of their personal universe. Not only is their work of high quality, but high quantity as well. As a result, they make more money than the three other groups.

Those individuals who have a balance between work and home rarely do anything else. Their management decisions are not as prejudiced as those who prefer either home to office or vice versa. They are managing their time in a way that gives them the best of both worlds. Research suggests both work at home and office is characterized by both quality and quantity, with little differentiation.

Finally, there are those who organize their life with little thought of home or office. These people set priorities sporadically, based on scattered social obligations. No one place forms the center of their world. They express neither high-quality nor high-quantity time at home or work. They float and prefer to organize their time around numerous social activities that are spontaneous. Generally speaking, this group tends to be less content with their life than any of the others. Because there is no single focus, priority, or base, these people tend to have more of a problem managing time.

No matter how much you enjoy your office or work, it is a good idea to end the day with some type of diversion. The brain and mind need to take a "mental-health break." This will give you space and the extra momentum you need for tomorrow.

To understand thinking more accurately, you may want to discover three things. First, what is your time perspective? Do you have past-, present-, or future-orientation? Next, identify why certain beliefs make you react? Have you consciously decided what to think or are you acting on other's beliefs? Are you filled with prejudice or fear and have no idea where these ideas came from or why they are in your head? Finally, implement behavioral changes that maximize your understanding of how you think. If you get angry every time the conversation turns to money, examine your beliefs about money and be creative with actions that will free you of this burden. When you deposit money into a savings fund and feel good about it you may gain insight into one kind of behavior that nourishes your stability. Watching reactions and thoughts to actions informs us of basic core beliefs. The natural state of thinking is to be like a boat floating on the ocean. We are meant to be relaxed and happy.

Breathing

Breathing is an important part of maintaining vibrant health. Yet we never think of it. It is the most important ingredient for our nutrition. We get proteins, vitamins, carbohydrates, and fats from food, but without air, we would not get much value from the foods that we eat. Without the oxygen that is found in air (about 20 percent), food will not energize our bodies, just as fire, without air, will not burn. Oxygen combines with the carbon and hydrogen furnished by food. These reactions generate heat and provide the living organism with energy for physical work, as well as for the many other processes essential for life, such as digestion, growth, and brain function. Breathing exhales carbon dioxide, which if not eliminated, builds up in the body, causing the tissue fluids to be too acid. To live, we must breathe.

This fundamental need begins from the day we are born. Since then we have continuously inhaled and exhaled hundreds of millions of times. Breathing is a natural part of living. The body is equipped, without effort, to breathe. Breathing means survival. It is a wonderful system. We inhale oxygen from the external environment, which comes from plants and exhale carbon dioxide, which plants thrive on. The environment creates air. Plants and living creatures need the opposite to survive. We need each other. It is important to have nature around us.

Have you ever noticed the three distinct parts of breathing and their effects? They are inhalation, exhalation, and the space between. When you are absorbed in the suspense or drama of a film you find yourself holding your breath. This is the space between.

Three Divisions of Breathing

Action	Result
Inhale	Tension/Contraction
Hold	Concentration of force
Exhale	Relaxation/Expansion

Breathing and the Causes of Illness

Deep breathing is the best way to maintain health. A long, deep, full inhalation and exhalation will expand and contract the lungs. These two opposite motions make a balanced breathing rhythm. The breath is a combination of yin and yang forces in cooperation. It is the balance of the autonomic nervous system with the sympathetic and parasympathetic branches that affects the functions of the internal organs. It is breathing, to a large degree, which affects the nervous system and therefore the functioning of all the other internal organs. Breathing affects the quality of blood through digestion and assimilation. Breathing is also tied to elimination. Abdominal breathing and exhalation are connected with blood circulation. The long, deep, rhythmical breath supplies both essential oxygen to body cells and mental stability. Only when the breath is calm can the mind be calm.

Inhalation expands the lungs creating a degree of tension within the body. This activates the nervous system. Our exhalation contracts the lungs, thereby relaxing nerve activity and loosening a tense body. Holding your breath makes for mental concentration and forceful body movement but at the same time it can create rigidity. If you feel tense often, emphasize your exhalation more—consciously make it a little longer than the inhalation. Make it longer and stronger. You can do this at any time. If you can control your breathing you can become really free.

Abdominal Breathing

While lying flat on the floor on your back put your right hand on your abdomen and left hand on your chest. While slowly inhaling, push out your abdomen (like a pregnant woman) and let your right hand visibly rise. Then exhale through pursed lips and slowly press your abdomen in toward your backbone. Repeat exercise while slowly raising and lowering legs, one at a time, to strengthen the abdominal muscles.

The daily practice of breathing exercises will improve general well-being. Try to spend time practicing each day. Practice deep breathing while walking and working. But, first, become consciously aware of your breathing by practicing the following exercise. You can then integrate this correct breathing into your daily life.

Sit with your back straight either in a chair or on the floor with your legs crossed in any posture that is comfortable. Relax your thinking and let the thoughts just drift off. Let your shoulders, then your arms, neck, and head become relaxed. Keep your eyes only half open with your gaze about five feet in front of you on the floor. Breathe only through your nose. Make your inhalation and exhalation the same length. Mentally, you can feel your whole body breathing, not just the nose and lungs. Practice this for as long as you like, up to twenty minutes at a time.

We cannot live without air for more than six or seven minutes. With deep breathing, we get over seven times the normal volume of oxygen. This means that we enrich the blood with oxygen and vitality, which, in turn, brings even more energy and essential life-force. In the case of cancer, abnormal cells do not like oxygen. According to Dr. Otto H. Warburg, winner of the Nobel Prize in medicine, cancer results from the increase of carbon monoxide due to oxygen insufficiency (hypoxia). Cancer cells thrive in an unclean environment. Cancer patients feel much better when they combine proper diet, breathing, exercise, and physical movement. Even if they do only a little while lying in bed, there are positive effects.

Heart disease and high blood pressure are also linked to how we breathe. Insufficient oxygen makes the pulse rate increase. Hold your breath for one minute taking your pulse before and after to discover the truth of this. The lack of oxygen will cause an instant change in the way your heart works. In the long term, our ability to obtain and deliver adequate amounts of oxygen to the cells, tissues, and organs is the main determinant of just how long we can expect to live. Of all the factors contributing to life span, lung function has the best positive correlation, greater even than the correlations of blood cholesterol levels or smoking with longevity. This documented finding suggests that oxygen deficiency currently is the measurable factor that most limits length of life.

Breathing and Emotions

For centuries the breath, body, and mind connections have been recognized by healing systems. In India yogis taught the importance of breath control for mind control and longevity. In Japan focus on the breath is used extensively to calm the mind while performing traditional arts such as calligraphy, Judo, archery, Aikido, tea ceremony, and Zen meditation. In China the Taoists taught breathing practices not only to focus, which would extend life but also to strengthen sexual power.

Because we are humans we think. There seems no end to our worries, jealousies, and negativity (unless of course the thinking process is in order). The welling up of emotion instantly creates a response in breathing. It changes from normal and relaxed to irregular and health threatening. When we are worried, our breathing is shallow, coming only from our chest. At this time we emphasize inhaling. When we are angry, our breathing becomes rough. When we are surprised, power goes into our inhalation, and when relaxed, the exhaling breath becomes long. When we disagree, we take short breaths. Rapid breathing is a signal that something is wrong; both our physical and mental powers are weak at this time.

Emotion and breathing are inseparable. If we are trained to breathe correctly, when times of stress arrive, we will be prepared to calm the emotion and mind with the breath. The violent emotion will subside, leaving us in a state of calm and clarity. Laughing is the best way to loosen up. When you feel unhappy, force yourself to laugh. As ridiculous as it sounds and as uncooperative as you will be at the time, try it. The strong exhalation of laughter changes the emotion.

The richness of the blood is the basis of the entire body's health, and the blood can be called rich only if it contains the necessary amount of oxygen and other nutrients. This comes from proper breathing, whole natural foods, and exercise.

Eating

At some level we realize that the purpose of maintaining a healthy lifestyle is to enjoy the unlimited opportunities afforded us on this planet. Each of us has a destiny—things we would like to do this lifetime. Of course, this requires a body to do them. Like any piece of equipment or machinery a fuel is needed. The prudent mechanic is aware of the quality and quantity of the fuel he uses. Our physical body requires at least as much consideration.

Unfortunately the question "why do we eat?" has to be raised. I say "unfortunately" because our choices in food have created pain, discomfort, and disease. Without grasping why we choose to eat the way we do, we are doomed to suffer. It is estimated that 70 percent of cancers are linked to diet. Almost 100 percent of heart and vessel disease is caused by the things we eat. If we include arthritis, asthma, allergies and so forth, we are beginning to speak of large numbers of people with chronic, degenerative, and life-threatening illnesses, most of which are related to diet. If you understand why you eat you may be in a position to prevent these troubles. If you do not understand, you will not be able to change.

There are two reasons for eating. The most basic reason is survival. If we do not eat, we do not live. The body has an appetite so that when the fuel reserves run low a message will remind you to refill. All creatures share this basic level. The second reason we eat is for pleasure. Variations of eating for pleasure are: to satisfy cravings for taste and texture, for emotional connections (such as chocolate from a lover), to satisfy frustration or celebrate success. Each of these categories in a straight forward or distorted way brings pleasure. If we eat only for pleasure, making healthful changes is extremely difficult.

From the study of the structure of human teeth, scientists have hypothesized that humankind has eaten a combination of foods. People are mixed eaters. The majority of our thirty-two teeth display a fondness for vegetables. The eight incisors cut carrots and cabbage while the twelve molars and eight premolars chop and grind onions and brown rice. In a minority position are the four canines whose function is best suited for ripping and tearing flesh and meat. Apparently, even as a mixed eater we have survived to the present day on a diet consisting of a large percentage of vegetables supplemented with much smaller amounts of meat.

Long surviving cultures, such as the Persian, Jewish, Chinese, and Indian, developed dietary and eating regulations to support and prolong life. These cultures used food in two ways, day-to-day eating—which serves to prevent illness, and eating to adjust an imbalance—which serves to cure illness. If the first, preventive eating, is successful, there is no need of the second. However, if you eat for pleasure alone, you will be in great need of curative eating.

Food Is Sacred

The combined energy of sun, earth, water, and seed power join to materialize as food. The source of this energy is from infinity. Energy is processed and packaged by nature. Condensed yin and yang energy allows us to survive.

- Food meets our physical needs. The calories, protein, and so forth keep the body functioning.
- Food meets our mental needs. Thinking clarity, memory, and alertness result from correct type and volume of foods.
- Food meets our spiritual needs. The fact that we eat and survive instills gratitude and thankfulness that we are provided for. This realization of dependence frees us. It generates a compassion to help others.

Food Classification

In the realms of both preventive and curative eating there is a classification system that we use. The yin and yang system comes from the Oriental experience beginning with ancient China. The medical quality of each food is described from several points of view. Food is analyzed by its nature, taste, movement, meridian it affects, yin-yang balance, organ it affects, and elemental influence it possesses.

Nature: hot, warm, cool, and cold
Taste: salty, pungent, bitter, sweet, and sour
Direction: ascending, descending, floating, and sinking
Meridian: enters one or more of the fourteen meridians
Yin-Yang Balance: each food is predominately yin or yang
Organs: affects one or more of the hollow and solid organs
Element: water, metal, fire, earth, and wood

It is a wonderful system with great attention to detail. But, it has the draw back that it is complicated, sometimes contradictory, and usually confusing for the inexperienced. The effects of food can be to strengthen, cleanse, nourish, and accumulate energy. By combining different qualities we can set a direction to stimulate the internal function, thereby correcting imbalance. The energy of preventing and healing illness comes from a variety of factors including diet. It is of little use to think that health is secured by one element, nutrient, or food. In other words, when you read that sea vegetables nourish the hair, do not limit this to mean that if you ate only *nori* seaweed that your hair would be wonderful. What it means is that within a balanced lifestyle, nori, together with other fundamentals of health, influences hair in a positive way.

Macrobiotic Eating

Macrobiotics has reduced, condensed, and greatly simplified the ancient teachings of Oriental medicine. The qualities of individual foods are summarized into a yin-yang classification. For the public comprehending and correctly using the details of the Oriental system are overwhelming. The macrobiotic system, when applied at the family level, is easier to use. Like any system, to become proficient, we must become avid students. We also must guard against repeating information that we do not know to be true. We must discover for ourselves what is true.

Foods recommended in the macrobiotic way of eating encompass a variety of textures and tastes. Variety in your choices should bring complete satisfaction in your eating. Delicious dishes can be prepared using the ingredients listed below.

Whole grains are the most important foods in a macrobiotic diet. Also included are beans, root vegetables, round vegetables such as pumpkin and squash, and hardy, green leafy vegetables. Soups, nuts, seeds, sea vegetables, fruits, and fish are also included.

Whole grains: whole wheat, millet, brown rice, rye, barley, oats, buckwheat, and corn. These can be used in their whole form or as flour in foods such as breads, tortillas, chapatis, and noodles.
Vegetables: Brussels sprouts, kale, watercress, mustard and collard greens, Chinese cabbage, red and green cabbage, bok choy and sprouts, string beans, broccoli, cauliflower, beans (e.g., lentils, garbanzo, navy, pinto, *azuki*, and black), winter squash, pumpkins, acorn and buttercup squash, leeks, scallions, onions, turnips, carrots, rutabagas
Soup: miso, *tamari* soy sauce, vegetable, or bean soups
Sea vegetables: dulse, nori*, wakame, kombu, arame, hijiki*, agar-agar, Irish moss and sea palm

Fruits: apples, cherries, pears, strawberries, chestnuts, berries, and others
Nuts: walnuts, almonds, hazelnuts, and others
Seeds: pumpkin, sunflower, sesame, squash
Fish: sole, snapper, cod, trout, and other white-meat fish
Beverages: nonstimulating teas such as twig, barley, toasted brown rice and corn, mild herbal teas, vegetable and fruit juices

The emphasis of whole health eating is on fresh, unrefined foods. Foods that do not fall into this category should be reduced or eliminated. Refined foods include white flour and sugar. Refined foods are without essential power. Even with sophisticated laboratory technology it is impossible to isolate all the vitamins and minerals necessary for life. However, eating a balanced diet of whole foods, which are natural sources of all vitamins and minerals, assures us of all our requirements. Wholesome foods should be ones grown in the climate in which you live. Temperate zone people, as in the United States and Europe, should be eating carrots, cauliflower, turnips, kale, onions, squash, garbanzo beans, apples, pears, strawberries, and so forth, bananas, papayas, and other foods that are tropical in origin are therefore not suitable for people living in temperate climates.

Animal proteins like beef, chicken, pork, lamb, turkey, and eggs, also all forms of dairy products (milk, cream, butter, cheese, cottage cheese, ice cream, yogurt, and kefir), should be minimized or avoided. The high-fat content, as well as the antibiotics that the animal has received, is damaging to humans.

Besides the animal fats found in beef and butter, other forms of fat are best avoided. These include lard, shortening, and margarine. Poor-quality blended or refined oils should not be used. These fatty items create a stickiness that causes red blood cells to lump together. Clumps of cells have less surface area than individual cells and therefore, less opportunity to carry oxygen and nutrients to the body's internal organs. A common symptom of sticky blood is fatigue.

Artificial foods should be avoided. This includes the flavoring, coloring, and preserving agents that are in all instant foods. Artificial sweeteners, as well as sugar, brown sugar, turbinado sugar, honey, molasses, and corn syrup, should be avoided.

Alcoholic beverage consumption should be limited and occasional. Soft drinks and artificially sweetened juices and drinks should be completely avoided. Care should be taken with the use of stimulating teas and coffee.

Effects of Alcohol
- Alcohol is a sedative-depressant of the central nervous system.
- It is capable of rupturing veins.
- It does not warm you up in the long run, but causes you to feel colder by increasing perspiration and body heat loss.
- It destroys brain cells by causing the withdrawal of necessary water from them.
- It can deplete the body of vitamin B_1, B_2, B_6, B_{12}, folic acid, vitamin C, vitamin K, zinc, magnesium, and potassium.
- Four drinks a day are capable of causing organ damage.
- It can hamper the liver's ability to process fat.

The Effects of Coffee

The daily cup or in many cases cups of java has become a worldwide routine. Without this ritual morning eye opener much of Western civilization may grind to a halt. The aroma and mystique of coffee drinking is often associated with leisure days lounging in European or bohemian coffee shops at a time when life left more space to ponder its mysteries. Or for some coffee drinking has become an addictive substance that is as much a part of living as breathing. For those who are confirmed coffee drinkers, this subject is certainly not neutral. Since many are going to drink coffee anyway they may as well learn what it is doing to them.

Caffeine and the Body

Although one of the world's favorite beverages, caffeine can be considered a drug. Caffeine acts directly upon the central nervous system. It brings about an almost immediate sense of clearer thought and lessens fatigue. It stimulates the release of stored sugar from the liver, which accounts for the "lift" coffee, cola, and chocolate (the caffeine big three) give. But these benefits may be far outweighed by the side effects. The release of stored sugar places heavy stress on the endocrine system. Heavy coffee drinkers often develop nervousness or become jittery. Coffee-drinking housewives demonstrated symptoms typical of drug withdrawal when switched to a decaffeinated beverage. Caffeine intake has been linked to benign breast disease and prostate problems. Medical research reports there is a strong relationship between coffee consumption and cancer of the bladder and the lower urinary tract.

People who drink five cups of coffee daily have a 50 percent greater chance of having heart attacks than noncoffee drinkers. Caffeine consumption can initiate symptoms of loss of appetite, weight loss, irritability, insomnia, feelings of flushing, chills, and sometimes a low fever. Scientists have shown that caffeine can interfere with DNA replication. Studies have shown that the amount of caffeine contained in about four cups of coffee per day causes birth defects in test animals.

Eating Guidelines

Common sense tells us that we should eat smaller portions and eliminate junk food if we are serious about maintaining vibrant health and preventing illness. A well-balanced meal mixes well in the stomach, digests easily, and is distributed rapidly throughout the system. For this reason macrobiotic food feels light and energizing.

Confirming the macrobiotic view, a growing body of medical evidence points to seed foods as a significant protection from disease. The National Academy of Science has stated that the incidence of breast cancer, colon cancer, and prostate cancer could be cut substantially if Americans ate more "seed foods." Other scientific studies corroborate these findings. Seed foods include all whole grains such as whole wheat, brown rice, and barley; beans such as kidney, lentils, and chick-peas; and commonly known seeds such as sesame, sunflower, and pumpkin. Studies have shown that seed foods contain protease inhibitors that appear to have a protective, anticancer effect.

Eat when hungry, drink when thirsty: If we eat or drink too much or when the body has no need for food or drink, then we are not responding to our inner voice. Instead, we are indulging our sensorial appetite. Overindulgence in anything is harmful to one's well-being.

Choose and eat only natural whole foods: Use whole, unrefined foods as much as possible. Choose vegetables that are fresh and chemical-free. Avoid processed, canned, and frozen foods. Vegetables from the sea are rich in minerals and are very healthful.

Chew well: Good food tastes better the more you chew. Brown rice, for example, becomes sweeter when chewed well, whereas meat quickly loses its flavor. In this way, chewing also helps you distinguish between good and bad food. When you are sick, chewing well is essential. Digestion of complex carbohydrates begins in the mouth—so the more you chew, the better absorption and assimilation you will have. To develop spirituality and sensitivity, it is also necessary to chew well. Mental clarity and judgment improve with mastication. Also, complete chewing leads to satisfaction after a meal, and lessens the desire to overeat. Chewing well does not mean chewing slowly! One who chews well should finish the meal with everyone else.

Eat only to 80 percent capacity: Never eat until you are full. Overeating creates excess, which, if it is not discharged, will cause imbalance. Overeating clouds the mind, makes you feel sleepy, and hinders your capacity to be active. A person who eats only to 80 percent capacity has a greater chance of success.

Enjoy your meals: All food should be eaten with the spirit of gratitude and enjoyment. Cooking, which is an art, and the presentation and consumption of the food should be a joyful experience. It can be one of life's greatest pleasures.

Do not eat when upset: If you are very tired, do not eat. If you are having emotional difficulties, do not eat. At these times, the body is not prepared to receive food or to digest it properly. Take a walk to calm down before you eat.

Your kitchen is your pharmacy: Our daily food is our medicine. Thus, the proper selection and preparation of daily meals is essential to the maintenance of health. Most illness, then, can be avoided with proper nutrition. Studies say that 70 percent of illness is diet-related. The importance of cooking cannot be overstated. Good macrobiotic cookbooks and cooking classes are essential in mastering the art of healthy food preparation.

What Has a Front Has a Back—Elimination

The harmony of natural balance teaches that each cycle must have two parts. There is always a yin and a yang aspect to every situation. Elimination is the second half of eating and digestion. The by-products of elimination have been kindly referred to as "Old Gold and New Gold." "Old Gold" meaning the stool and "New Gold" meaning urine.

Old Gold

The goodness of digestion is balanced with the waste that remains after useful elements are extracted. The ability of the internal organs to separate the useful from the waste is a sign of proper function and good health. This waste must be eliminated from the body for the cycle to be complete. Babies have bowel movements after each feeding. Most adults have bowel movements one time each day. Observation of the stool gives valuable information regarding digestion and health. The color, texture, and odor indicate the quality of digestion. If particles of undigested food linger in the stool it is obvious that digestion is not good. A good stool is one piece of light golden color material with little odor that floats in the toilet. If the stool is dark either there has been animal products such as beef consumed or there is blood in the stool. Blood in the stool can be a serious problem. A good stool floats because of the fiber content that it gets from whole grains and vegetables. Good bowel movements give you a feeling of lightness and of relief. Toxins are eliminated from the body by this system. This process extends the quality and quite possibly the quantity of life.

New Gold
Like the stool the color, volume, and odor of urine indicates the health condition. Urination usually occurs four or five times per day. If you urinate more than this either you drink excessively or there may be kidney or bladder trouble. Excessive urination depletes the body of valuable minerals. The color is best when it is golden yellow, not too light or clear nor too dark. Of course there should be no pain when urinating nor should you find a rust color that normally means blood in the urine.

Summary
An ancient Chinese quotation sums up the value of food in healing, "First try food; resort to medication only when food fails to effect a cure. Food is the first line of defense." The principle involved in food therapy is to create and maintain balance. Each meal should strike a fine balance not only in flavor, aroma, texture, and color, but also in the energies and essences they impart to the body when digested.

Movement

The rotation of the earth on its axis creates the patterns of day and night. The cycle of the moon around the earth creates the lunar phases of waxing and waning. The earth's yearly journey around the sun creates the dramatic and beautiful change of the seasons. These cycles move in harmony through space creating the physical foundation for life. Movements supporting each other, perfectly choreographed, allow an exquisite reality to exist. The constant travel of the solar system through space produces pervasive results—movement and change. From these undeniable facts it is no mystery why movement is a key factor in life. The result of celestial movement is life. On a smaller level, what is the result of the way we move?

The way we use our bodies and move has broad effects. Movement can support our dreams by allowing us to accomplish our goals. Or it can create an avalanche of problems, pains, and deformities. The all too familiar example of arthritis, the effects of wear and tear, demonstrates in a tangible form, how we have used our bodies throughout a lifetime. We undervalue our ability to move, until this gift is endangered. Sit in a wheelchair for a day and you will begin to see the precious gift that you possess.

Labor or movement is instinctive to human beings and plays an important role in life. In the ancient Chinese classic *Su Wen* it says, "Excessive leisure and ease cause circulatory problems and a subsequent loss of health. However, too much work exhausts the *Qi* and blood and injures the sinews and bones." Our bodies are made to move and be active. From birth until death, this process goes on. Modern people do not physically move as often as in the past. Formerly the majority of people worked on farms, which are physically demanding. Walking, bending, and lifting are activities that were a natural part of the farm day.

With technology, very few people are required to do strenuous work. It looks as though we will be required to do even less in the future. The word *chore* has virtually gone out of use. Office work uses the brain but leaves the body sedentary. This lack of movement creates serious problems including circulatory problems and weak, atrophied muscles. Ancient peoples had to work hard to forage for food—it was not so easy to get. They were active in obtaining the food and, as it was not so abundant, they ate less. Wild animals also must expend energy through stalking and hunting to feed themselves. We, on the other hand, have very little difficulty in obtaining food. We can go to the market, restaurant or coffee shop anytime we want. We eat too much and do not walk enough.

Modern people never completely use their bodies. We always do the same repetitive routines. We drive to work or sit at a desk all day. Some sit at a computer using only wrists and fingers for hours at a time. From these routine patterns we can see why imbalance is produced. Recently, laws are being made to protect office workers who do such singular tasks as data processing. The number of hours spent at a computer is regulated because chronic painful injuries, such as tendinitis and carpal tunnel syndrome, result from using only one part of the body. Modern life and culture easily make imbalances. The physical rigors of farm life, while using the whole body, often overused it, creating an opposite type of imbalance. Imbalanced activity of any nature always produces disharmony.

Muscles, aided by the joints and bones, make every motion possible. They also push food along the digestive tract, suck air into the lungs, and tighten blood vessels to raise blood pressure when you need more pressure to meet an emergency. The heart itself is a muscular pump. While technological advances have changed our way of living, the needs of the human body have not changed. Muscles are meant to be used. When they are not used, or not used enough, they deteriorate. If we are habitually inactive, we must pay the price in decreased efficiency.

The main recipients of the movement of the muscles are the joints and spine. Observe a person's joint and back condition and you will discover their real age and flexibility. Because of stiffness they appear sometimes older than their recorded number of years. By loosening and stretching vertebrae and relaxing the associated spinal muscles, you may restore optimum nerve and energy impulses to the vital internal organs. Tense spinal muscles not only block nerve and energy channels, they also deplete vital energy because it takes a lot of energy to keep these muscles tight.

Specific Benefits of Movement

An obvious effect of regular exercise is the firming and toning of muscles. Internally all organs and systems are affected with most noticeable changes in the heart, lungs, and circulatory system. The heartbeat becomes stronger and steadier, breathing becomes deeper, and circulation improves.

Research shows many strength and quality of life improvements with regular exercise. The following results were noted after a group of sedentary people began a systematic conditioning program:

- Increased strength, endurance, and coordination
- Increased joint flexibility
- Reduction of minor aches, pains, stiffness, and soreness
- Correction of some posture defects
- Improvement in general appearance
- Increased efficiency in performance of physical and mental tasks
- Improved ability to relax and reduce tension
- Reduction of chronic fatigue

Fatigue is one of the most voiced complaints. Chronic tiredness can stem from a problem such as *chronic fatigue syndrome*, a debilitating illness. But in many people it is the result of gradual deterioration of the body for lack of enough vigorous physical activity. Continual inactivity produces muscular weakness that results in inability to do daily work easily and efficiently. An important benefit of increased muscle strength and general endurance provided by exercise is an increase in the body's capacity for carrying on normal daily activities and pushing back fatigue. A fit person uses less energy for any given movement or effort than a flabby or weak person.

The Importance of Posture

Humans are built to stand, sit, and walk erect. Correct posture is essential to another of the fundamentals of health, breathing. When you slump, you squeeze your lungs into a cramped position and seriously limit the operation of your diaphragm. When you sit bent over a desk, at study or work, you rob your body of oxygen, impair circulation, hamper the functions of all vital organs, and stretch your muscles and bones into unnatural positions. No wonder you are fatigued! You probably sit with your legs crossed ensuring that circulation to the legs is blocked, preparing the way for broken capillaries and varicose veins.

Correct Posture

For correct posture, align your body with an imaginary plumb line from the center of the top of your head through the center of your pelvis to midway between the arches of your feet. Stand up with your feet parallel, about six inches apart. Pull your abdomen up out of your hips, your chest up out of your abdomen, and your neck up out of your chest. Set your shoulders back easily and comfortably. Stand tall but relaxed.

When you sit, keep your trunk in the same position. Sit on your hips, with your feet flat on the floor or ankles lightly crossed. You can work for hours at your desk in this position without fatigue, stopping now and then for a good stretch. Hold the same basic posture when you walk, letting your arms swing naturally in rhythm with your stride.

Many physical movements, particularly sport activities such as swimming, basketball, tennis, gymnastics, ballet, and the martial arts, flow artistically when performed by an experienced enthusiast. The key to a stunning physical performance depends on the performer's ability to relax. Physical relaxation is a prerequisite for proper breath control and energy circulation. Vital energy flows more efficiently when you are relaxed, thus feeding all cells, tissues, and organs. Relaxation also affects mental clarity and links body with mind, energy with spirit.

Lack of exercise, especially the lack of walking, predisposes a middle-aged person to heart disease and arteriosclerosis. Aging begins in the feet. Thus walking is the best exercise. In general the average person walks 3,000 to 6,000 steps a day. The ideal is 10,000 steps a day. Walking increases both breathing and pulse rates. On the average a person's pulse rate should be 50 to 60 at rest, 80 to 100 when walking, and 120 to 130 when jogging. After trotting, a person over sixty will have a rate of about 110. Of course, no one should exercise beyond their physical capacity. It is important to adjust the speed of one's walking with the pulse rate and to walk everyday or at least every other day.

If we are living naturally there would be little need to do special exercises. But, we do not and exercise is a necessity for both physical, emotional, and mental health. Some extraordinary kinds of exercise such as Yoga and Dô-In (a form of self-massage), systematically coordinate the body, breath, mind, and spirit. They are also important in teaching economic use of energy. They improve posture, which significantly affects not only the nerves, but also every major system in the body. A balanced program of exercise, including some rigorous action and some controlled stretching, is very helpful.

Sleep

One of the most natural and enjoyable activities that we all do is sleep. Sleep is that period of inactivity where we are unaware and generally unresponsive to our environment. It is the time to release all the day's tensions. It is a time of rest and renewal.

Although most people dream, it is not a particularly good sign of health. This statement may shock some people. But consider the purpose of sleep is to rest and renew the system. Dreaming is a working function, not one of rest. During sleep the body and mind should be in a resting state. Healthy people do not normally dream. Dreaming is the body's way of processing either physical or psychological residues. If during the day, emotional snags are dealt with completely, there will be no residue that needs to be processed during sleep. In a similar way, when no agitating materials are circulating in the brain's bloodstream (such as fats, sugar, beef, coffee, and chemical stimulants), no pictures or dreams will be perceived by the brain's nervous system. However, true dreams can occur for healthy people, which can serve as predictions of things to come or contact with spiritual vibrations.

Sleep is our body's house cleaning time. If you are eating properly and exercising, then the recovery time for your organs and systems occurs quickly. This means that a healthy body sleeps less. Not eating three hours before bedtime will promote sound sleep. Besides a shorter sleeping time, a healthy person has very deep sleep, the body is soft and the breathing slow. During sleep there should be very little body movement. Movement during sleep is a corrective mechanism by the body. If there are imbalances, the body will make adjustments to try to correct and eliminate these abnormal conditions while you sleep. Unfortunately, long-term bad habits inhibit complete correction during sleep therefore they must be dealt with during daytime.

Sleeping Materials

The bed, sheets, pillows, and bed clothes are the tools of sleep. You will enjoy sleep and recover from the toil of the day if the bed is not too soft nor too hard. Cotton sheets are best. During sleep the body throws off waste products and water. The bed clothing and sheets absorb this waste. A good body scrub before bed and changing the bed linen regularly allows the pores of the skin to breathe. It is a good idea not to wear jewelry, especially metal objects to bed. False teeth, contact lens, and any other artificial device should be put aside for the evening. A healthy sleeping posture is flat on the back with the arms relaxed at the sides. Generally, sleeping on the sides or on the stomach shows troubles.

Necessary Conditions for Sleep

Sleep is very much like death except that breathing and vital organ functions continue at a minimum rate. It is during sleep that the body's self-healing mechanism functions. During this time new cells are constructed and old cells recycled.

The body produces sleep-inducing substances. Healthy, active people have no trouble falling to sleep. Yet, many people experience insomnia. Reducing stress and correcting the diet are helpful in solving this problem. An amino acid, tryptophan, is responsible for stimulating the production of serotonin—the sleep-inducing agent. If the body cannot absorb or does not have enough tryptophan then serotonin will not be produced and insomnia will result. Tryptophan is found in all meat and dairy products such as hamburger, turkey, and the famous bedtime beverage, milk. It has been recommended that sleepless individuals eat Dagwood-style ham, turkey, and cheese sandwiches and drink warm milk before bed. This is not a good idea. The problem is these protein-rich foods supply many other amino acids that stimulate the body, therefore inhibiting sleep. They also stimulate digestion at a time it should be resting. Researchers discovered that volunteers who had eaten a high-carbohydrate meal at night were sleepier than those who had eaten a high-protein meal. Apparently, the insulin released after a high-carbohydrate meal serves to take up amino acids other than tryptophan into body tissues, freeing the tryptophan for uptake into the brain. My suggestions of including whole grains and vegetables in the diet supply abundant carbohydrates.

The following are four conditions of sleep:

1. When the body and mind are evenly tired, then sleep naturally comes quickly.
2. If you have done little activity and are not tired enough, then sleep will not come. Your body has no need of it.
3. When there is an imbalance between the body and the mind, normal sleep will not come. For example, when the brain is overworking from the artificial stimulation of coffee or other stimulants and/or you are worried and mentally concerned about something, the mind will not let you sleep even when the body is tired.
4. When physical troubles are present, especially a stiff painful neck or hips, natural sleep is difficult in coming.

Pre-sleep Ritual

Preparing yourself before bedtime increases the body's natural healing process and decreases sleeping time. Many people start with some relaxation exercises to unwind from the day's tensions. Including a hot salt bath before bed is an excellent way to relax. Soak in the warm water, perhaps scented with pine or another aromatic oil, for ten to twenty minutes. Give your body a full scrub with a luffa sponge, brush, or a wet towel. The scrub removes the day's dirt and grime, and also old skin cells. It brings blood and nutrients to the skin's surface. While you sleep this blood will refresh surface tissue and keep your skin flexible and young looking. If you have trouble falling to sleep sip a warm cup of chamomile tea. Try reading an uninteresting book such as one on taxes, it is a guaranteed cure for insomnia. It is better to go to sleep before midnight.

Mentally reviewing the day's activities helps to clear up any loose ends and unfinished business. Thinking about your activities before you go to sleep lessens the likelihood you will worry about them in the dream state. Chanting and meditation before bed clean vibrations from the body and open the central, spiritual channel. These techniques prepare you for the next day. If you have a problem or project, ask for guidance from the world of nature as you sleep. Teach yourself to tap into the information stored in the invisible world that is useful to you in accomplishing your purpose on earth. We have come from infinity, and in sleep, we temporarily go back to infinity. If you are eating well you will enjoy between five and seven hours of sleep.

Ideally, when you awake from sleep, you should feel happy and clearheaded. You should have positive thoughts and an optimistic attitude. You should feel prepared to start another exciting day. A healthy person awakens alert without any aches or pains. The body should feel flexible and not stiff. Sleep is the great refresher and energizer.

Relationships and Sex

Yin and yang create every void and fill every vacuum. Yang energy's drive for harmony leads it to the receptive, smoother yin energy. Each of these unsettling forces seeks, and simultaneously defends against, being neutralized by the other. This antagonistic attraction is as true in relationship as it is in the formation of weather.

The innate nature of being male or female is to be complete and, at the same time, incomplete. Yin and yang produce dualistic, two-sided responses to every life situation. It is no wonder that the interaction among men and women is frequently referred to as the "battle of the sexes." The fact remains all people need relationships. These relationships must possess both complementary elements and opposite energies to be interesting and satisfying. Without a spark of opposition, a sameness prevails that leads to dullness, lack of interest, boredom, and eventually conflict and separation. A separation fueled by the natural tendency of both yin and yang to seek to dissolve one into the other.

Many people feel they cannot find the right mate. You do not have to look far to find people unhappy with the quality of their relationships. Divorce and separation, once rare, is now the norm. It appears that people are correct, they are not finding partners to share a satisfying and lasting relationship. Many women find men insensitive, sometimes violent, but usually weak without a strong direction in their lives. Contemporary men's eating habits of steak, hamburger, and eggs (excessive yang energy) and alcohol, coffee, sugar, and desserts (excessive yin energy) may contribute to these observations. Man on the other hand often find women domineering and too strong and demanding. Women's current habit of eating as much meat, poultry, and eggs (yang energy) as men may contribute to the display of unlady-like strength from many men's point of view. It is difficult for male-female attraction to be strong when the energy is much the same.

The fear of personal commitment as well as the fear of AIDS and sexually transmitted diseases dampens the prospects of beginning open and happy relationships. Singles are wary of each other and if they could each would request sworn testimony about sexual partners for the last seven years to determine the possibility of HIV exposure. Additionally, most adults are children from divorced families without exposure to a model of successful relationship. They are often fearful as adults to develop lasting, meaningful relationships themselves having seen the difficulties involved and the failure of their parents' marriages. They have a low self-esteem and are afraid of being an inadequate partner and mate. The major difficulty is that while there is resistance to and avoidance of developing relationships, each person longs for companionship and the pleasures of sex.

Over 2,000 years ago, Confucius said, "Food and sex are natural." These two items, food and sex are the only two indispensable requirements for the survival and propagation of the species. If we look at the advertising media apparently Confucius was not wrong. Food and sex sell, which means we have interest enough to buy. They are the strongest natural instincts and the most basic functions we have. As such, food and sex are also the most fundamental indications of health and disease and the best means of working toward longevity.

Food, above all, is a constant cure and forms the foundation of preventive health care. If proper dietary habits are cultivated, even when disease does strike, its effects are far less debilitating, and recovery is quick. For us, food is medicine. But it is the need for relationship that finds its fullest expression in sexual contact that truly fuels and feeds the species.

Testing Yin and Yang

If you would like to see the movement of vital energy responsible for our basic drive to seek opposite forces you can do a test that will show an obvious fact— every person has yin or yang energy. Traditional healing teaches that males are governed by one type of force while females are governed by another. These forces come before any social or cultural training that we may learn when we are young. Each social group teaches boys and girls how they are supposed to behave. This instruction is limited to that particular group. The innate forces of yin and yang are not limited to national boundaries nor to geographical locations. There is a maleness in every male animal or plant and a femaleness in every female animal or plant. Here is the test. From a mixed group of friends, have a woman sit in a chair. The person who demonstrates stands behind. Dangle a pendulum over the center of the woman's head. A pendulum can be made by tying a two foot piece of string or sewing thread to the end of a metal fingernail clipper. Hold the device as still as possible. Shortly, the tool will begin to move in a circular motion, carefully note the direction. After a couple of minutes test another woman. The nail clipper moves in the same direction for all women. Ask for a male volunteer and hold the clipper over a man's head and observe the movement.

While this test is a simple, party game, you can see a distinct difference in the electromagnetic fields of female and male. Do the test several times with different people so that you are assured of this truth—each person has yin or yang energy. Female energy makes the pendulum swing in a clockwise direction, while male energy produces an opposite counterclockwise direction. Now, have a woman and a man sit in separate chairs next to each other. Repeat the test one more time over each person. While holding the pendulum over the woman's head ask the man to touch lightly the woman's hand. What happens? The pendulum stops moving. Her yin energy is balanced by his yang energy. Momentary harmony is established. When he removes his touch the pendulum again swings and her female yin energy reestablishes its dominant nature. If we had reversed roles and had the woman touch the man the results would be the same. Yin and yang energies each have the power to balance. If, on the other hand, two women or two men touch there is a very different response. Instead of the pendulum stopping, the swing will increase in intensity. This signifies an addition of the same kind of energy in the electromagnetic field. In other words, when a man and a woman meet their energies neutralize and balance each other. When two people of the same sex meet the energy increases to double yin or double yang.

Human Development

Historical Oriental literature concerning sex treats it as any other activity that either enhances health and longevity or detracts from it. Unlike the standard Western view that sex is evil until matrimony, sex was viewed as either performed in healthy or unhealthy ways. Its purpose, besides bringing pleasure and a sense of closeness, is to generate and circulate energy. If sexual activity increases vital energy it is considered healthful, if it decreases energy, it is viewed as harmful.

In the Chinese system vital-essence *jing* is produced by the transforming effects of *Qi* on digested food and drink in the stomach and small intestine. This makes up the creative force inside the body and takes two forms: life essence and semen essence. Life essence is stored in the kidneys, which secrete it into the bloodstream as needed. It controls growth, development, decay and death. From a Western perspective, "kidneys" mean the renal and suprarenal glands, the glands sitting on top of the kidneys. "Life essence" refers to the hormones secreted from these glands, such as adrenaline, which control many body functions.

Semen essence refers to semen in men and the ova in woman. Embryos formed from the union of male and female semen essence are nourished by the life essence also formed by this union. After birth, the child produces its own life essence by digestion. The sexual *jing* in girls matures at two times seven years, around age of fourteen, and deteriorates at seven times seven, around age of forty-nine. For boys *jing* matures at two times eight years, age of sixteen, and begins to lose potency at eight times eight, age of sixty-four.

Female Superiority

Today in modern society women and men are recognized as equal concerning legal rights and responsibilities. Formerly in a male dominated society women were treated as second class citizens. The truth is that laws change but people's minds and behavior are not as fast. We experience a lag time. Fortunately, there is a growing maturity among people that recognizes while women and men are very different, each possesses human qualities that are beyond a superior-inferior classification. Since society's survival is dependent on its physical protectors, the warrior men have had an illusion of superiority. Nothing can be further from the truth. Deep inside men have always known this fact for a couple of important reasons. Women live longer, do not get sick as often, recover quicker when they become ill, need fewer calories and less sleep to survive, and most frightening to men, can have repeated sex without loss of energy. Every man knows that in spite of male boasting and the popular illusion of conquest, every woman can outlast any man. In the heart of the untrained man is the knowledge that in the realm of sex, one of his strongest desires, he can be defeated by woman.

It is for this reason, the vulnerability of men, that sexual advice and practices developed in ancient China and India. The essential difference between the sexual nature of man and woman lies in the different nature of male and female orgasm. When a man ejaculates, he ejects his semen essence from his body. When a woman reaches orgasm, she produces sexual secretions but they remain in her body, she does not lose a thing. For both men and women, sexual essence is an important source of vital energy. This vital energy supports and nourishes the body's life-sustaining functions including immunity. The ancients felt that if a man ejaculates each time he has sex this practice robs him of his primary source of vitality and immunity. This leaves him weak and open to disease. He can expect to shorten his life. The link of decreasing physical and mental capacity and ejaculation is casually recognized, but not given much emphasis, in the West. One common example is the advice to serious athletes and students not to have sex before an important event or examination.

Every time a man ejaculates he loses his yang essence. To protect men and to increase the satisfaction of women, sexual habits were promoted to help men conserve their vital essence. Because sex is such an important aspect of living and communicating, practices were developed to have frequent sex without the harmful, negative side effects that lead to physical and mental exhaustion and depression. This is called the *Tao of Yin and Yang* or the *Tao of Sex*. Tao means "Way" or "Path." Discipline and training teach men to conserve their semen and have sex without regular ejaculation. Through breathing and internally circulating yang energy it is possible for men to maintain a peak drive, performance level, and pleasure. The long-term pleasures associated with ejaculation control outweigh the short-term pleasure experience. Men regularly fall asleep after intercourse, sometimes have weakness in the legs and lower back, especially as men age, and some men even have a difficult time mowing the lawn the following day! If orgasm were the source of these conditions women would feel them also. But they do not. The cause is the loss of semen and yang essence. Ancient literature promises that if a man guards and regulates his ejaculation his body will grow strong, his mind will be clear, and his vision and hearing will improve. One of the greatest promises is that his love for his woman will greatly increase. He will feel as if he could never get enough of her. And importantly, he will have the capacity to act on this love.

In the 1600s in Japan, *Yôjôkun* (the Secret of Health Preservation) was written by Ekiken Kaibara (1630–1714). He wrote about the art of long life and the role of sex. Kaibara agreed that sexual contact may be enjoyed regularly if the man follows the Tao of Yin and Yang. The prudent male should conserve his essential vitality by regulating the frequency of ejaculation. Seminal emission was regulated according to season, and age and physical strength of man. Warm months allow for greater frequency of ejaculation and colder months less. Younger were permitted release more than older man. Of course the more vitality a man possessed the more his body could tolerate a loss of vital essence. According to Kaibara, "If a person who is extremely vigorous and healthy suppresses the urge too long, this can cause trouble. If a person allows sexual desire to get the better of him, sexual gratification will become a bad habit that will be hard to break."

In the Chinese text *Precious Recipes* Sun Simiao tells us, "A man can live a healthy and long life if he carries out an emission frequency of two times monthly or twenty-four times yearly. If at the same time he also pays attention to wholesome food and exercises, he may attain longevity." Dr. Sun lived to the age of 101 by following his own advice. His personal schedule of emission was once every hundred sexual encounters, though he considered this too strict a regimen for the average man.

The conservation of the man's semen during intercourse is given great importance. When a man ejaculates, this loss must be compensated by absorbing the woman's sexual secretions. Without this compensation the loss of yang essence has no counterbalance. For this reason ejaculation through masturbation or homosexual relations was regarded as harmful to the yang essence and energy. There is no moral judgment, it is a matter of enhancing vitality or not. Because there is no loss of essence, female masturbation or homosexual relations are not considered to be harmful.

Food and Sex

While many foods, concentrated sources of yin and yang energy, are used to encourage a strong sex drive, certain foods create an excessive drive. One obvious cause is the consumption of concentrated animal protein. The eating of beef, chicken, eggs, and other animal foods can create over-stimulation of the sexual organs, as can overeating of any food. This may create excessive sexual preoccupation and abnormal sexual tendencies.

Seed foods have been thought to replenish the seed (sexual) essence. These foods include grains, beans, and seeds. If planted these seeds will produce a new plant. Seeds carry the sexual essence and transmit the ability for a species to continue.

Prepared side dishes containing root vegetables such as burdock root and carrot promote strength in the lower part of the body where the sex organs are found. Warmth from cooked foods generates a smoother flow of energy within the system, assisting in the distribution of energy and power. The properties of ginseng root as a boost to immunity and sexual power is well known. Other herbal favorites include: codonopsis (*dang shen*), astragalus (*huang qi*), dioscorea (*shan yao*, mountain potato), atractylodis (*bai zhu*), and glycyrrhizae (*gan mao*, licorice). Nourishing the body's vital energy by supplying nutrition is a direct way to enhance sexual power. For this reason, food and cooking should be given high priority if one is serious about building up sexual vitality, the foundation of relationship.

Sex and Immunity

The aim of food and herbal preparations is to tonify and strengthen the system. Not only have these practices of prescribing food and beverages been used effectively to maintain health and prolong life but their underlying medical principles have also been confirmed by recent scientific research in the West. The hormonal secretions the body produces during sex affect the system as a whole, especially the immune system.

In a study conducted in 1974 at the Max Planck Institute of Psychiatry in Munich, researchers discovered a significant increase in testosterone levels in the blood of 75 percent of men who were shown a mildly erotic film. German scientists subsequently discovered that men with high-hormone levels, high-sperm count, and dense semen have unusually high resistance to some diseases and absolute immunity to others.

A delicate balance lays the foundation for the proper functioning of the body's systems and therefore immunity. This balance is the result of the correct amount and kind of nutrients coupled with emotional stability that includes self-esteem and compassion for others. Securing health takes a commitment to the development of better relationships. In a perfect world everything goes smoothly and there is no hurt or pain. But that world does not exist yet. Until then the practice of honest communication between partners will minimize misunderstanding and distortion of truth. Living a life filled with love lightens the heart. The pleasure and intimacy of sex can serve as a centering device, a focal point to help to coordinate body, mind, and spirit. If our relationships do this, we reap the joy, satisfaction, and intimacy that we all deserve.

Blood and Immunity

All creatures have essential fluids that allow the inner processes to function properly but animals have a unique material that separates them from plants— blood. Blood is a warm fluid tissue composed of two parts. The intercellular substance is a fluid called *plasma*, in which float formed elements—blood cells. The total volume of blood forms about one-twelfth of the weight of the body or about five liters (about five quarts). About 55 percent, a little over half the volume, is fluid, the remaining 45 percent of the volume being made up of the blood cells. This packed cell volume or hematocrit ranges from 40 to 47 percent in healthy people. A higher or lower percentage means trouble.

Blood plasma is made up of 91 percent water, 8 percent protein, and almost 1 percent mineral salts. Elements such as oxygen, carbon dioxide, internal secretions, enzymes, and antigens are found in the plasma. This serves as a transportation system. The blood cells come in three types: red blood cells (erythrocytes), white blood cells (leukocytes), and platelets (thrombocytes).

Red Blood Cells

Red blood cells are a pale buff color when viewed alone but as a group they appear red giving blood its color. There are about five million red blood cells in each cubic millimeter of blood. Red blood cells need protein for their structure derived from the amino acids; they also need iron, so that a balanced diet containing these substances is necessary for their replacement. Women require more iron as some is lost in the menstrual flow. Western medicine teaches that red blood cells originate in bone marrow, especially in that of the short, flat, and irregular bones, at the ends of the long bones and in the marrow in the shafts of the ribs and in the sternum.

In the process of development in the bone marrow the red blood cells pass through several stages. At first they are large and contain a nucleus but no hemoglobin. Next they pick up hemoglobin, and finally lose their nucleus and are then passed out for circulation in the blood. The average life of a red blood cell is about 120 days. The cells then wear out. Worn-out cells are screened by the spleen and liver and are removed from circulation.

White Blood Cells

White blood cells are transparent and not colored. They are larger and fewer than red blood cells. They average eight thousand in each cubic millimeter of blood. White blood cells play a very important part in protecting the body from microorganisms.

Functions of Blood

Blood acts as the transport system of the body conveying all chemical substances, oxygen, and nutrients required for the nourishment of the body so its normal functions may be completed. It also carries away carbon dioxide and other waste products. It is the red blood cells that carry oxygen to the tissues and remove some of the carbon dioxide. The white blood cells provide many protective substances and functions against microorganisms such as bacteria. The plasma distributes proteins needed for tissue formation. It is the medium by which all cells receive nourishment and by which cells eliminate their waste buildup. Finally, the blood system is the means how internal secretions, hormones, and enzymes are transported from organ to organ.

Our central computer, the brain, needs an adequate supply of blood. If deprived of blood for longer than three or four minutes irreversible changes take place and some brain cells die. Uncertainty, cloudy thinking, and indecision may be encouraged not only by lack of blood but by the quality of blood that reaches the brain. Besides the mechanics of blood production, we must be concerned about the quality and distribution of that blood.

Blood Quality

Naturally blood quality includes the red blood cells' abilities to hold iron, oxygen, and nutrients, as well as its ability to remove waste from other body tissues. The material source of blood comes from food. Adequate nourishment allows the body to function properly and supply its needs. Basic to meeting these needs are whole foods. Refined foods always require nutrients they do not possess in order to be processed by the body. Common sugar is a good example. Sugar requires calcium to be processed. Unfortunately sugar contains no calcium as it is superrefined. Where does it get the calcium? From calcium in the blood that was intended to build bones, teeth, and regulate chemical reactions such as digestive enzyme production. If the depletion is long term, calcium will be stripped from the bones and teeth directly. Excessive amounts of protein also add ammonia and other toxic substances that pollute and alter the blood's quality.

An easy measurement of the blood is to look at the acid-alkaline relationship. Blood is always alkaline. The degree of alkalinity depends on the hydrogen ion concentration and this is expressed as the pH of blood. A pH of 7 represents a neutral solution like water. The pH from 7 to 1 signifies an acid solution, while from 7 to 14 is an alkaline solution. The pH of blood is 7.35 to 7.45. This figure is constantly maintained. Only a very slight variation on either side is compatible with life. The maintenance of the constant degree of alkalinity of the blood therefore is most important and this is controlled by the elimination of carbon dioxide (an acid gas), excretion of acids in the urine, and the alkaline reserve property of the blood. The body's mineral reserves buffer the blood against rising acid levels that result from normal metabolism.

In addition to the material factors related to blood, we want to consider the energetic quality that blood has. In the ancient teachings there has been a strong connection between blood, body fluids, and energy. They are the essential substances within the human body. The body's energy is a reflection of the combined functions of the internal organs. This energy must be nourished by blood. The moisture of the internal organs is supplied by the body fluids. And the normal structure and function of the organs rely on energy. The production and distribution of energy depend on the normal physiological activities of the internal organs. These circular relationships of requirement and supply reflects the spiral nature of nature.

Blood originates through the transformation of food in the stomach and spleen area where it is received and digested. The essence that is extracted is transported up to the heart and lung areas. By the action of the heart energy and the lung energy it becomes blood. Food is the material foundation of blood. A secondary source of blood comes from the bone marrow, which is produced by the kidneys. The kidneys are regarded as very important as they influence the energy of the stomach, spleen, lungs, and heart. The heart and lungs are responsible for the distribution of blood. This is accomplished by breathing.

Fig. 3 Production of Blood

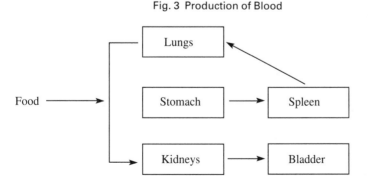

Immunity

Blood feeds every organ and tissue in the body. How we maintain good quality blood is the key to survival, because blood lays the foundation for the immune function. The immune system also known as the *reticuloendothelial system* has several components. Throughout all the tissues and organs of the body there are certain cells that ingest foreign particles and bacteria. They are particularly concentrated in the lymph glands, spleen, liver, and bone marrow. These cells have great powers of multiplication and are related both to lymphocytes and to the blood-forming organs. They are concerned in protecting the body from infection. The main contributors to immune function are: bone marrow, spleen, lymph nodes, thymus, liver, intestines, and stomach.

Factors that Weaken the Immune System

Eating Meat: Meat is high in protein. The main nutrition of microbes is protein. Increased protein levels create acid in the blood. This breakdown of protein makes an excellent environment for microbe growth. Meat creates an acid blood condition. Many kinds of microbes and fungi favor a slightly acid condition that is toxic for our body cells. Meat overloads the kidneys and liver. Protein contains nitrogen. In the liver the nitrogen breakdown is removed to make ammonia. Ammonia is toxic and is turned into urea. It also contains many purines. Uric acid is made from the breakdown of purines. Sulfur and phosphorus in meat turn into sulfuric and phosphoric acids in the body. The kidneys receive and filtrate this blood, reabsorbing useful materials and excreting useless or harmful substances. If the kidneys cannot filter all the wastes, the body has trouble from the excesses. Meat does not contain enough minerals, vitamins, or dietary fiber. Meats contain microbes that cause disease in humans. Ordinary cooking does not destroy the germs in meat. They are killed only by a temperature of 240° F. Oven heat does not penetrate to the interior of the roast. This means it is possible to get diseases caused by eating meat, whether raw or cooked.

Eating Sugar: Because of the difficulty in processing sugar from cane or beets it was once thought of the most developed food. In Japan it was used as a medicine. Americans consume 140 pounds per person each year. Men (primarily in teenage boys) consume more than women in the United States.

While sugar temporarily raises body temperature, long term it cools it down. This inhibits internal functions. Consuming sugar depletes mineral reserves. Sugar needs many kinds of nutrients and enzymes to be processed. Sugar makes the body tired and lacking in energy, creating a craving for meat. This creates a meat-sugar cycle. It removes calcium and other minerals, depletes our stores of protein, and consumes important nutrients like vitamin B_1. Calcium is found in bones (98 percent), teeth (1 percent), and throughout the body (1 percent) for the regulation of muscle function especially the heart, the clotting of blood, nourishment of cells, release of energy, and transmission of nerve impulses; in the stomach, calcium restrains excessive acid secretion and neutralizes various detrimental food additives. Calcium ion protects our body from the virulent character of sodium and potassium ions, copper and other metals, and also helps to regulate body temperature. When you eat sugar you become more thirsty and drink more water. This causes you to void minerals via the urine. This creates dental caries and bone loss. Sugar cools down the sexual desire, leads to frigidity, impotence, and sterility. Sugar causes blood diseases such as hemophilia and other blood clotting troubles.

Early Warning Signs of Immune System Dysfunction
1. Fatigue and Malaise
2. Weight loss
3. Fever and chills
4. Headache and confusion
5. Shortness of breath, night sweating
6. Severe muscle aches and/or sore throat
7. Swollen lymph nodes (glands)
8. Abnormal bleeding
9. Skin rashes
10. Persistent diarrhea
11. Lesions in the mouth, nose, or anus

Circulation of Blood, Lymph, and Energy

The movement of the body's essential fluids and energy is critical to proper maintenance of immunity. From the previous explanations you can understand how the material in blood and fluid production and their liquids defend the body. The quality of the body's organs and fluids is important. When stagnation occurs you can now see why it can harm the system. The buildup of toxic materials pollutes the internal environment. If the volume of pollution remains long enough the body adjusts to survive. An active adjustment produces cells that can survive in such a toxic condition. If the system is strong they become malignant cells. These cells are mutant, abnormal cells and tissues, but they continue to function. If the body is not strong the cells degenerate and do not function. This is the beginning of fatigue, allergies, and eventually immune system collapse.

Everyone has some buildup of waste material. When the circulation is processing this material the body keeps on top of the volume and little harm is done. Breathing and receiving shiatsu sessions promote a strong stimulus for circulation and the elimination of toxins. These techniques positively affect the three main organs responsible for the production and movement of the body's fluids—kidneys, lungs, and spleen.

The body's ability to separate the useful substance from the waste material is at the core of successful cleansing. In the Oriental medical model the kidney action of separation sends the useful portion up to the lungs to nourish and moisten them and waste products to the bladder. The bladder eliminates the fluid as urine. The spleen also separates the useful from the waste and sends the vapor of useful material from digestion to the lungs to nourish them. The lungs then distributes this energy throughout the body. This is done because of the pumping action of breathing. Whatever waste the lungs generate is pushed down to the kidneys which then eliminates

Fig. 4 Fluid Production and Circulation

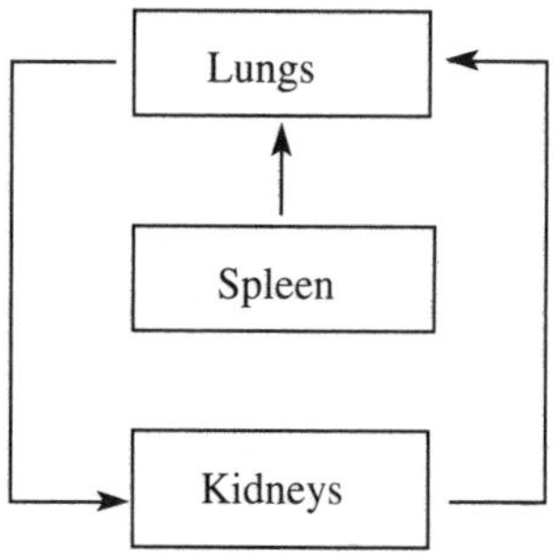

it. In this way the kidneys maintain a close relationship with the lungs and spleen and direct fluid production and distribution within the body.

How to Strengthen the Immune System
- Eat grains and vegetables.
- Do not eat meat, eggs, dairy products, or processed foods.
- Do not eat sugar, honey, syrups, or other sweets.
- Chew very well (50 to 100 times per mouthful) and do not overeat.
- Breathing is extremely important, breathe deeply everyday.
- Receive regular shiatsu treatments.

Beginning of Conception

The Beginning of Creation

The ancient mythology of Chinese folk religion describes the Oriental version of the West's creation story. According to historical sources, "We learn that chaos was like a hen's egg. Neither Heaven nor Earth existed. From the egg P'an-ku was born, while of its heavy elements Earth was made and Sky from the light elements. P'an-ku is represented as a dwarf, clad in a bearskin or a cloak of leaves. For 18,000 years the distance between Earth and Sky grew daily by ten feet, and P'an-ku grew at the same rate so that his body filled the gap. When he died, different parts of his body became various natural elements. His body fleas became the human race." Humankind's search for an explanation of life and creation occurs in all cultures. The older Western view of God working for six days and resting on the seventh with a follow-up of creating Eve from the rib of Adam, to the modern theory of creation beginning with a "big bang," an explanation of how we as humans have come into existence has persisted. Without knowing how at least we know that heaven and earth came into being, but can we learn how do the fleas of P'an-ku become humans?

Conception and the Process of Biological Development

From an ancient mythological or modern scientific point of view, movement and life begin with conception. It is one of the most marvelous processes. The union of the female's egg with the male's sperm is the physical reason that species continue. Simultaneously, there is an energetic exchange that goes on in this production.

The developing baby depends on its mother for care and nourishment before the actual delivery. At the moment of conception support from the mother begins. In the Japanese culture it is believed that education begins at this time. This is called *Tai Kyô*. The best education occurs when the parents love each other and the forthcoming baby. If mother and father are in a happy relationship, this vibration is felt within the womb.

The internal environment of the womb is the baby's world for nine months. It is best if the environment can be made to be peaceful and serene, an atmosphere conducive to study, happiness, and growth. It is best if the mother does not smoke, drink alcohol, or use medications or drugs during this embryonic development period. Alkaline quality blood is essential for the baby's best interest. The nervous system develops best if it is not over-stimulated by emotional swings or loud music. Babies seem to like soft music and gentle activities.

How the Baby Develops

The female yin energy produces an egg (physically yang in structure) while the male yang energy produces sperm (physically yin in structure). The male's yang energy, transmitted through the sperm cell, meets and joins with the feminine yin energy found in the egg cell. The joining of these two energies creates a new energy. It is at this point that life starts. This new group of cells attaches to the uterus. While attached to the uterus it receives nourishment from the mother through her bloodstream and the newly formed placenta. This new life has two energies. Yin and yang energies are inherited from each of the parents.

Of the two energies, yang energy is quicker. It spirals downward from infinity contracting as it moves. When it reaches the body it is an active condensed form of energy. This energy creates the materially compact nervous system, which develops up the body in a yin direction. Eventually this becomes the central nervous system, the autonomic nervous system, and other nervous systems. This upward movement forms the brain and later it creates the hollow organs.

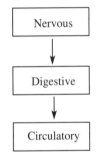

Fig. 5 Oriental Theory of Formation of Systems

Yin energy is slower. Its expansive tendency makes the digestive system (beginning at the mouth moving toward the anus) and later it creates the solid organs.

Yin and yang together create the circulatory system. This is done with the combined efforts of the Heart and Heart Governor meridians. The circulatory system begins to form in the center of the body.

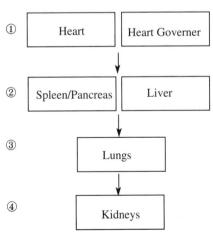

Fig. 6 Oriental Theory of Formation of Internal Organs

We become full humans when the digestive system is capable of making blood. Blood is then circulated to the entire body. Beginning in the center it moves both to the upper and lower segments. The heart and a system develop to accomplish this task efficiently. This is the circulatory system. As the digestive system energy goes up, it spreads out. This forms the lungs. The example of a water hose can be used to illustrate the movement of *Ki* or vital energy. Strong force (traveling in yang meridians) makes the water go straight. Less or slower force (flowing through yin meridians) makes things spread out. Here the slow, spreading energy forms the solid organs like the lungs.

The spleen/pancreas organs receive initial growth from leftover Heart energy (fire element) of the circulatory system. The pancreas is then completed from the yin-yang energy that spreads out (earth element). At the same time the Liver is formed (wood element). These energies then goes up to form and nourish the Lung (metal element). From here energy then goes down to form the Kidneys (water element).

Birth Facts

In the United States, 80 percent of American women receive at least one drug during delivery. The 30 percent of the infants born vaginally are dragged into the world with forceps. While another 15 percent of all deliveries are done by Caesarean section.

Caesarean section has increased by 200 percent in the last twenty years. Mostly because of the fetal cardiac monitor, which provides an ongoing reading of the child's heart rate and breathing during birth. Obstetricians say that it helps them spot troubles sooner and do something more quickly. However, others feel that it needlessly exposes increasingly large numbers of women and their children to the hazards of surgery.

It is best not to remove the child from the mother after delivery. Nature wants this time together to bond the child with the mother and vice versa. Some authorities say the mother is tired from the birth experience and would be better off resting. If you have ever experienced a birth, you know that there is a great deal of electricity in the room and the last thing the mother wants to do is sleep. The mother wants to watch and be with the baby. Hundreds of recent studies confirm this view. Both mother and child do not need sleep or food, but to stroke and snuggle and to look at and listen to each other.

Summary

The Asian culture has always been concerned about progeny, and one of the main purposes of preventive medicine is to strengthen the genetic plasma passed on to their offspring. Healthy, robust parents usually produce healthy, robust children. And children born healthy and robust go through life with less disease, greater vitality, and healthier minds. By keeping themselves in optimum health through preventive care, especially around the time of conception, these people continually seek to improve their genetic stock.

There are several stages that we pass through from birth to death. We visit infancy, childhood, adolescence, adulthood, and old age. It is important to keep up our training throughout our lives to survive in good order. We are supposed to live to be over one hundred years of age. We should die of old age of natural causes. The best natural cause is that all the organs wear out at the same time. If we follow natural order we should know when we are going to die. There should be no struggle as we know energy continues on infinitely after death. Throughout life our moment-to-moment time should be happy. Wondering if we are going to come back to this planet again in some reincarnated form should not be that important to us because our focus is on living in the present not the future. As humans we should make ourselves and the environment better. In this way our life will be filled with positive, beneficial activities that bring happiness to us and to others.

Food and Cooking

The human race has developed sophisticated cultures yet on a biological level we remain animals with the survival needs and abilities of other animals. All creatures must eat. But humans have a great diversity concerning what and how to eat.

Focusing on the structure and function of teeth gives us insight into our past and perhaps into our needs. When teeth arrive in an infant, the baby is then equipped to eat food besides mother's milk. This is true of all mammals. Humans have thirty-two teeth. There are twenty molars and premolars for grinding, eight incisors for cutting, and four canines for tearing. The teeth show that we are mixed eaters, that is, we can eat almost anything. This contributes to our survival. It is my opinion that this is why we developed a complex brain. From observing the teeth and the length of the digestive system, humans are meant to eat mostly vegetables, particularly whole cereal grains. Curiously, eskimos have longer, sharper canine teeth, a structure produced by eating meat.

In preparing food, attention must be given to such details as how the dish looks, its color, and of course, its flavor and taste. Attendance at cooking classes is essential to learn the best and most nutritious way to make and display whole natural foods. In these classes you will learn about quality, using only the best ingredients, organic when possible, and vegetables without chemical residues. We all already know about quantity. It is important not to overeat. We feel best when we eat only to 80 percent capacity. Always remember to chew well. These simple tips cannot be overemphasized. My experience has shown that women feel best when approximately 5 to 10 percent protein is included in the diet. For men slightly more, 10 to 15 percent, is good. Protein stays in the system longer than carbohydrates. Men are yang on the outside and yin on the inside, therefore a fuel that stays longer benefits them. Women have a stronger digestive system therefore they can assimilate carbohydrates for some of their protein needs. You may want to remember a few simple guidelines.

Seven Guidelines for a Healthy Diet

1. Increase complex carbohydrates: Eat plenty of whole grains, vegetables, sea vegetables, legumes, and fruit. Complex carbohydrates can help you lose weight because they are naturally low in calories, high in dietary fiber, provide plenty of vitamins and minerals, and create a natural feeling of fullness and comfort. Processed and highly refined foods contain sugar, refined salt, and fat—all enemies to good health and nutrition. They also decrease your vitality and energy levels.

2. Eliminate refined and processed sugar: The average American consumes more than 140 pounds of refined sugar a year. Packaged foods are full of disguised sugar. Sugar's many names include sucrose, corn syrup, maltose, or lactose. Sugar promotes tooth decay and actually robs the body of vitamins and minerals it would otherwise receive from complex carbohydrates. Once you have eliminated sugar from your diet, the taste of sweetness in other foods increases.

3. Reduce fat: Fat comes in two forms: saturated fat (like butter and other fats derived mainly from animals) and unsaturated fat (monounsaturated and polyunsaturated, which come from plants and fish). Excess saturated fat can be deadly. A high-fat diet combined with red meat results in high-cholesterol levels and elevated blood pressure —two symptoms that contribute to heart disease.

4. Reduce cholesterol: A high-cholesterol level can lead to serious health problems including atherosclerosis, a heart disease characterized by the accumulation of fat debris inside the heart's arteries. The body makes its own cholesterol therefore you should restrict outside sources. Cholesterol is only found in animal foods. Watch out for eggs, hamburger, bacon, cheese, and shrimp.

5. Eliminate refined salt: Most Americans consume too much salt—between six and eighteen grams per day. Much of this comes from snack foods such as pretzels, potato chips, and salted nuts. Naturally occurring sea salt should replace refined salt in small to moderate amounts. The body needs approximately five grams a day. Moderate amounts of salty seasonings such as miso and tamari soy sauce can be used unless blood pressure is high. If you are uncertain how much sea salt you need, skip salt for a while. Your body will tell when it is time again to season your food. The longer you are a vegetarian the larger volume of unrefined sea salt your body can utilize.

6. Avoid junk food: Fast foods may be convenient and even to some, it may taste good, but most commercial fast food is high in fat, sodium, and calories. Plan your meals and pack a lunch so you are not tempted by the smell of deep-fried foods. Regarding calories you can eat one Big Mac at 541 calories or three cups of cooked brown rice at 189 calories each.

7. Exercise: Walking is one of the best exercises you can do. Move your body and feel the difference.

Energy, Carbohydrates, and Hypoglycemia

Energy and food are inseparable. Diet and its effects on the mind also are inseparable. They relate to each other in a sort of double feedback way. What occurs psychologically affects the diet in many ways. And then, the resulting change in nutritional status has important effects in psychological function. This means that a continuous interplay exists, and that this can, if allowed to run haywire, carry you to great heights or depths of mental and physical disorder. On the other hand, understanding this connection can promote total health.

An uneven and irregular alteration of the blood sugar can be most disrupting to psychological functioning. When the blood sugar climbs abruptly, one will usually feel a surge of energy, but when it drops, equally abruptly, there is a feeling of weakness, irritability, anxiety, and often a sense of being out of control.

Though large amounts of sugar in the diet will inevitably run up nutrient debts and eventually result in the breakdown of some system of the body, it need not be carbohydrate metabolism that fails. Not everyone suffers hypoglycemic attacks from eating sugar.

Some people who are subject to large drops in blood sugar, or hypoglycemic spells, have this problem because they are unable to regulate insulin secretion properly. After eating a meal heavy in sweets, insulin is slow to appear, so glucose cannot move from the blood into the cells and blood sugar begins to soar. Finally, when insulin secretion does come, it comes in full force, and so much glucose is removed from the blood that blood sugar drops drastically and one begins to experience the characteristic weakness and shakiness.

Food absorbed from the intestines is taken up by the portal vein and goes directly to the liver. Here all blood is filtered and nutrients are sorted out, some put in storage and others released for immediate use. If the liver is healthy and is able to separate nutrients and to store glucose, then excessive amounts of this sugar are not dumped into the blood. Poor liver function triggers hypoglycemic attacks and the accompanying mental distresses.

The liver also serves to provide a constant internal environment in which the nervous system can function. A smooth function ensures a sense of calm and peace of mind. When the liver fails in this function, because of overeating, eating excess protein, fat, and refined carbohydrates, and chemical exposure, toxic materials remain in the blood and are circulated throughout the body. This causes a sensation of heaviness, achiness, and soreness. These waste products remain in circulation and affect the nervous system as well as the brain. This creates a feeling of apathy, lethargy, and often depression.

Dietary Fiber

Fiber is what we used to call roughage. It is an important part of healthy eating. The human digestive tract is unable to digest fiber, or plant materials such as cellulose and pectin that are found in unrefined flour, cereals, fruit, leafy vegetables, and legumes such as lentils.

Fiber is, however, of great importance to your diet. It provides bulk to help the large intestine efficiently carry away body wastes, and it may also help prevent diverticular disease and cancer of the large intestine. Some physicians believe that because fiber affects the way the body uses fats, a high-fiber diet may even help to reduce the development of atheroma (patches of fatty tissue which damages the vessel walls) by lowering the levels of the fats (including cholesterol) in the blood.

Some of the most famous fiber sources are oats, rice, wheat, and psyllium. Actually, all whole grains, vegetables, sea vegetables, and fruit contain fiber.

Bread

When it comes to bread, we were better off in the Stone Age. Back then, grains of wheat were crushed between stones to make flour, and most people made whole grain "peasant" bread.

In 1870, a new invention made it possible to grind flour 100 times faster. The steam-powered roller mill was initially hampered by one problem. When heated by the high-speed grinding process, the oil-rich wheat germ gummed up the steel rollers.

Millers solved this problem by sifting out the germ, and in their eyes, the process reaped additional benefits. Without the oily germ, the shelf life of the flour was greatly increased because it could not go rancid. What is more, the brown coating of the wheat, called *bran,* was sifted out with the germ during the grinding process. Previously, it had been painstakingly removed by sifting the flour through a fine cloth. Now the snow-white flour prized by the upper classes could be enjoyed by all. Unfortunately since the presence of vitamins in food was not yet discovered, the millers who brought white flour to the masses had no idea they were robbing consumers of the most nutritious part of the wheat.

There is a dramatic difference between whole wheat flour and white flour. During refining about 70 percent of twenty-one essential nutrients is removed with the bran and germ. These nutrients include all the fiber (helpful in preventing constipation and colon cancer), most of the vitamin E (protects cell membranes and other vitamins) and a host of trace minerals, whose important role in health has just recently become clear. (Examples are copper and chromium, which may protect against heart disease.)

White flour, which consists of the starch endosperm of the wheat groat, is "enriched" with three vitamins and iron to bring it to the level of whole wheat, but the remaining seventeen nutrients are not replaced.

Unfortunately, to find a truly whole grain bread in most stores is not an easy assignment. Far too few are available, and many breads touted as whole grain with names like "honey wheat" or "dark and grainy" are impostors—full of white flour but darkened with caramel coloring or a brown wrapper.

To tell if a bread is whole grain, look at the ingredient list. The only flour listed should be whole wheat, whole rye, whole barley, and so on. Whether it is stone-ground makes little nutritional difference.

"Wheat flour" or "enriched wheat flour" simply are names for white flour (made from wheat as opposed to other grains).

Another type of whole grain bread is made by sprouting and chopping grains such as rye, barley, and wheat rather than grinding them into flour.

"Bran" breads have slightly more fiber than whole wheat but usually are made with white flour so they lack the benefits of the germ.

Types of Flour

Bread is principally made from wheat. There are three classifications of wheat: winter, spring, and duram. Spring and winter wheat name the season following planting. Duram is a very hard wheat that is not satisfactory for bread making because it will not rise; it is used for making pasta.

Protein quality is the most important aspect of flour for bread making. This is what builds the structure of the bread. Terms such as hard wheat and soft wheat indicate protein quality. Hard wheat is high in protein, it yields a "strong" flour and is used in bread making. Soft wheat is low in protein, yields a "weak" flour and is best suited to making cakes and cookies. Gluten forms when flour protein (glutelin) is combined with water and kneaded. Elasticity of bread dough results from this gluten formation.

Whole wheat flour: Ground from the whole wheat kernel, this contains the bran and the germ which hold most of the grain's vitamins and minerals. It also contains more protein than enriched white flour. It should be refrigerated so the fat (from the wheat germ) does not become rancid.

Hard spring wheat flour: A whole wheat flour that is high in gluten and protein. It is a high-quality flour for bread making as it allows the dough to rise well and hold its shape. It contains 12 to 14 percent protein.

Winter wheat flour: Lower in protein and gluten so this is not as ideal for bread making. It contains about 10 percent protein.

Whole wheat pastry flour: Made from soft winter wheat this is best suited for preparing tender pastry, cookies, and baked goods. It makes a very heavy loaf if used alone in bread, but can be mixed with hard wheat flour for satisfactory bread making.

Unbleached wheat flour (unbleached white): This flour contains all of the germ and part of the bran. It is less nutritious than whole wheat flour and produces lighter colored and textured baked goods with more nutrition than bleached white flour.

Bleached and/or bromated enriched white flour (all purpose flour): The most prevalent flour on the market today. It is nutritionally inferior to other wheat flours and contains only the endosperm of the wheat kernel. To make the flour whiter it is treated with chemicals such as chlorine dioxide and acetone peroxide. This process destroys vitamin E and B vitamins that may have survived the milling process. After bleaching the flour is often bromated or phosphated (dough conditioner) which reduce the need for kneading. The enriching process adds thiamine, riboflavin, niacin, and iron to about the level in whole wheat flour. It does not add the other essential vitamins and minerals removed during the processing.

Self-rising flour: Refined, bleached flour which is combined with baking powder.

Graham flour: A coarse ground whole wheat flour.

Rye flour: This flour is low in gluten and is unresponsive to commercial use. For this reason it generally is mixed with other flours higher in gluten such as wheat flour.

Triticale flour: The first human made grain. It was produced by crossing several different species of wheat and rye. It has more protein and B vitamins than either wheat or rye. Its flavor is slightly sweet in taste.

Gluten flour: A starch-free, high-protein flour. It is washed from hard wheat, dried, and ground. With water and kneading it forms an elastic dough that stretches making it useful in baking with low gluten flours such as rye and soybean.

High-quality Vegetable Protein

It is sometimes thought that beef is king. When it comes to protein, common thought has been that animal sources are best. Well, times have changed. By all accounts the leading cause of death, heart disease, is almost 100 percent diet-related. And, you have guessed it, the major culprit is beef. But American farmers have come to the rescue. Over the years, the United States has developed a large base of agricultural products. One of the most successful and unusual has been the soybeans. This country is the planet's largest soybean producer. And while soybeans may be one of the largest cash crops almost all of the crop is exported, primarily to Asia, the home of the soybeans. Just a small percentage remains in this country for use. While the soybeans have been in use in the Orient for over 4,000 years a Gallup poll taken in the United States showed that over 50 percent of those questioned have neither seen a soybean plant nor tasted soybeans, whether fresh (green), dry, or sprouts. It has only been since the 1970s with the macrobiotic and natural foods movements that the soybeans have gained some reputation in America.

The soybeans are a high-yielding and easy to harvest plant crop. They can be produced more inexpensively than any other grain. The American annual harvest is sufficient to provide every person in the United States with 165 pounds of pure, high-quality protein, enough to fill the average adult protein requirement of every American for a couple of years.

In this country, soybeans are known for their by-products in the form of cooking oil, vegetable shortening, margarine, soy sauce and, more recently, *tofu* or bean curd. Soybean meal, which contains two-and-a-half times as much protein by weight as steak, rarely makes its way onto our tables. Of the nation's soybean crop, only 3 percent of what is not exported is used for human consumption; the remainder is fed to cows and chickens, mixed into pet food, or used industrially to make caulking components and printing inks among other things.

In macrobiotic or vegetarian diets soybeans are used primarily in three forms. The most commonly known preparation is as tofu, sometimes called *soy cheese*. This preparation is made from soymilk with the addition of a solidifying agent. It can be added to soups, marinated with soy sauce and baked or fried, or sprinkled on salads. It has a neutral almost tasteless flavor that blends well with whatever seasoning it is prepared with.

Miso is another popular soybean product. Miso is a cooked, fermented preparation that is between several months to several years old. It has a variety of flavors, all delicious. It can be prepared with any grain but most commonly it is made with barley, brown and white rice. It is principally used as a seasoning for flavorful soups.

The third use for soybeans is in the form of tempeh. Originally from Indonesia, this soybean product makes a wonderful addition to the diet. Whole soybeans are cooked and a bacteria is introduced that makes the beans stick together in something like a burger. These patties can be marinated and baked, barbecued, fried or added to soups.

Each style of soybean preparation is unique and has a particular role to play in a nutritionally balanced diet. They are all extremely easy to digest so the nutritional contents are readily and easily absorbed and assimilated by even the most fragile digestive systems.

Diet and Emotions

Food affects the functions of the internal organs. Emotions also affect the functions of these organs. For example an angry, tense person will not product sufficient digestive enzymes. This retards digestion and absorption. The stomach is easily affected by emotional states. Feelings of worry, hopelessness, depression, and inadequacy may be caused by and also be the cause of indigestion. The opposite is also true. The function of the organs affects the emotions. The pain of a peptic ulcer breeds a feeling of inadequacy and a doubting attitude of your abilities. The following are examples of some common emotional connections.

Organ	Emotion
Lungs	Grief, melancholy, sadness
Intestines	Nervousness, overwhelming anxiety
Stomach	Worry, hopelessness, dependency, inadequacy
Pancreas	Weakness, anxiety, introversion, insecurity, lethargy, apathy, irritability
Heart	Excitability
Kidneys	Fear, terror
Liver	Depression, anger, hate

Health and Spiritual Awareness

To live a good life good judgment is necessary. Whole Health Shiatsu stimulates the physical body to function efficiently. Because of the body-mind connection the mind too is influenced in a positive way. Our human ability to grasp elusive, non-concrete concepts adds a depth of understanding and meaning to living.

Infinity is extremely difficult to comprehend. Ancient Oriental Buddhist literature spoke very eloquently about the nature of the unfathomable. It is recorded in the Heart Sutra (*Maka Hannya Hara Mitta Shin Gyô*). This sutra was condensed from the teachings of Buddha that were recorded in thousands of volumes. Because of its importance it is chanted often by Buddhists. The title translates as "The Great Teaching Which Reveals Supreme Judgment." The translation by Herman Aihara is that one who reaches supreme judgment perceives that all matters and minds are manifestations of Oneness, Infinity and thus overcomes all sufferings.

> Ladies and gentlemen:
> Matter is not different from Infinity, Oneness, God.
> Infinity is not different from matter.
> Matter is Infinity.
> Infinity is matter.
> Sensations, emotions, desires, and intellect are infinity.
> Ladies and gentlemen:
> All matters and minds are the manifestations of Oneness, Infinite world.
> In Infinity, nothing is created nor destroyed,
> Nothing is dirty nor unclean,
> Nothing increases nor decreases.
> In Infinity, there are no sense organs which are changing.
> There are no sensations, emotions, desires, nor consciousness.
> There are neither eye, ear, nose, tongue, body, nor mind.
> There are neither color, voice, smell, taste, flesh, nor mental activity.
> There are neither visible world nor conscious (invisible) world.
> There are neither autonomic intuitive action nor end of intuitive action.
> There are neither old age nor death.
> There are neither eternal youth nor eternal life.
> There are neither security nor disciplines.
> There are neither knowledge to learn nor things to acquire, because there is every
>   thing here.

One who attains the supreme judgment has no bondage. Because of no bondage, he has no fear. Because of no fear, he can transmute all emotional, illusional thinking to eternal joy and happiness.

In past, present, and future, all wisest men understood, understand, or will understand this supreme judgment—the dualistic constitution of Oneness, Reality—and thus embrace, love, and enjoy everything (whatever comes to him).

Therefore, this teaching of supreme judgment is the most miraculous mantra, brightest mantra, highest mantra, greatest mantra.

> This mantra can transmute all sufferings.
> This is the teaching of truth.
> Now, you have reached supreme judgment.
> Here is Infinity, Oneness and Nirvana.
> You are Buddha, Eternal Oneness.

From other religious teaching it is said, "When you look at the mysteries of life and can appreciate the natural blessings given to you by the power of God, you will be free from illness." The natural medicine and healing power within human beings comes from the food consumed and the body organs that digest the food and turn it into energies for the body. Buddhist scriptures explain this healing power with the story of the bodhisattva (enlightened teacher) named Yakushi Nyorai. Yakushi Nyorai is considered the Master of Medicine. This teacher's legacy is given to each of us as our everyday food. Food provides humankind with essential material necessary for survival. When you realize that all food and drink are the products of nature, it reminds you of the care that our creator has for us. It also will prevent you from abusing your body through excessive consumption. Food is another form of divine healing, it must be respected and treasured. One example that we can display as an act of appreciation and as sign of understanding is to chew food well. It is a universally known fact that thorough chewing of food is necessary to aid proper digestion.

The Mind and Diet

Positive thinking and proper diet are essential for the preservation of health. What is positive thinking? It is the ability to recognize and appreciate the true significance of situations. True appreciation is to be able to also accept adversities as valuable life experiences.

Many people are unaware of the makeup of their consciousness, nor of the interacting spiritual forces that exist. They merely attribute their misfortunes to bad luck, occupation, environment, other people, and so on. While people entertain this popular notion, they will be unable to attain true happiness in life.

Source Energy in Cooking

There are many sources of heat that have been used in food preparation. For centuries stories have been told of a Garden of Eden like environment where all people's food needs were supplied by picking fresh fruit directly from an abundant tree. We recognize this first cooking style as solar heat. It has become the dream of every busy person who does not have time to spend in the kitchen. However, a different story of humanity has developed based on archeological findings. In these pre-civilization times the number and types of food available were limited, survival was dangerous and time-consuming. Most root or tuber vegetables are inedible without cooking of some sort. For the ancestors of cave dwellers, before the use of fire became routine, tough inedible root vegetables were not eaten. Scientists explain the arrival of speech when humans were capable of uttering more than grunts and groans. They say that when humans used fire and cooked formerly inedible root vegetables it supplied a new source of necessary vitamins and minerals for the physical development of the vocal cords. Cooking softened and pre-digested the tough cellulose and freed the proteins, carbohydrates, vitamins, and minerals locked in the root vegetable's cells. These elements encouraged the vocal cords to develop to what we have today. This allowed a greater range of sound to be produced. The combinations of these sounds create the complexity and richness of language. We can assume with the ability to communicate the depth of human experience, humanity's consciousness took a giant leap forward. All this became possible with an expanded food source that cooking provided.

The use of a heat source in food preparation also lengthened life span by purifying the food. The frequent sources of illness such as dysentery from bacteria as well as viral, yeast, and parasitic infestations are eliminated when foods are sterilized by cooking. The practice of not allowing these bugs to enter the human digestive system is a major historical step in humanity's conquest of disease and movement toward the goal of longevity. To this day the long lasting cultures of India and Asia rarely use raw food.

The sources of heat are solar, wood, coal, oil, gas, electricity, microwave (electromagnetic), and irradiation. The first set of two, solar and wood, are the most ancient and have been used the longest time. They need no preparation. They can be used immediately. The first style, solar, requires no work while the second, wood, requires that somehow you ignite a couple of sticks and viola! you have a fire. The second set of two, coal and oil, were used later in society's development. It took sometime to discover that coal would burn. Oils had to be pressed from plants or stored from animal fats so there is some preparation before they can be used, but, people discovered these talents early and these two have also been used for centuries. The third set of two, gas and electricity belong to the modern era of fuels. Gas must be extracted from the earth and contained that means a technology to do so, while electricity must be generated, stored, and delivered. This also demands a technology only available in the twentieth century. Each source of heat gets further away from the primary origin—fire. The final set of two, microwave and irradiation, are products of the ultramodern age. While they possess the ability to heat, there is no visible reminder of fire. Neither possess a flame. The latest in food preparation is purposely irradiating foods for a longer shelf life. Foods are bombarded with radioactive residue. Because there is no radioactive readings in the final product this process is considered safe. I feel this is extremely shortsighted and dangerous. The radioactive material used in this process comes from the nuclear industry. They have ingeniously found an additional use for their waste. Nuclear power is used in many countries essentially to boil the water that is used to produce steam that turns the generators at a power plant that produces electricity. It is considered to be a clean, energy efficient fuel. However, when you factor in the thousands of years life span of the spent fuel and the dangers associated with its use and storage, it is hard to defend this as a clean and safe heating source. Equally so, is the use of radiation in food preparation.

Microwave Energy

The modern kitchen includes an appliance that did not exist a couple of decades ago. It is the microwave oven. Because it is so common it deserves some discussion. I am often asked why microwave cooking is not recommended, especially when a serious illness is present. There is no denying the convenience of this kitchen appliance. Even with the rush of modern life, I cannot recommend its use. Here is what microwave manufacturers tell us about how the appliance works. Electrical energy is transformed into electromagnetic energy or microwave energy by a tube called a magnetron. This tube is like a broadcasting station sending out waves of high-frequency energy in the cavity of the microwave oven where they are reflected off the metallic side walls, floor, and ceiling of the oven and are eventually absorbed by the food. This electromagnetic energy causes the molecules of the food to agitate. This agitation produces friction that in turn causes it to cook. Microwaves penetrate about 1/2 to 1 1/2 inches, depending on the density of the food and after that heating occurs through transference or conduction. Because all the heat is produced in the food itself no heat is wasted in preheating the oven or heating the utensils. Microwaves are high-frequency radio waves, supporters say they cannot cause a chemical change or a breakdown in your foods.

Microwaves pass through certain substances, such as paper, plastic, glass, and ceramic, as light passes through a window. These materials may warm up eventually, as heat transfers from the food to them.

There are certain precautions the manufacturers warn against. The principal precaution is "do not allow yourself to be exposed to the microwave energy." Exposure is regarded as harmful. They suggest you do not operate the oven if it is damaged. It is particularly important that the oven door close properly and that there is no damage to hinges and latches, door seals, and sealing surfaces. With such strong recommendations it is apparent that the slightest leakage or malfunction is potentially dangerous. It is also unknown what the long-term effects of microwave cooking are. We do know that the water molecule agitates because of the magnetic charge it carries. Each water molecule inside food has a positive and negative charge. The microwave's magnetic strength moves these water molecules swiftly, banging them around. This movement creates the heat that cooks the meal. Some researchers have stated that the final cooked product leaves all the north poles (the positive charges) aligned in the same direction in what was once a random order. Connoisseurs claim this new arrangement destroys the flavor and taste of the food. I feel the swift agitation method disturbs the harmony of the food and increases the likelihood of agitating the consumer. Many people who use microwave cooking live a hurried, stressful, and agitated lifestyle. They do not feel the effects of this style of cooking. But for sensitive people or those with damage to their immune systems like cancer patients, this style of cooking can only make matters worse.

The Energy of Cooking

Cooking is unique. Not only can flavor be affected by preparation but so can the energetics of foods. Someone who is ailing with a yin condition will do well to include some yang cooking styles into the menu plan. On the contrary, someone who is excessively yang can temper their passions with more yin styles of cooking. Energetically speaking, we can see that the use of pressure, salt, heat, and time will make the energy of the food more concentrated. Quick cooking and less salt preserves a lighter energetic quality of the food. Essentially there are five cooking styles: steaming, boiling, sautéing, deep frying, and baking. These affect the five movements: stable, downward, upward, gathering, and dispersion.

1. Stable energy cooking uses any of the cooking styles in a balanced way. Round vegetables are used, and the use of sea salt and other salty condiments is moderate.
2. Downward energy cooking emphasizes a longer cooking time with root vegetables and beans. Baked beans are an example of an earthy dish.
3. Upward energy cooking is on the light side. Green leafy vegetables are steamed to lighten the body and allow energy to move upward. Boiled salad also has the same effect.
4. Gathering energy cooking is strong, slightly salty cooking. Sautéed vegetables including hijiki concentrate energy, gathering it to a center. A moderately long cooking time accomplishes this task.
5. Dispersion energy cooking is a quick style of cooking like boiling or short time quick sautéing with oil. Leafy vegetables as well as ginger, brown rice vinegar, and small amounts of raw salad move energy outward.

Practical Cooking Styles

To give you a firm basis to explore the world of cooking, I have included a list of the most practiced preparation styles in cooking. Please note that these are descriptions of cooking techniques, not detailed menus.

Pressure Cooking: Grains or beans are placed in a pressure cooker with water. The cooker is brought up to pressure with a lid on a medium flame. The flame is reduced to medium-low and the ingredients are then cooked for the required length of time.

Steaming: There are three main ways to steam.

1. *Lightly steamed:* Vegetables or fruits are placed in a pot with a small amount of water. The pot is covered and the ingredients are steamed for two to three minutes on a medium-high flame.
2. *Steamed with a steamer:* Leftovers, bread, vegetables or fruits are placed in a steamer. The steamer is put into a pot with a small amount of boiling water. The pot is covered and the ingredients are steamed for the required length of time.
3. *Long steam:* Vegetables are cut into large chunks and placed in a pot with a small amount of water. The pot is covered and the ingredients are brought to a boil on a medium flame. The flame is reduced to low and cooked until the vegetables are soft.

Stew: Beans or vegetables are layered in a pot. Water is added to almost cover the vegetables. The pot is covered and the ingredients are brought to a boil on a medium flame. The flame is then reduced to medium-low and the ingredients are cooked until soft. The lid may be removed at the end of cooking to allow any excess liquid to evaporate.

Sautéing: There are three main ways to sauté

1. *Short sauté:* A skillet is placed on a high flame and allowed to warm slightly. Oil is added and heated. The vegetables are then placed in the skillet and moved back and forth for approximately one to two minutes. If more than one vegetable is used, each variety can be sautéed separately, one after the other.

2. *Long sauté:* Vegetables are sautéed as above and then a small amount of water is added to the skillet. The skillet is covered and the flame reduced to low. The ingredients are cooked until soft.

3. *Waterless sauté:* A skillet is placed on a high flame and enough water is added to cover the bottom. When the water begins to boil, the vegetables are added and sautéed as in the short sauté.

Boiling: A pot of water is brought to a boil on a medium flame. Vegetables are immersed in the water and cooked until soft.

Blanching: A pot of water is brought to a boil on a medium flame. The flame is turned up high and vegetables are immersed in the water for less than one minute. The vegetables should be crispy and brightly colored.

Refreshing: Vegetables are placed in a strainer. The strainer is either dipped in boiling water or boiling water is poured over the vegetables.

Marinating: Vegetables or bean products are submerged in a liquid made from water and either salt, tamari soy sauce, or umeboshi. The ingredients are left for at least one hour.

Pressing: Vegetables are placed in a bowl or pickle press. A small amount of salt is worked through the vegetables. If using a bowl, a plate and a heavy weight are placed on top of the vegetables. If using a press, the lid is secured. The vegetables are then left for the required time. Before serving, the liquid from the vegetables is discarded.

Pickling: Vegetables can be pickled in many different ways. The length of time varies from three days to a year.

1. *Brine pickles:* Vegetables are submerged in a liquid made from water and either salt, tamari soy souce, or umeboshi. They are then left to sit for at least three days.

2. *Pressed pickles:* Vegetables are pressed as in pressed salad. However, extra salt is needed, and they are left for at least a day.

3. *Miso pickles:* Vegetables are immersed in a crock or miso and left for at least one week.

4. *Nuka pickles:* Vegetables are immersed in a crock of *nuka* bran, salt, and water, and left for at least two to three days.

Deep Frying: Oil is heated in a pot. Vegetables, grains, bean products, *seitan*, or *fu* (a wheat product) are submerged in the oil and cooked until golden brown.

Tempura: Oil is heated in a pot. Vegetables, bean products, seitan, or fu are dipped in batter and cooked very quickly in the oil. The outside should be crispy.

Baking: Grains, beans, bean products, vegetables, or fruits may be baked in an oven.

Raw Salad: Fresh vegetables or fruits can be eaten raw.

Dry Roast: Seeds or grains are placed in a warmed skillet. The ingredients are moved back and forth in the skillet over a medium-high flame. The flame may be reduced to medium-low if the ingredients need to be roasted for a long period of time.

Barbecue: Foods are cooked on a grill over direct flame.

Cooking for Different Body Types

There are four body types. Each of these types require a slightly different approach to cooking as their needs are individual. The four types are Yin-Fat, Yin-Thin, Yang-Fat, Yang-Thin. The yin or yang aspect describes the individual's general energy level and internal organs' function characteristics.

There are types of people who are very active, the first to try or do something; those who respond quickly to challenge, and do not get sick often. Their bone structure and muscle development is larger and more defined. These characteristics describe yang inherited traits. For individuals who have a smaller bone structure and less developed muscles, they exhibit yin inherited characteristics. Whether someone has the fat or thin aspect is obvious.

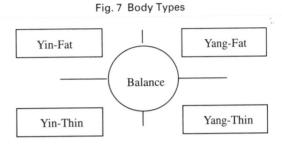

Fig. 7 Body Types

The aim of cooking is to create balance. By using various foods and preparation methods we can bring the energy to a middle way, thereby enhancing our strengths and tonifying our weaknesses. When these methods are used in the diversity of the family, make the menu in a composed way with a good balance of yin and yang so that all members will find balance in the food. If we do not eat in a middle way we will become extreme in both health and behavior. A whole health macrobiotic counselling session is useful to point out balance to those who are unfamiliar with these techniques of balance. However, counselling advice is useful only for a short time. The client must develop an understanding of the process of maintaining balance or their health will never be secure.

Yin-Fat

Tendencies: People of this body type are easy to get sinus and upper body trouble. This includes brain troubles. Their blood is on the thin side. They feel cold easily. Their body is too loose and expanded. They should eat regularly and not fast. The Yin-Fat type represents morning, spring, and the very young stage of development up to the age seven.

Cooking and Menu Suggestions: They should be careful with sweets including sugar, honey, fruit juice, cookies, and cakes. Pressure-cooked organic brown rice should be a mainstay in their diet with the addition of other grains also included. Their rice however, should not be cooked with too much water, nor should it be too soft. Eating rice balls help keep up the energy between meals. Cooked vegetable side dishes should make up approximately 30 percent of the diet. It is important not to eat or drink excessively watery items. It is a good rule to remember to drink only when you are thirsty. The food should always be warm. Sautéed vegetables are a welcome part of the menu. Cut vegetables in medium-sized pieces and prepare with a longer cooking time. The salt flavor can be prominent in cooking as can the use of stronger condiments such as *gomashio* (sesame salt) and *tekka* (a root vegetable preparation). This person needs animal protein regularly in the form of fish and may enjoy the special fish dish *koi-koku*, which is a mixture of carp (*koi*) or other fishes like snapper or cod, and root vegetables.

Short hot salt baths will warm the body and increase circulation. The bath should be followed by the drink, *ume-sho-bancha*, to replenish minerals.

Yin-Thin

Tendencies: The body of this type is overly contracted. Their digestive system has a difficult time absorbing food, therefore it is very important for them to cook well. They need both salt and oil, however, if they receive too much the body cannot process it. The Yin-Thin body type represents night, winter, and the old-age years.

Cooking and Menu Suggestions: Pressure-cooked brown rice may be too strong for them. Rice cream or a softer, moister version of cooked rice, *kayu*, is good. The grain can be cooked for a long time in a clay pot. A slower, gentler cooking style is best. Whole grains should be the main food with a 30 percent or less portion of cooked vegetables. Tiny cut vegetables are appropriate. The smaller cuts push potassium out of the vegetable and replaces it with sodium. Gomashio should be ground a lot so that it is a fine powder and easy to absorb. Tekka is O.K. to use. Cold foods including salads are not recommended. Long hot baths are not good for this body type, but short salt baths to warm the system and increase circulation are O.K. Because of the difficulty with digestion, fasting is not recommended.

Yang-Fat

Tendencies: People of this type eat and drink to excess. Their body is puffed up with water retention. They have excess sodium in their thicker than normal blood and need more potassium. Because of their excessive nature drinking more liquid than required is O.K. for a while until the blood thins down a bit. They can also freely take long hot baths and fasting may be beneficial for them. The Yang-Fat type represents the time around noon, summer, and the teen-ager of development, from the ages of seven to eighteen.

Cooking and Menu Suggestions: They do not need much grain in their diet. What grains they do eat should not be pressure cooked. They can boil the grains. As they have a tendency for constipation the fiber-rich quality of grains are welcome but in smaller than normal amounts. They may find soups with brown rice, rye, wheat, or other grains added tasty and light. Flour products like breads, pastries, and noodles should be minimized. They are welcome to enjoy as much vegetable side dishes as they please. They should eat plenty of vegetables. Boiling, sautéing, raw, pressed salads, and vegetable soups are useful cooking styles for this body type. Vegetables can be cut in large pieces. Seasoning should be light on both salt and oil. Less cooking time with a simpler taste help to create balance. Gomashio should be used moderately. Tekka is unnecessary to use. The sour flavor of plum vinegar (*ume-zu*) can be enjoyed. Unless there are complications of arthritis this body type can usually tolerate fruit such as apple, orange, and strawberry, as well as the nightshade family of vegetables like potato, tomato, eggplant, and bell pepper.

Yang-Thin

Tendencies: People who have been eating macrobiotic food for a long time generally develop into this type of condition. Their body is slim while the organ function is firm and toned. The Yang-Thin body type represents the evening, the autumn season, and the ages between thirty-five to fifty-five.

Cooking and Menu Suggestions: A wide version of the standard macrobiotic diet that includes grains, vegetables, soup, beans, pickles, nuts, seeds, fruit, and fish is recommended. The grain should be cooked until soft. Vegetable dishes should make up approximately 25 percent of the overall diet. The seasoning can be mild. Liquid can be consumed as the body requires it. Warm food should be the mainstay with the addition of specialty items like fried rice and a Japanese favorite, shredded *daikon* with *kampyo* (dried gourd) prepared in a *nishime* style. Gomashio should be used moderately. The use of salt and oil can be to taste for those eating. Vegetables should be cut in medium-sized pieces and cooked al dente, not too long nor undercooked. A hot salt bath can be taken whenever the Yang-Thin person feels like it.

Flavors and Energies

The taste and smell of foods and herbs correspond to the "five tastes" and " four energies." The five tastes are pungent, sweet, bitter, salty, and sour while the four energies are cool, cold, warm, and hot. Pungent food and herbs disperse and promote circulation. Sweet foods nourish the body and harmonize the stomach. Bitter foods and herbs solidify and purge. Harsh, sour flavors astringe and solidify; and salty ones soften and purge. Cool foods treat fever diseases. Hot foods remedy cold diseases.

The Five Flavors and Tastes:
1. Pungent flavors such as fresh ginger, perilla (*shiso*), mustard, and mint are used to disperse external toxins. This flavor positively affects the Lung/Large Intestine organ set.
2. Sweet flavors have a tonic and soothing effect. For example, ginseng nourishes energy and strengthens the system while licorice works as a paregoric that relieves intestinal pain. Sweet foods include corn, sweet potatoes, winter squash, peas, and dates. This flavor positively affects the Spleen/Pancreas/Stomach organ set.
3. Bitter flavors like burdock root and bitter melon, have drying and purging actions. Rhubarb regulates the bowels and purges fevers. The skin of pomegranate, sour and harsh, stops prolonged diarrhea, and heals anal prolapse. This flavor positively affects the Heart/Small Intestine organ set.
4. Salty flavors like kelp and sea salt soften, solidify, and moisten. The salty flavor is used to treat stagnant sputum and swollen glands. This flavor positively affects the Kidney/Bladder organ set.
5. Sour flavors disperse energy. Foods include olives, salted plums (*umeboshi*), whole grain sourdough bread, and vinegar. This flavor positively affects the Liver/Gall Bladder organ set.

Bland substances, those with no taste such as agar-agar (a sea vegetable used for thickening) or poria (a medicinal mushroom) are diuretics.

The Four Energies of Food:
1. Cool natured foods include pears, oranges, watermelon, bitter melon, crooked neck squash, eggplant, green lentils, tofu, and raw salads.
2. Cold foods include ice cream and iced beverages.
3. Mild, warm foods are chicken and beef.
4. Hot foods include wine, chili, curry, mutton, and eggs.

In a mostly vegetarian diet you can see that none of the warm or hot foods are included. If you are a cold-natured person how do you satisfy your need for warmth without such extremes as hamburger, chicken, eggs, and wine? In a word—cooking. The use of cooking styles becomes extremely relevant. Which do you think has the greatest amount of potential heat for the consumer, steamed or boiled rice; pressure-cooked rice; or seasoned fried rice? The most cooling style is steamed or boiled rice, with fried rice being the most warming. For the long-time vegetarian, pressure-cooked short-grain, organic rice is the most balanced. Thus to maintain one's health, a person chooses suitable foods according to his individual physical condition.

Causes of Some Common Problems
The following is a list of some conditions that arise when excess food or too much of a particular flavor is eaten.

1. Eating and drinking without restraint injures the Spleen and Stomach and changes the metabolism, predisposing one to disease. For example, frequent consumption of fatty food causes damp fever, stomach problems, heartburn, congestion, and chest stagnancy that in turn cause carbuncles, rashes, and abscesses.
2. An excess of pungent food causes fever in the gastrointestinal tract, stomach upsets, and hemorrhoids.
3. Too much sour food injures the Spleen and Pancreas.
4. Too much bitter food injures the Liver.
5. Too much salty food injures the Heart.
6. Heavy drinking of alcoholic beverages damages the Ki and blood and causes mental instability.

Chapter 3
Traditional Wisdom

In the Jewish book of civil and religious laws known as the Talmud is written, "Everyone whose deeds are more than his wisdom, his wisdom endures. And everyone whose wisdom is more than his deeds, his wisdom does not endure." This statement is just as true for societies as it is of individuals. Investigating traditional knowledge can be useful. It gives a foundation to start from, experiment with, and add to. The foundations of the natural healing and treatment techniques contained in this book originate from Asia and particularly from China. In our studies however, we should be vigilant not to believe everything that the past presents to us. We should be attentive to universal principles that are practical, useful, and easy to apply. In this way, we contribute to the long history of investigation, I hope, elevating humankind to a higher quality of physical and spiritual living.

One of the first contributions came from China with the inventions of a character-based written language and something to record it on—paper. With these inventions, experiments and research in the fields of medicine, herbs, acupuncture, and agriculture were not limited to oral repetition. The foundation of traditional medical thought for the first time could be recorded, in a series of ancient classics. Each dynasty added new resources as it drew from the past. With a country as old and active as China's, this promoted a rapid spread of ideas, theories, and practices. It was during the early Han dynasty that the theories and exploits of the Yellow Emperor were written down in *Huang Di Nei Jing* (The Internal Book of Huang Di). The following excerpts from this classic explain the underlying thought basic to the Oriental healing arts and its understanding of cause and cure of imbalance. The book begins with the emperor asking his chief physician about the state of his people's health. The emperor asks, "I've heard that ancient people were able to live to one hundred years and still be the same as when young. But nowadays, when fifty years old our activities decrease. How is this? Is it due to the times, or have humans lost something?" The physician answers, "The ancient people knew the way, the Tao, and the rule of yin and yang. The ancient people could control their eating habits. They knew the rules of life, walking, and sitting. They didn't overwork. For these reasons, they were healthy and balanced in body and mind and were able to live to one hundred years. But today, people are not like this, they drink too much alcohol and think about sex and after drinking will go to bed and lose their vital essence according to their sexual desire. At the same time as losing their vital essence, they lose and disperse the truth. They don't know how to keep the body healthy. They don't know how to control their mind and cannot control their desires. They are against the living pleasure, the Tao." Later the physician continues, "The four seasons and yin and yang are the beginning and ending of everything, the root of birth and death. If one goes against this rule one can get injury, creating general catastrophes, like a flood, which affect all others as well. If one doesn't go against the rule disease doesn't occur, this is the Tao."

Ancient research continued with another classic, *Shen Nong Ben Cao Jing* (The Pharmacopoeia of Shen Nong), that lists all known herbal plants with which to treat man's imbalances. Herbs are divided into three categories: an upper class of drugs that nurture life, a middle group that nurture "nature" or vitality and a lower group labelled "poisons" or medicines from toxic plants that were used to fight the most virulent diseases.

About the sixth century A.D. Chinese influence spread beyond its borders into Korea and on to Japan. Buddhist monks brought with them the Chinese writing characters as well as traditional medical practices, which included much information concerning food. History has it that Japanese delicacies such as tofu and miso were some gems Buddhist priests bestowed on the Japanese people.

Before Buddhism left China's borders China was, and still is, under the influence of Taoism. Embodied within Chinese medicine, physical health is an integral part of the whole body of law of Chinese spiritual and social life. The Taoist principles of balance apply as well to diet and medicine. Accordingly, food is taken not just for survival but also to constantly balance, regulate, and tune up both physical and mental health. Food and medicine became interrelated. Foods were chosen as much for their therapeutic qualities as for nourishment and taste. They were to be taken in moderation and adjusted to one's state of health. They were categorized according to the nature of their therapeutic value—"cold" foods such as fruit and certain vegetables, sliced pork, crab and fish were recommended to reduce "heat" in the body. "Hot" high-protein foods such as fatty meats, eggs, fried and spiced foods and ingredients soaked in wine, were taken to heat up and invigorate the system. The mainstay of the diet, rice and vegetables was adjusted with these specialty items for particular effects.

Diet alone was viewed as the principal sustaining agent for good health. As individuals suffered from direct illness, diet and medicine began to merge into more powerful medicinal curative diets. Tonics, soups, and stews mixed with particular flavors and tastes from distinctive herbs were used to deal with minor problems. Special preparations developed using everyday items like tofu and ginger to counteract fever or palpitations, or lotus root, daikon, or watercress soup to ward off bronchial infection and colds. The direction of food therapy was always the balancing of opposing forces within the metabolism, forces that were part of the crucial interplay of yin and yang. A thirteenth century physician stated, "To correct an imbalance, adequate diet is the first necessity. Only when this has failed should medicines be prescribed."

The Foundation—Ki

Science and the Western world view the universe from a materialistic outlook. We have searched for the smallest unit of matter to discover the basics of life. In the realm of health this thinking leads to the search for solutions to problems with a material basis. When this theory is applied this means if you have a headache you take aspirin, when you have a tumor you remove it.

The foundation of Oriental healing and natural medicine is based on an entirely different premise. The underlying thought is everything comes from infinity, it is all from nature, therefore the basis of the universe is the energy that comes from nature. The gathering together of Heaven's forces mold humans, animals, plants, and mineral creations. From the invisible infinite universe comes all that is visible. In Japanese this energy is called "Ki."

From birth Ki flows. Without any stagnation or hindrance to its flow we will not have many serious troubles. We will not have much sickness. If the quality of Ki becomes bad the opposite is true, we will become sick. In Japanese the word for sickness is *byôki*—imbalanced, sick, or bad Ki. Balancing the flow of Ki and creating a more harmoniously functioning body is the aim of natural healing. As an external solution we apply shiatsu. For an internal solution we adjust the diet. We cannot see Ki but it is always moving and creating everything. We are constantly receiving its influence. This is how we receive nature's power.

Ancient books record the movement of Ki. The *I Ching* or *Book of Changes*, says "infinity displays itself as opposing forces, yin and yang." Yin and yang mingle creating a product of their interaction. This result minglings with another and the process continues. So it is said that from the one (infinity or nature) comes two (yin and yang), from the two come many (everything). How the many show themselves is regulated by five essential motions of change. The five stages of development are known as the Five Transformations or commonly as Five Elements. I call them the Five Phases of Energy.

Ki

Ki is life-force, vitality. Generally speaking there are two types of Ki. The first is material Ki. This is the essential material foundation constituting the human body. Its sources are Ki from food (literally translated from Oriental characters as grain and water). The second is Ki from breath (literally the atmosphere). Nowadays we call this type of Ki as oxygen. It is referred to as "clean Ki." This Ki is functional Ki. This Ki is found in all organs and meridians. While Ki itself is a universal force, it has many names. Each of the names describes Ki depending on its source of origin, location, or current function.

Understanding Ki by Source of Origin

1. *Hereditary Ki:* A primary Ki. It is an original Ki that is formed in the embryo. This is considered congenital Ki and comes from our parents. After birth this Hereditary Ki (*Yuan Qi* in Chinese) continues to exist but it must be replenished by Ki from food. It is stored in the Kidneys. For this reason it is sometimes called Kidney Ki or Ki of Kidney Yang. A deficiency of Hereditary Ki refers to congenital weakness and is considered the cause of birth defects. Ancient classics state, "The Kidneys are the origin of the human body before birth." Their function is to store the essence that dominates growth, development, and reproduction. Only when the internal organs are activated by Hereditary Ki can they do their formal functions. Hereditary Ki can be considered the prime motivating force in the body. The more sufficient the Hereditary Ki, the more vigorous the organs function, therefore healthy you are. If your Hereditary Ki is exhausted all types of illnesses can occur.

2. *Central Ki:* Ki produced by the combination of breathing "clean Ki" inhaled

by the lungs that is mixed with the Ki of food. Central Ki (*Zhong Qi* in Chinese) is stored in the chest. This Ki flows out by way of the throat and dominates the breathing as well as speaking and the voice. A strong voice indicates there is sufficient Central Ki. A weak voice points to a deficient state. Central Ki also nourishes the Heart and Lungs. It influences the blood vessels thereby promoting blood circulation.

3. *Ki from the Essence of Food and Water:* An extremely important type of Ki. This Ki is digested and absorbed by the Stomach and Spleen. This Ki is transported upward to the Lungs where it is mixed with oxygen (clean Ki) and becomes Central Ki. The Lungs are related to all the blood vessels. The normal functions of the Ki from the Essence of Food and Water are to insure normal life activities and provide the material source for these activities.

Fig. 8 Energy from Food

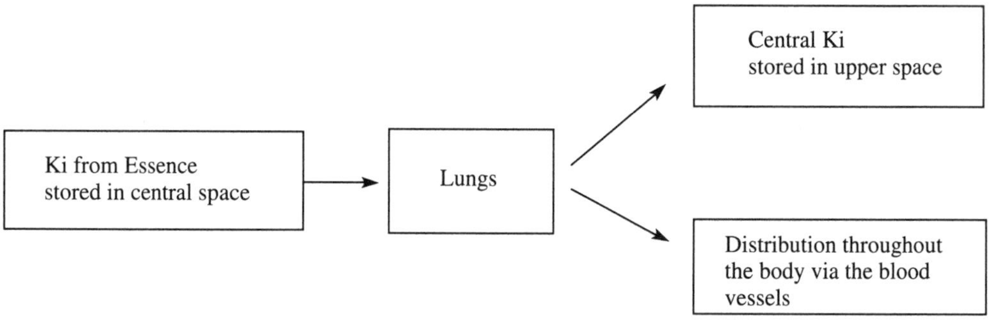

Understanding Ki by Location

1. *Nutrient Ki:* This Ki supplies all internal organs with energy to survive. Nutrient Ki (*Ying Qi* in Chinese) also supplies the meridians with this energy. This mainly flows within the blood vessels with the blood. Nutrient Ki comes from the Ki from the Essence of Food and Water and its function is to produce blood and nourish the whole body. It propels blood circulation.

2. *Defensive Ki:* This Ki acts something like antibodies and protects the organism from external factors including disease causing factors. Its job is to protect and resist against disease. This Defensive Ki (*Wei Qi* in Chinese) also comes from the Ki of the Essence of Food and Water like the Nutrient Ki. It flows mainly outside the blood vessels through the sweat glands, pores, muscles, connective tissues, and skin region on the surface of the body. Defensive Ki also is very active by adjusting the opening and closing of the pores. This allows entry and exit for both health benefitting and disease causing elements. This action also regulates body temperature. Defensive Ki has another function of warming up the body and nourishing the tissues and organs. Both the Nutrient Ki and Defensive Ki influence the physiological functions of the body.

Fig. 9 Five Types of Energy—Ki

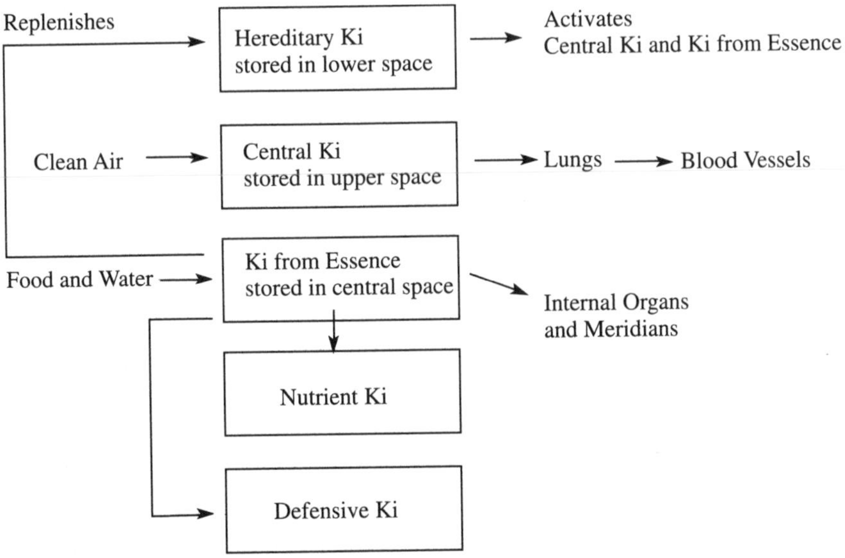

```
Replenishes                ┌─────────────────────┐    Activates
      ┌──────────────────► │ Hereditary Ki       │ ─► Central Ki and Ki from Essence
      │                    │ stored in lower space│
      │                    └─────────────────────┘
      │                    ┌─────────────────────┐
Clean Air ───────────────► │ Central Ki          │ ──► Lungs ───► Blood Vessels
      │                    │ stored in upper space│
      │                    └─────────────────────┘
      │                    ┌─────────────────────┐
Food and Water ──────────► │ Ki from Essence     │ ──► Internal Organs
      │                    │ stored in central space│    and Meridians
      │                    └─────────────────────┘
      │                              │
      │                              ▼
      │                    ┌─────────────────────┐
      │                    │   Nutrient Ki       │
      │                    └─────────────────────┘
      │
      │                    ┌─────────────────────┐
      └──────────────────► │   Defensive Ki      │
                           └─────────────────────┘
```

Functions of Ki

Inside the human body Ki performs many functions. It has a propelling function that promotes circulation of blood as well as nutrient substance throughout the body. This promotes growth. Ki has a warming function that helps to maintain normal body temperature and also provides energy to the internal organs. It has a defensive function by traveling on the surface of the body. It is responsible for protection against invasion of external disease causing factors. Once disease enters the body they are resisted by this Ki. It also helps with an early recovery.

Ki has a function of making changes occur easily. The body's ability to adjust to physical, psychological, and emotional challenges is enhanced by Ki. This function helps with the production and transformation of Ki, blood, and body fluids. It also helps the internal organs maintain a better function. The final function of Ki is its restraining function. The ability to restrain is seen in the body's ability to keep blood inside the blood vessels, to keep urine in check, and to control the sweat glands and other body secretions. Propelling and restraining functions describe Ki in blood circulation. When it fails to propel, then blood stagnation occurs. When it fails to restrain, hemorrhage occurs. Stagnation and bleeding are two signs of Ki deficiency.

There is traditional Oriental medical saying that is often repeated. "Ki is the commander of blood. Blood is the mother of Ki." Ki must be fully nourished by and is dependent on blood for it to do its jobs properly. At the same time, Ki is involved in blood production and transportation. So Ki produces blood and blood circulation relies on the propelling function of Ki. Ki leads blood throughout the body, while Ki needs blood to continue its functions. Each is dependent on the other.

Ki Diseases

There are two principal problems that are observed in the body when Ki is out of balance. Discovering the cause and making corrective adjustments in the organs or systems involved sets the direction for recovery.

The first cause of change: Deficiency of Ki is due to hereditary weakness, prolonged illness, or malnutrition. Clinical symptoms of Ki deficiency include yin signs like lack of concentration, easily tired, low spirit, and weakness. When the deficiency occurs in particular organs you will find the following signs:

> Heart—palpitation, shortness of breath
> Lungs—shortness of breath, cough, low voice
> Spleen—loss of appetite, watery stool or diarrhea
> Kidneys—weakness of lumbar region and knees, seminal emission, and bed-wetting
> Liver—dry painful eyes, headache, restlessness

The second cause of change: Stagnation of Ki occurs when there is obstruction in some part of the body. It can be caused by emotional factors, such as depression; improper diet, external factors such as damp and cold; and accident or trauma. Some symptoms are a moving, distensive pain that comes and goes. The pain can be limited to one location or it can be body wide.

Symptoms of Ki Diseases

"Ascending Ki" describes the common occurrence when opposing symptoms of extremely cold hands and feet and a hot, flushed face are seen. It is thought that Ki is trapped in the upper body. Corrective applications should aim to treat ascending Ki by normalizing and regulating its flow.

"Obstructed Ki" describes when Ki is stagnated in the lower portion of the body. The main subjective symptom is the sensation that a foreign object is stuck in the throat. Other symptoms are chest discomfort, shortness of breath, and palpitations to the extent that the heart is pounding and the person feels that it is going to stop beating altogether. Obstructed Ki also causes an irregular pulse that intermittently stops.

The origins of Ki diseases are very hard to diagnose. People with no serious physical symptoms may suffer from these diseases along with those who display symptoms of every type of degenerative condition. However, since Ki diseases are always linked to the seven emotions, it seems appropriate to discuss them. The seven emotions are: pleasure, anger, anxiety, pensiveness or brooding, sorrow or grief, fear, and shock or terror.

Ki diseases affect the nervous system, the meridian system, the blood, and the mind. Such diverse conditions as schizophrenia and Parkinson's disease are included in this category.

> Pleasure calms Ki.
> Anger stimulates Ki.
> Anxiety obstructs Ki.

Brooding coagulates Ki.
Grief reduces Ki.
Fear suppresses Ki.
Shock disturbs Ki.

In the simplest terms, knowing the theory and existence of Ki and how it displays itself in the creation and function of the body, is extremely important in understanding how to treat someone with shiatsu and diet. Being attentive to the body's energetic subtleties gives valuable insight in the restoration and maintenance of health.

Spirals of Change—Yin and Yang

In the West we are accustomed to taking medications when we are ill. The power and strength of medicine cannot be denied. What price do we pay for power and convenience. Over the counter cold remedies always suggest recommended doses. Many people feeling the remedy must be safe or they would not be able to be purchased it without a prescription often exceed the doses. In macrobiotics there is a saying, "What has a front, has a back; the bigger the front, the bigger the back." The back side is that unfortunately dozens die needlessly each year from these simple cold tablets and syrups. They either took too much or their body did not have the ability to process the drug safely. All drugs are potentially dangerous. The liver must break down and process all substances that enter the bloodstream. Drugs cause side effects and damage this vital organ. Ironically, cold medications only suppress symptoms. In the end it is the body that cures the cold.

Natural healing does not use drugs. We adjust the body through living patterns including diet, breathing, exercise, sleep, special food and herb remedies, and shiatsu. The decision to adjust these patterns is based on the relationship of yin and yang. Yin conditions display deficient symptoms. This is called *Kyo* in Japanese and *Xu* in Chinese. Yang conditions display symptoms of excess or fullness. This is called *Jitsu* in Japanese and *Shi* in Chinese. Our medicine then is to apply yang treatments to yin conditions and yin treatments to yang conditions. To make more sense let us take at look at yin and yang more deeply.

The Yin-Yang Theory

The theory of yin and yang pervades every aspect of traditional Oriental medicine. The balance between these two primordial cosmic forces is viewed as the key factor in all natural phenomena and life processes.

Facing the sun is considered yang. Having your back to the sun is yin. The sunny side of the mountain is considered yang, while the shaded side is yin.

The interplay between yin and yang sparks all change and movement in the universe. Yin represents the negative, passive force. It is the female in nature, dark, and is symbolized by water. Yang symbolizes the positive, active force. It is male in nature, bright, and is represented by fire. Yin and yang are always a relationship of two things. These two are opposite qualities within a single entity. Everything is an integral entity that is at once in conflict and interdependent. In mathematics for example, this is addition and subtraction, multiplication and division. In physics there is action and counteraction. In chemistry there is composition and decomposition. In biology there are the opposite acting parasympathetic and the sympathetic nervous systems, complementary branches of the autonomic nervous system.

Of the two forces, ancient Taoists believed yin to be superior and stronger as it is the major nourishing force. On the other hand, many present day natural lifestyle enthusiasts take an opposing view and emphasize yang believing this to be the source of power. I think it is well to remember that whole health is found in balance.

History of Yin and Yang

The familiar *Tai Ji* symbol represents the interaction of yin and yang. This interaction is visible with one portion of darkness gradually becoming lighter with a bright part remaining within the darkness. The other half of the logo moves in a contrary pattern with darkness in the light's center. For years this symbol has represented change.

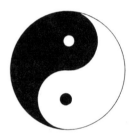

Fig. 10 Taiji—Yin-Yang

Chinese sources claim that in the Spring, Autumn, and Warring States dynastic periods (770–221 B.C.) in China's long history, the yin-yang symbol first appeared. At the same time the trigrams and hexagrams of the popular classic *Book of Changes* (*I Ching*) appeared. This book explains how yin and yang change and interact with one another. The theory takes the process of change and development in the material world as its base. Its popularity remains because this agrees with observable fact.

George Ohsawa said, "Theory without practice is useless. Practice without theory is dangerous." China must have listened because in 1954 the combination of traditional medicine (theory and philosophy) with Western medicine (practice and power) was initiated. Yin-yang and the Five Element theories contribute greatly to medicine and healing. Traditional practice uses them to explain the physiology and disease process in the human body. For our purposes they can serve as guides to diagnosis and treatment in shiatsu practice.

Describing Yin and Yang

Basic to the understanding of this principle is the assumption that the elements of nature are temporary and changing. Recognizing this, human beings who want to follow nature must conduct their lives accordingly; that is, they must be prepared to adapt and change. These two forces are always opposite and antagonistic, and yet, while, they are complementary, for they are always combining and cooperating. These two tendencies, constantly interacting, were understood in ancient China to create balance. This happens both inside the body and outside in the world.

With the predominance of one tendency giving way to the dominance of its opposite, and vice versa, everything therefore is constantly changing. Although always changing, each thing still contains both yin and yang. This fact creates a wholeness that is con

	YIN	YANG
Everyday Observations	Rest Dark Moon Cold Large Up	Action Light Sun Hot Small Down
Body Structures	Front of body or head Soft parts Expanded organs	Back of body or head Hard parts Compact organs
Body Location	Peripheral parts Upper position (e.g., head)	Inner parts Lower position (e.g., legs)
Function	Nervous function Female function Mental activities Eliminating function Ascending movement Expanding movement Exhaling function (relaxation) Physical inhalation (expansion) Flexible Slow	Digestive function Male function Physical activities Consuming function Descending movement Contracting movement Inhaling function (tension) Physical exhalation (contraction) Inflexible Rapid

stantly evolving. Bound together, yin and yang unify. Yang is the inward movement that creates contraction. Yin is the outward movement that creates expansion. The chart above will give you an idea of yin and yang qualities.

Yin and Yang Relationships

Within yin and yang there are four relationships. They are opposition, interdependence, inter-consuming/supporting, and inter-transformative.

1. *Opposition.* For every condition there exists an opposite condition. For health the opposite is illness, for wealth there is poverty, for hot there is cold. Each of these conditions exists because of the struggle between yin and yang. This points out the relative character of life.

2. *Interdependence.* Each of two opposing aspects depends on the other for its existence. There is no temperature without hot or cold. There is no daily cycle without daylight and nighttime. Change occurs not only because of opposition and conflict between yin and yang but also due to their relationship of interdependence and mutual support.

3. *Inter-consuming/supporting.* This is a gaining and losing relationship. One part gains while the other part loses. When you buy a new television your entertainment capacity gains while your bank account loses. Another way of explaining this relationship is the common saying, "You can't have your cake and eat it too!" As one weakens the other strengthens, one consumes the other supports, one decreases the other increases. If yang gains, yin loses and vice versa. When a function is performed it takes nutrient substance to accomplish the task, a function gains while substance loses.

In the West we feel that disease is caused by microbes that invade the body. Oriental healing attributes disease causing factors to weather changes, humidity, wind, cold, heat, and dryness. The classification of disease producing factors depends on the patient's symptoms. There are four combinations that pinpoint the cause and determine the specific aim of treatment. There are either excess or deficient symptoms that originate from either the inside or the outside. These combinations produce the yin or yang symptoms. The internal sources always leave a deficient condition while the external sources always create a condition of excess.

Yang Symptoms:
Internal Source—The body is deficient of fluid that shows as yang-heat symptoms.
External Source—The yang disease causing "evils" invade the body and consume the body's yin-cooling factors with the result of having imbalanced yang and fever symptoms.

Yin Symptoms:
Internal Sources—The body's weakness in yang energy leads to an excess of yin that displays cold signs.
External Sources—The yin disease causing "evils" invade the body and exhaust body's yang energy with the result of having imbalanced yin and cold signs.

Fig. 11

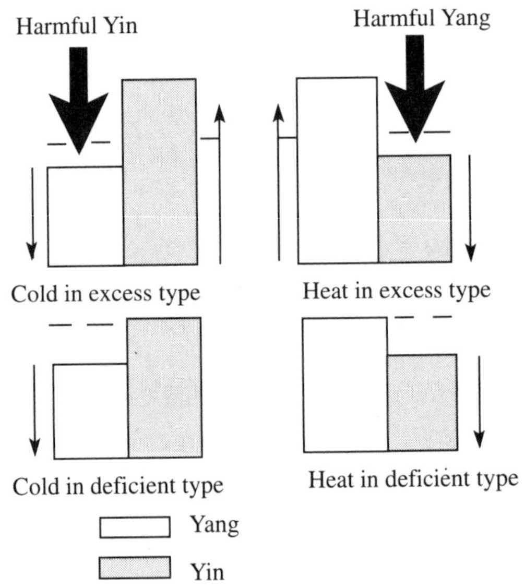

4. *Inter-transformative.* This relationship occurs when certain limits and conditions are reached. At that time yin and yang turn into their opposites. This illustrates how the universal law of change is governed. As the season changes, for example, at the peak of midsummer when it is its hottest the weather begins to change toward autumn. This also can explain the changes of disease in quality, as when yang symptoms change into yin symptoms. Hepatitis is a good example. During acute infectious hepatitis there is the

jaundice stage with yellow complexion, nausea, pain, and loss of appetite. This is an excess condition. If it continues it can turn into chronic hepatitis or cirrhosis with lassitude, dizziness, not very severe rib pain, and an accumulation of fluid in the abdomen (ascites). These are deficient condition.

The Six Stages of Disease

One of the older Chinese text books, *Treatise on the Treatment of Acute Disease Caused by Cold* (*Shang Han Lun*) written in the second century A.D. records the stages that disease caused by cold from an outside source pass through. It points out the changing nature of illness and reminds practitioners to respond correctly so illness does not settle deeper in the patient. If not turned around the final stage, Absolute Yin, precedes death. In the past the complications of fever killed many. Oriental medicine has been in a continued search for understanding and treatment for this condition. From the second century until the introduction of antibiotics, the Six Stages theory has played an important role in the training of medical personnel.

Be warned however, that not every illness begins at stage one and passes on to stage six. This six stage process is true in acute fever diseases of outside origin.

Yang diseases are:
1. Greater Yang disease occurs when an external "evil" attacks the body. The main symptoms are stronger than normal pulse, headache, fever, and chills.
2. Lesser Yang disease is characterized by a bitter mouth, dry throat, giddiness, and vomiting. This state begins to involve the nervous system.
3. Sunlight Yang disease always is characterized by feelings of extreme heat. There are periods of constipation or diarrhea due to the disease toxin invading the stomach and other internal organs.

Yin diseases are:
4. Greater Yin disease has the main symptoms of chills, diarrhea, vomiting, and dysentery.
5. Lesser Yin disease which exhibits the cardinal symptoms of weak pulse, anemophobia (fear of wind) or chills, fatigue, and cold hands and feet.

Fig. 12

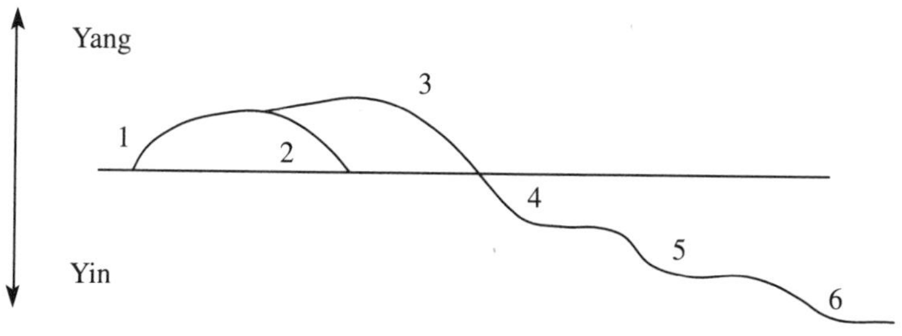

Stage 1=Greater Yang   Stage 4=Greater Yin
Stage 2=Lesser Yang   Stage 5=Lesser Yin
Stage 3=Sunlight Yang   Stage 6=Absolute Yin

6. Absolute Yin disease which has the symptoms of thirst, scanty urine, and exhaustion.

Summary

The terms *yin* and *yang* are regarded as relative and complementary, and not as absolute and mutually exclusive. The nourishing systems support and build up body heat and strength while the other exchange systems regulate and secrete liquids for lubricating the body. The kidneys, the liver, and the pancreas in particular are regarded as secreting important fluids for balancing the systems.

Macrobiotic philosopher and teacher George Ohsawa taught Oriental culture, philosophy, and medicine in Europe and around the world. The story goes that he found Europeans to have difficulty understanding the traditional versions of yin and yang, so he reversed them but only in some categories. Ohsawa felt the Oriental mind grasped intangible concepts more easily than Europeans. Oriental philosophies had taught these people to be familiar with the spiritual world. For them spirit and energy were parts of life. The languages reflect this. The Japanese words for weather, illness, and wellness are *tenki* (heaven's Ki), *byôki* (disturbed Ki), and *genki* (harmonious Ki). Europeans have a more material thinking process. For Orientals, Infinity (intangible) is "the Great Yang" and the earth is yin. Ohsawa felt things you could touch fit better into the European concepts of solidness, so he called the earth yang, and spaciousness yin. The major differences between the traditional Chinese system and Ohsawa's macrobiotic system occur in the yin-yang naming of the internal organs, the up and down movement of energy, and the naming of the surface location versus internal location. Traditional Chinese medicine names the active functioning of solid organs, like the Liver, Heart, Spleen, Kidneys, and Lungs as yin. While the nourishing, supporting, hollow organs like the Gallbladder, Small Intestine, Stomach, Bladder, and Large Intestine are described as yang. Also Oriental medicine describes the top part of the body and the head as yang and the bottom part and the feet as yin. It classifies the internal, deep (soft) parts of the body as yin and the surface as yang (hard). The basis for these classifications is determined by the movement of energy. Remember that yang is function and cannot be touched.

In contrary fashion Ohsawa termed the solid organs as yang (solid and tangible) and the hollow organs as yin (physically empty, storage places, not as active as their mates). He felt the top of the body was yin and the bottom part yang. He described the surface of the body as yin and the interior as yang (energy concentrates as it moves in a tighter spiral inward, centripetal). In my opinion there is justification for both systems. Both systems say fire is yang and water is yin. In this we have agreement. The Chinese system further explains that fire burns up, therefore upward movement is yang. Water flows down, therefore downward movement is yin. The Ohsawa system explains that light entities rise (light in physical density), like cream in milk or hot air, so therefore upward movement is yin. Heavy things sink like a rock thrown into a lake, therefore the downward movement is yang. The Chinese system is based on energy, while the Ohsawa system emphasizes a more material approach.

Ohsawa's reversal remains in the macrobiotic system. Many people have difficulty understanding how one system can describe the Heart as yin while another can describe it as yang. Remember that these systems are created by people as models to understand natural, universal forces. No system perfectly describes reality. The ultimate paradox is that with Ohsawa's input we now have a yang version of yin and yang in comparison to the original yin version, or is it yang? Oh, well!

Yin and yang are tools. Study them, play with them, and try to apply them. Because of the complexity of the ancient yin-yang system it can be confusing. Sometimes the more you study the more confused you become. In your mind simplify this material into a working model for yourself. Use it as a guideline. Based on this historical information develop your own understanding. When you are doing a shiatsu treatment this information should be in the back of your mind, not the front. Your attention should be on the receiver. Allow your intuitive ability based on empirical study to guide you to successful shiatsu sessions.

Often the use of external treatment methods such as acupuncture, shiatsu, moxibustion, and herbs are not enough to create a permanent balance. The person may feel better temporarily only to revert to their original condition. We must always think about a more permanent solution. In our treatments I have continually come back to dietary adjustment. For me this is the most important point. If we eat wrong food or too much food, we will get into trouble. We must change the diet to be healthy. Because the body is made from physical material and the world is also material, dietary change is the only truly fundamental method to survive in this world. While the mind and the spirit may need no body to exist, if we want remain as a physical entity on this planet we do. In Japan there is a saying, *Chôshin Chôsoku Chôshin*, it means "regulating body, breath, and mind." If you can regulate these in your everyday life, you will be O.K.

Life on the Move—Five Phases of Energy

The Five Phases of Energy, also known as the Five Elements and Five Transformations, always go along with yin and yang. Their functions and relationships were documented by the fourth century B.C., but the framework was probably around for a long time before. The five representatives of movement are named *wood, fire, earth, metal,* and *water.* Water and fire are essential in order to grow, prepare, and eat food. Metal and wood are basic tools for carrying out production and survival. Earth is necessary for the growth of everything. These elements are considered indispensable for the life of all people. The physical nature of an entity is at the foundation of the classification system. This is determined by observation of natural facts and is determined by the shape and quality of the thing viewed. The Five Phases are used to generalize about everything in the universe and are not limited solely to solid elements. They have a broad, extensive meaning.

There is an interesting and definite relationship between the Five Phases that can be summarized with the following: Inter-promoting, interacting, overacting, and counteracting relations.

Inter-Promoting—Mother-Son Relationship

Each phase is in a position of being inter-promoted and promoting. Promoting means to encourage growth. Fire promotes earth, earth promotes metal, and so on. The promoting element is considered the "mother" element while the element being promoted is considered the "son." This forms the "Mother-Son" relationship. Metal for example is promoted by earth, which is the mother of metal, while water is the son of metal, being promoted by metal.

Interaction—Controlling Relationship

In this phase each segment is being acted on and is acting on another part. This relationship exerts control or resistance. There is an ancient saying, "Without growth there is no development. Without control, hyperactivity will lead to harm."

In the promotion of growth resides control, and in control there exists promotion of growth. They are in opposition and also cooperation. Normal growth and development is protected by this relative balance established between promoting and acting.

In cases of either excess or deficiency there are abnormal relations and instead of interacting, the elements begin to overact or counteract.

Fig. 13

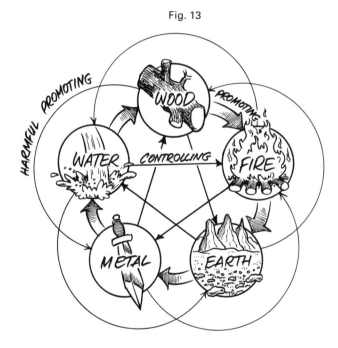

Overacting Relationship

Overaction implies invasion or bullying of one element by another. This occurs because of weakness by the receiver of the action. For example normally wood acts on (controls) earth, but because earth is so weak it is acted on with double force.

Within the organs there are either excess (hyper) or deficient (hypo) conditions.

These five elements are each related to the paired *Zang-Fu* (solid-hollow) organs. The effects of these relationships extends to the partner organ also. What this means is that if the wood phase (Liver/Gallbladder) is overacting on the earth phase then either the Spleen/Pancreas and/or the Stomach systems are being affected.

Counteracting (Harmful Promoting) Relationship

Because wood is too strong, it will overact on earth. Simultaneously it will counteract on metal. If wood is too weak, the reverse direction would occur. The Liver Ki (wood) overacts on the Spleen (earth) because the Spleen is too weak. This makes the Spleen even weaker. A counteraction on the Lungs could occur because of weakness. This could be seen as tuberculosis or dilation of the bronchioles.

Fig. 14

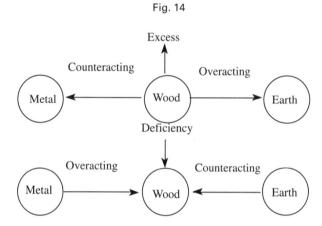

The Origins of the Five Phases Theory

The first recorded information regarding the Five Phases goes back as far as between the tenth and fifth centuries B.C. It is explained in detail as a complete system in the classic *Nan Jing*. In today's medical schools in China it is taught that the origin of yin-yang and the Five Elements began in Chinese history during what the Chinese refer to as the slave society period. Its development progressed during the feudal society period and has been fairly stable since.

As nothing is perfect, there is a weakness with the Five Phases system because it does not explain all pathology and disease patterns of the Zang-Fu (internal) organs. It also cannot be used to explain all the patterns of imbalance that you will encounter in shiatsu sessions. On the brighter side, it does have value by adding specific information con-

Properties of the Five Phases	
Wood	Develops and grows, upward expanding motion
Fire	Inflames and ascends. active motion
Earth	Produces crops, stable, condensation process
Metal	Killing and shrinkage solid state
Water	Downward direction, floating state

Correspondences Associated with the Five Phases

Five Phases	Human Body					Nature				
	Solid	Hollow	Senses	Tissues	Process	Seasons	Environment	Color	Taste	Dire
Wood	Liver	Gallbladder	Eye	Tendon	Birth	Spring	Wind	Green	Sour	East
Fire	Heart	Small Intestine	Tongue	Vessel	Growth	Summer	Heat	Red	Bitter	South
Earth	Spleen	Stomach	Mouth	Muscle	Transform	Late Summer	Damp	Yellow	Sweet	Middle
Metal	Lung	Large Intestine	Nose	Skin/Hair	Harvest	Autumn	Dryness	White	Pungent	West
Water	Kidney	Bladder	Ear	Bone	Storage	Winter	Cold	Black	Salty	North

cerning distant relationships in the body and the universe, and most importantly, it reminds us of the interconnectedness of all things.

These properties will help you understand the movement of energy and the functions of the Zang-Fu organs. The classification of the Five Phases reflects our dependence on nature. It also explains adaptability of both man and nature. The system is based on environment, climatic changes, and geographical influences and their effects on the functions of the human body. Based on these points, you can more easily understand physiology and illness states.

The Five Phases system presents an organized, systematic way to realize the sacred relationships between Heaven, Man, and Earth. Heaven's force is represented by yang and Earth's force by yin. Man suspended between the two receives influences from both. The energies of Heaven and Earth have specific and general effects on the energies of Man. This idea is the central focus of natural healing applications. All things in the universe are seen to interact, therefore nothing can exist independently of anything else.

If you understand the interconnectedness and the orderly relationships this system describes, you will be able to understand unusual diagnostic subtleties and be able to suggest appropriate treatment routines. For example when low back pain and knee weakness are complaints, which major organ needs treatment? If a woman is losing hair, a young person their teeth, or vision is blurred or fading prematurely, which organs are responsible? If someone is pale, they cough frequently and have a runny nose, which organ is weak? Using the Five Phases system you can figure out the solutions to these and other problems.

Five Phases Applied to Emotional Traits

Organ	Positive Attitude	Negative Attitude
Heart	Tranquility/Peace	Excitability
Spleen	Comprehension/Friendliness	Worry
Lungs	Security/Happiness	Grief
Kidneys	Confidence/Courage	Fear
Liver	Patience/Understanding	Anger/Irritability

Summary
The Five Phases Theory leaves us with an historical insight into the thinking of people who sought patterns of harmony in nature. While it is logical and orderly, up to a point, it is not entirely consistent with reality. There are many observations found in nature and in a treatment situation that do not conform to the physical nor emotional connections described and promoted by this theory. Even in China as far back as the fourth century B.C. at its introduction, criticism pointed out its shortcomings. As usual, our purpose is to learn for the past, blend this information with observable fact and intuitive insight. With this perspective, and if it is not taken literally, this theory has a place in Whole Health Shiatsu.

The Point and Meridian Theory—*Tsubo* and *Keiraku*

All internal organs and body functions depend on energy. How does this energy get distributed throughout the system? The answer is simple, through the meridians or channels (*keiraku* in Japanese, *jing* in Chinese)—the body's pathways of energy. This energy transportation system is the ancient explanation by which blood and energy get to the organs and also how the organs communicate with the surface of the body. Simply stated a slight reduction in the flow causes illness; complete lack of flow causes death.

There are special locations found along each meridian. We call these places acu-points (*tsubo* in Japanese, *shuwei* in Chinese). These points cover the entire body and extend their influence to the internal organs. Acu-points are not actually points. They are more like a hole or volcano. They are the entry and exit places for the body's energy as well as natural forces of health and illness. It is at these locations that the body's energy can easily become sluggish and stagnant. Many acu-points occur in places that are vulnerable and slightly weak. The bends of the wrists, elbows, and knees, the depressions of the muscles, and places where nerves emerge from muscles are common sites. In these spots any internal disturbance produces powerful reflex actions. The effects can be seen while the acu-points themselves are invisible. Trouble along the meridians at the acu-points is sensed as pain, numbness, a sense of pressure, stiffness, chills, flushing, spots, small discolorations, and color changes. Each organ has an area that is changed when disease is present. The Lungs and Heart show changes on the forearms, the Liver in the armpits, the Spleen on the inside of the thighs, and the Kidneys at the back of the knees.

Development of the Point and Meridian Theory

Hole—*Tsubo*
The word *tsubo* or *acu-point* derives from the Oriental characters meaning hole or orifice, and position—the position of the hole. Traditionally, the word *hole* was combined with other terms such as hollow, passageway, transport, and Ki. This suggests that the holes on the surface of the body were regarded as routes of access to the body's internal cavities. The acu-points are spots where Ki comes out.

There are three phases in the historical development of the concept of these holes or acu-points. In the earliest phase people would use any body location that was painful or uncomfortable. Because there were no specific locations for the points, they had no names.

In the second phase, after a long period of practice and experience, certain points became identified with specific diseases. The ability of distinct points to affect and be affected by local or distant pain and disease, became predictable. As the correlation between point and disease became established, names were given to these points. For example "wind pond" (Gallbladder 20) was named because this is the site where flu or cold producing factors (wind) lodge in the body. When you have symptoms this spot is sore.

Fig. 15 Tsubo

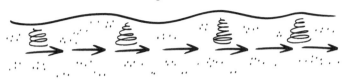

In the final phase, many previously localized points, each with a singular function, became integrated in a larger system that related and grouped diverse points systematically according to similar functions. This integration is called the *meridian* or *channel system.*

In most shiatsu styles there is great emphasis on learning the locations and functions of the acu-points. As a study, this is useful. My style of treatment however, does not emphasize treatment of individual or groups of points. My primary aim is to stimulate Ki flow to be harmonious and balanced. When you apply the techniques in the following chapters you will discover the effectiveness of this overall approach in comparison to stimulating isolated points. Treating the whole body balances the whole person.

Meridians—*Keiraku*

The meridian or channel theory developed from observing the effect from stimulating acu-points on the surface of the body. Many of these points were discovered accidentally such as when a man received a wound in battle that relieved his asthma (Lung 1). Ocassionally it was observed that a woman's menstrual pains diminished after accidentally brushing a heated rock at the fireplace that touched a spot on the inner ankle (Spleen 6). In a more direct way while probing the skin surface for symptoms of disease, it was discovered that certain locations reacted when illness was present. For example it soon was realized that every back injury had related pains located at the knees and calf muscles. Massaging these related pains would sometimes lessen or eliminate the original trouble altogether. So it was discovered that a connection, the meridian system, existed between the surface of the body and its internal organs.

Fig. 16 Meridian Connections

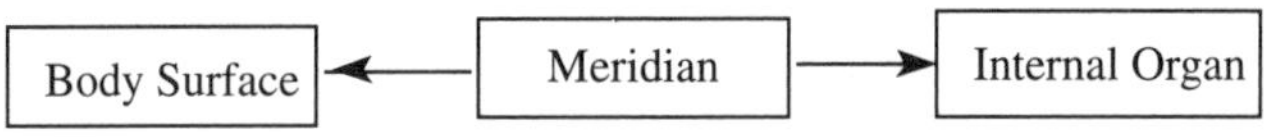

Body Surface	←	Meridian	→	Internal Organ

As time went on these connections were noted, recorded, and named. Often the use of individual points affected areas nearby and at a distance, including the functions of the internal organs. It began to be surmised that these points somehow were joined together. The idea of isolated acu-points affecting individual areas was replaced with the notion of extensive connections or channels. This comprehensive view explained many formerly unexplained facts. One example is how stimulating the feet can affect headaches. This development led to the formation and mapping out of the twelve regular and two central meridians.

The functions of the meridians are to circulate Ki and blood, warm and nourish the tissues, and to link the whole body so as to keep the internal organs, limbs, skin, muscles, tendons, and bones intact in structure and to make the body function as a whole.

There are two sides to a coin. On one side, the meridian transportation system brings life-force from the surface of the body to deep into the interior and from the depths back to the surface of the body, accomplishing the job of warming and nourishing. On the other side of the coin, the meridians are responsible for the occurrence and transmission of disease. When the function of the meridian is impaired, the organism is open to attack from outside disease causing forces. Once these forces enter the body they are transmitted deep into the interior through the meridians. When external disease factors enter and block the channels, superficial symptoms appear such as chills, fever, and headache. When these forces drive deeper into the body through the meridians, organs and systems begin to decline. This is how the external disease factors influence the internal organs. Each of the meridians flow in a definite part of the body and each of the twelve regular meridians connects with a different internal organ. Tenderness or other abnormal reactions along the areas the meridians pass through or at certain acu-points also aids correct diagnosis. Pain on the upper back below the shoulders indicates trouble in the lungs, hot flashes suggest a disorder in the liver, and so forth.

Modern Research

Many studies have been conducted by biophysicists in Japan, China, and France. They postulated that a measurement of acu-point electricity would be a biophysical index that would illustrate the objective existence of the meridian system. They discovered that acu-points have a lower skin resistance. When an electrical current is passed through a classical acu-point, it has a higher electrical conductance which is a lower resistance, than the surrounding area. They also discovered that when disease or illness is present, pathological changes take place in the body while changes are found in the resistance of relevant meridians and acu-points. Similar internal changes are also reflected by the unbalanced resistance of the acu-points. In other words, imbalance in the organs affect the acu-points, imbalance in the acu-points affect the organs. Researchers also found that the external environment such as temperature, season, and time of day, changed the resistance of acu-points.

In the Lanzhou Medical College in China a test of the acu-points of the Stomach meridian showed significant variations in conductance when the stomach lining was stimulated by cold or hot water, either before or after eating. In Beijing, ear acu-point research learned that low resistance points on the outer rim of the ear were elevated either in the presence of disease or following long-term stimulation of a corresponding internal organ.

Individual Meridian Characteristics and Functions

Each of the classical meridians has a distinct flow pattern. Each also has associated duties, jobs, and responsibilities in the maintenance of the entire body system. This information was discovered thousands of years ago, yet its practical value continues. Much of what you are about to learn is useful in understanding the diagnostic connections of the body. It also points to the marvelous construction and precision of the human body. With a thorough understanding of the foundations of natural healing, the most important aspect of health—prevention—can be more easily secured.

The Chinese call the relationship of the meridians and paired organs Zang-Fu. The concept of organs in Oriental medicine is very different from our Western ideas. If you try to understand the Chinese model with Western concepts you will not grasp its deepest meaning and will probably also be less effective in your treatment. For example the traditional meaning of Liver in Oriental medical terms does have some relationship to the physical liver but mostly it is a concept to understand patterns of energy and how this energy is expected to behave in both healthy and disturbed conditions. The greatest difference between the Eastern and Western view is that the organs do not emphasize the physical nature of the organ. The organ names do not refer to specific types of tissues and cells but to concepts that describe patterns of integrated functions. Thousands of years of clinical observations rather than surgery revealed these functions. Therefore there has always been a lack of emphasis placed on the physical structure with a greater emphasis placed on function and relationships.

The organs are divided into two principle groups: yang (solid) and yin (hollow). Each solid organ (Zang) has a mate, a hollow organ (Fu). For example the liver (solid) is paired with the gallbladder (hollow). Zang organs produce, transform, and store the vital essence—Qi (Ki in Japanese). Fu organs serve as a passageway to receive, digest, and transport the nutrient essence within the body and to excrete the waste residue. The solid organ is more active and therefore considered more important to survival. It is also for this reason that much more is written about the functions of the solid organs.

LUNGS AND LARGE INTESTINE

Lungs

In traditional Oriental medicine, the Lungs correspond to the metal phase, the westerly direction, the season of autumn, the dry climatic condition, the color of white, the emotions of sadness and worry, the pungent taste, and the sound of crying. Their opening is the nose, and they govern the skin.

The function of all organs in classical medicine is based on clinical observations of patients over hundreds of years and not necessarily the physical structure of the organ in Western medicine. Most of the Lung functions have a common character: they are dispersing and descending in nature, that is they send energy away in different directions and especially downward. The Lungs dislike cold.

When a Western anatomical description is explained the organ name is written with a lower case letter, for examle, "The liver filters the blood." When a Oriental medical description is given the organ name is written with an upper case letter, for example, "The Liver is responsible for an unrestricted flow of energy."

1. The Lungs govern Ki and respiration: The term *Ki* is often explained as vital energy. Although this term is not totally accurate, and there are different types of Ki, it is sufficient for this purpose. Governing Ki and respiration is the most important function of the Lungs, because it extracts "clean Ki," energy from the air for the body, which combines with "food Ki," energy extracted from food by the digestive system. These two forms of Ki combine in the chest where they form Gathering Ki.

The Lungs spread this newly formed Ki all over the body to nourish the tissues and promote all physiological processes. This Ki also aids the Lung and Heart functions, as well as promoting good circulation to the limbs and controlling the strength of the voice. The strength, tone, and clarity of voice are all dependent on the Lungs.

The Lungs are the most external of the yang* organs, they are the connection between the body and the outside world. Therefore the Lungs are easily affected by exterior pathogenic (disease-causing) factors, and are vulnerable to invasion by climatic factors.

2. The Lungs control pathways and blood vessels: While the Heart controls the blood vessels in traditional Oriental medicine, the Lungs play an important part in maintaining their health. The pathways refer to where energy flows in the meridians that help nourish the vessels along with the blood flowing with them. When the Lung Ki is strong, the circulation of Ki and blood will be strong, so the limbs will be warm. While if it is weak, the limbs, especially the hands will be cold.

3. The Lungs control dispersing and descending: The Lungs have the function of dispersing Defensive Ki and body fluids all over the body to the space between skin and muscles. This ensures that one's resistance to external illness is equally distributed all over the body under the skin, performing its function of warming the skin and muscles and protecting the body from external pathogenic factors. A common cold usually manifests as an impairment of the Lung dispersing action. If this defensive energy is chronically weak there are exercises, foods and herbs that can build up the body's strength.

The Lungs have a descending function because the Lungs are the uppermost organ in the body. The Lung Ki descends to interact with the Kidneys, while the Lungs direct fluids down to the Kidneys and the Bladder. If this function is impaired, cough, breathlessness, and stuffiness of the chest may result.

4. The Lungs regulate water passages: After receiving refined fluids from the digestive process, the Lungs spread them throughout the body in the area under the skin and controlling the bodies fluid loss through sweating. The Lungs also direct fluids down to the Kidneys and Bladder. An impaired Lung function could result in urinary retention.

5. The Lungs control skin and hair: The fluids that the Lungs receive from the digestive process and spread throughout the body under the skin gives the skin and hair nourishment. Thus if the Lung function is normal, the skin will have luster, the hair will be glossy, and the opening and closing of the pores and sweating will be normal. Also if this function of the Lungs is impaired, besides affecting the quality of the skin and hair, the pores are often open with symptoms of spontaneous sweating. A person with these symptoms is often more vulnerable to attack from external disease causing factors, like catching a cold.

6. The Lungs open into the nose: It is said that the nose is the opening of the Lungs to the outside world. If the Lung Ki is weak, or if the Lungs are invaded by an external pathogenic factor, the nose will be blocked, and there may be loss of the sense of smell and sneezing.

---

* The Lungs are classified as yang organs within macrobiotic teaching. They are considered yin organs by classical Oriental medicine. Both philosophies considered the organs to be solid.

Diet
Excessive consumption of cold and raw foods is said to affect the Spleen causing it to generate phlegm that ends up being stored in the Lungs. An excessive consumption of milk, cheese, butter, and other dairy products can have the same effect on the Lungs.

Emotions
The emotions that can effect the Lungs if they persist over a long period of time are sadness and worry. Prolonged sadness disperses Ki, which results in a deficiency of Lung Ki. Prolonged worry causes stagnation of Ki in the chest that affects the Lungs.

Posture
Sitting for long periods of time over a desk to read or write can weaken Lung Ki, because the chest is impeded and proper breathing is impaired.

The Lung Meridian of the Hand (Yin Meridian)

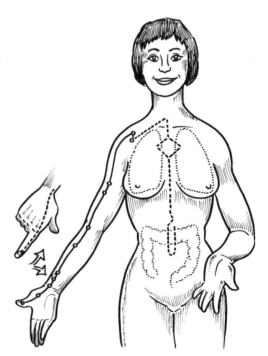

Fig. 17 Lung Meridian

There are eleven points on the Lung meridian. The Lung meridian pertains to the Lungs and communicates with the Large Intestine through the diaphragm. The channel also associates itself with the Stomach and the Kidneys.

● *Symptoms and signs:*
External—Meridian: chills, fever, hidrosis or anhidrosis, nasal obstruction, headache, pain in the chest or of the shoulder and the back, decrease in temperature, and pain of the forearm and the hand.

Internal—Organ: cough, asthma, dyspnea (difficulty breathing), fullness of the chest, expectoration, dryness of the throat, color changing of the urine, increase in temperature of the palm, and distress or hemoptysis (vomiting blood), accompanying occasionally with fullness of the abdomen and mild diarrhea.

Large Intestine
The large intestine is located in the abdomen. The upper end is connected with the small intestine by the ileocecum and the lower end empties into the outside of the body through the anus. The main function of the large intestine is to receive the waste material sent down from the small intestine and, in the process of transporting this waste to the anus, absorb any valuable part of its fluid content and then turn it into feces to be excreted by the body. The Large Intestine function can be summarized as that of transportation and transformation, typical of all Fu organs.

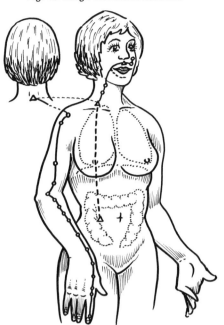

Fig. 18 Large Intestine Meridian

The Large Intestine Meridian of the Hand (Yang Meridian)
There are twenty points on this meridian. This channel pertains to the Large Intestine, communicating with the Lungs and connects with the Stomach directly.

● *Symptoms and signs:*
External—Meridian: fever, thirst, sore throat, epistaxis (nosebleed), toothache, redness and pain of the eye, swelling of the neck, pain of shoulder and the upper arm either redness and burning sensation or chills, and finger trouble.

Internal—Organ: pain of the umbilicus region or abdominal wandering pain, borborygmus (growling stomach sounds), and loose stools with yellowish mucus or complicated with dyspnea.

SPLEEN / PANCREAS AND STOMACH

Spleen
The Spleen corresponds to the earth phase, the center direction, the season of late summer, the damp climatic condition, the color of yellow, the emotions of anxiety and worry, the sweet taste, and the sound of singing. Its opening is the mouth, and it governs the flesh and muscles. The Spleen disperses energy upward and dislikes damp.

1. The Spleen governs transportation and transformation: The Spleen has the function of digesting food, absorbing its essential substances with a part of the fluid supplied, and transmitting them to the heart and the lungs from where they are sent to nourish the whole body. Normal functioning of the Spleen is required for good appetite, normal digestion and absorption, good nourishment, and normal transmission of fluid.

2. The Spleen controls blood: The Spleen has the function of preventing blood from escaping the organs and vessels where it is supposed to be. It has failed in this job when excessive bleeding during menstruation takes place or nosebleed.

3. The Spleen dominates the muscles: Strong muscles provide powerful movement and the four limbs will feel warm. The Spleen enables muscles to receive adequate nourishment from food essentials thereby maintaining muscle thickness and strength. Problems in this function result in weak muscles, cold limbs, fatigue, and atrophy.

4. The Spleen keeps organs in place: The Ki of the Spleen has the function of holding and keeping the internal organs in their normal positions. When the stomach, bladder, or uterus drops the Spleen is failing in this job.

5. The Spleen opens into the mouth: The Spleen function shows itself on the lips. The Spleen Ki passes through the mouth. This is how it influences the taste. The Spleen

and mouth coordinate in receiving, transforming, and transporting food.

The Spleen Meridian of the Foot (Yin Meridian)
There are twenty-one points on the
Spleen meridian. The Spleen meridian
pertains to the Spleen and communicates
with the Stomach, then it connects
directly with the Heart, the Lungs, and
the Intestines.

● *Symptoms and signs:*
External—Meridian: heaviness of the
head and trunk, general fever, weakness
of the extremities, pain of mandible and
cheeks, tongue trouble, and atrophy of
muscles of extremities. Coldness on the
medial aspect of the knee, and edema
(swelling) of the leg and foot.

Internal—Organ: epigastric pain,
diarrhea, indigestion, borborygmus
(intestinal noises), vomiting,
splenomegaly (spleen enlargement), loss
of appetite, jaundice, abdominal distension, hard lumps in the abdomen,
constipation, and dysuria (painful
urination).

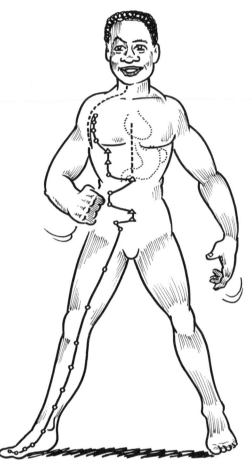
Fig. 19 Spleen Meridian

Stomach

The stomach is located very close to the center of the body in the mid-truck region
below the sternum (breast bone). The upper connection links with the esophagus and
the lower outlet connects with the small intestine via the pylorus. Its main function is
to receive and decompose food. The Stomach is called the "Sea of Food, Cereal, and
Water." The stomach receives and temporarily stores the food mass coming from the
mouth while partially digesting it and then sending it downward to the small intestine.
The Spleen receives the nutrient essence from the Stomach and sends it to the Lungs.
The normal function of the Stomach is to have a downward movement of energy. This
force drives the changing food mass to leave the stomach and travel to the small intestine. When problems occur the Stomach Ki ascends rather than descends. This "adverse
ascension of Stomach Ki" is seen as stagnation of food with its accompanying symptoms of abdominal fullness, distention, and loss of appetite. In severe cases there is
vomiting, nausea, belching, and regurgitation of stomach acid. Most of the stagnation
disorders that occur in the Stomach can be attributed to excess. Overeating and the
consumption of improper foods creates pain, burning sensations, irritation, bleeding,

Fig. 20 Stomach Meridian

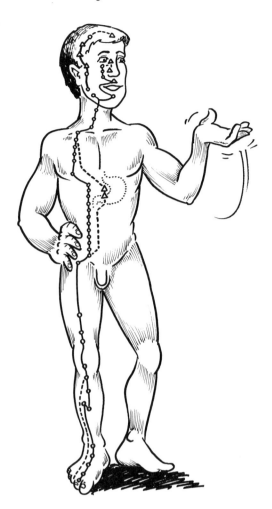

unusual hunger, halitosis, and other troubles. Moderation and correct food choice remedies these situations. Because of the strong working connection between the Stomach and Spleen with reference to digestion and absorption, it is said that these organs are the source of health.

The Stomach Meridian of the Leg (Yang Meridian)
There are forty-five points on this meridian. This channel pertains to the Stomach, communicating with the Spleen and connects directly with the Heart, Small and Large Intestines.

● *Symptoms and signs:*
External—Meridian: fever, perspiration, red face, cloudy consciousness, delirium, eye pain, dry nose, epistaxis (nosebleed), fever blisters, sore throat, swelling of the neck, deviation of mouth, facial paralysis, chest pain, swelling of the leg, and coldness of the lower extremities.
   Internal—Organ: abdominal distension, edema, disturbance of sleep, manic psychosis, discomfort when reclining, rapid digestion, excessive appetite, seizures, and yellow urine.

HEART AND SMALL INTESTINE

Heart
The Heart corresponds to the fire phase, the southerly direction, the season of summer, the dry climatic condition, the color of red, the emotions of excessive joy and excitability, the bitter taste, and the sound of talking. Its opening is the tongue, and it governs the blood vessels. The Heart disperses energy outward and dislikes heat. The Heart controls the blood vessels and is responsible for moving the blood through them. It also stores the spirit, and is therefore the organ most frequently associated with mental processes.
   1. The Heart dominates the blood and vessels: The Heart Ki has the function to prepare blood to circulate in the vessels. The vessels are the house for blood circulation. The Heart Ki must be sufficient or this will influence circulation. This can be seen on the complexion of the face. If the Heart energy functions well the person is full of vital-

ity with normal pulse beats that are harmonious, powerful, and regular. If this energy is deficient then he tires easily. This function is viewed through the complexion and the pulse.

2. The Heart houses the mind: Mental activity is involved with the Heart. "Spirit or Shen" is a general term of life activity of the body that can be seen by others. If there is abnormal Heart energy and deficient "spirit" then insomnia, lots of dreams, poor memory, restlessness, and mental disorders can be present.

3. The Heart opens into the tongue: The tongue is the mirror of the Heart. Heart energy passes through the tongue and controls its color, form, motion, and taste sensation.

The Small Intestine separates the waste material from the nutritious elements in food. The nutritious elements are distributed throughout the body, while the waste is sent on to the Large Intestine.

Almost all the disorders of the Heart are those of weakness.

> Deficient Ki—General fatigue, panting and shallow breathing, and frequent sweating
> Deficient Yang—Swollen face, ashen gray or bluish green complexion, and cold limbs
> Deficient Yin—Flushed feeling in the palms and face, low-grade fever, and night sweating
> Deficient Blood—Restlessness, irritability, dizziness, absentmindedness, and insomnia

The pattern Heart excess arises from an excess of Heart fire. This is marked by fever, sometimes accompanied by delirium, a racking pulse, intense restlessness, insomnia or

Fig. 21 Heart Meridian

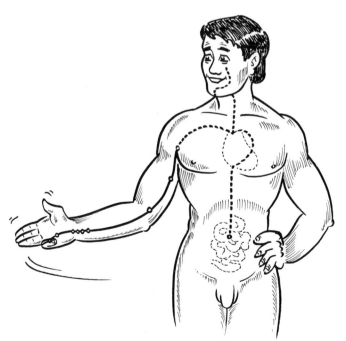

frequent nightmares, a bright red face, a red or blistered and painful tongue, and often a burning sensation during urination. The later symptom is considered to be the result of heat being transferred from the Heart to the Small Intestine, interfering with the Small Intestine's role in metabolism and the body's management of water.

The Heart Meridian of the Hand (Yin Meridian)
There are nine points on the Heart meridian. The Heart meridian pertains to the Heart connecting with the Small Intestine and has some connection with the Lungs and Kidneys.

● *Symptoms and signs:*
External—Meridian: general feverishness, headache, pain in the eyes, pain along the back of the upper arm, dry throat, thirst, hot or painful palms, coldness in the palms and soles of the feet, and pain along the scapula.

   Internal—Organ: pain or fullness in the chest and ribs, irritability, shortness of breath, discomfort when reclining, vertigo, and mental disorders.

Small Intestine
The small intestine is situated in the abdomen, its upper end connected by the pylorus with the stomach and its lower end connected with the large intestine through the ileo-cecum. The small intestine is an important site for absorption of nutrients that build blood. Its main function is to receive and temporarily store partially digested food from the stomach. It digests the food mass further and absorbs the essential substance and a portion of the water in food. The small intestine then transfers the residues with a considerable amount of fluid to the large intestine. In a similar way as the Kidneys, the Small Intestine can separate essential from waste substance.

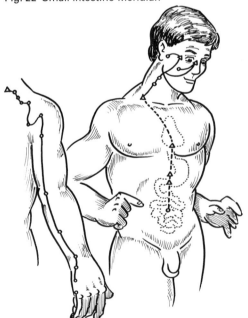

Fig. 22 Small Intestine Meridian

Problems in this function can be seen in the excretory processes especially in urination and feces production. Dysfunction stimulates urine to be plentiful while the stool may move excessively fast without time to have water-soluble nutrients removed. This makes a soft or watery stool. The reverse can also occur and may create constipation. A hyperactive Small Intestine may be caused by Heart fire that produces scanty red urine with a hot sensation during urination.

The Small Intestine Meridian of the Hand (Yang Meridian)
There are nineteen points on this meridian. The Small Intestine meridian pertains to the Small Intestine connecting with the Heart and has some direct connections with the Stomach.

● *Symptoms and signs:*
External—Meridian: numbness of the mouth and tongue, pain in the neck or cheek, sore throat, stiff neck, excessive watering of the eyes, and pain along the lateral aspect of the shoulder and upper arm.

Internal—Organ: pain and distension in the lower abdomen, possibly extending around the waist or to the genitals, diarrhea, and abdominal pain with dry stool or constipation.

KIDNEYS AND BLADDER

Kidneys

The Kidneys correspond to the water phase, the northerly direction, the season of winter, the cold climatic condition, the color of black, the emotion of fear, the salty taste, and the sound of groaning. The sensory organ is the ear. Their openings are the urethra and anus. They control the bones, marrow, and brain and their health is reflected in the hair of the head. The Kidneys dislike cold.

1. The Kidneys control growth: The Kidneys are the storage place for hereditary inheritance. The hereditary essence is the material foundation that allows the assimilation of acquired or replenished essence. Acquired essence is renewable and comes from food and drink. This energy must replenish the hereditary essence because only if acquired essence is present can development and growth take place. The Kidneys also regulate growth of females at seven year intervals, while males are regulated at eight year intervals. Kidney energy exerts a strong influence at approximately fourteen years old with the beginning of the reproductive cycle and menstruation; at four times seven years, twenty-eight years of age, the physical prime of life is near a peak; and at age of forty-nine, the cessation of menses and the child bearing years are over. For men, reproduction begins at approximately age of sixteen; the prime of life occurs around age of thirty-two (eight times four); decline begins at age of fifty-six, and the ancients felt that by age of sixty-four Ki declines to such a degree that the teeth and hair begin to fall out.

2. The Kidneys dominate water metabolism: The three main organs involved in water balance are: Kidney, Lung, and Spleen. The Kidneys have the ability to separate the useful liquid from the waste and to send the useful up to the Lungs (as moisture) and the waste to the Bladder (as urine). The Kidneys first separate the clean from the turbid and then eliminate the waste.

3. The Kidneys dominate the reception of Ki (air): The Kidneys mainly receive Ki. It is also in charge of breathing. The distribution of the clean Ki inhaled by the Lungs to the whole body depends not only on the descending function of the Lungs but also on the Kidney function of reception and control.

4. The Kidneys dominate the bones: Growth and development of bones comes from the Kidney essence. Kidney essence produces marrow. The upper part of the spinal cord connects with the brain, while the bone marrow nourishes the bones and manufactures blood. The supply to the brain, the solidity of the bone, and the adequacy of the blood are therefore all closely related to the condition of the essence of the Kidneys.

The Kidneys are the storage place of basal yin and yang of the body. Therefore, any disorder, if sufficiently chronic, will involve the Kidneys. Diseased Kidneys will affect other organs.

Fig. 23 Kidney Meridian

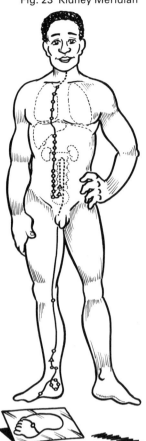

Symptoms of Deficient Kidney Yin
The lower back is weak and sore, there is ringing in the ears and loss of hearing acuity, the face is ashen or dark, especially under the eyes. Dizziness, thirst, night sweats, and low-grade fevers are common. Men have little semen and tend toward premature ejaculation, while women have little or no menstruation. This deficiency produces similar disorders in the Heart and Liver.

Symptoms of Deficient Kidney Yang
This pattern is generally seen as loss of warmth along with the previously mentioned symptoms. There is a feeling of fatigue and coldness. There is a notable weakness of the legs. Excessive urination is also present. And sometimes faint voice, coughing, puffiness in the face, and spontaneous sweating. This deficiency produces similar disorders in the Spleen and Lungs.

The Kidney Meridian of the Leg (Yin Meridian)
There are twenty-seven points on the Kidney meridian. This channel pertains to the Kidneys to communicate with the Bladder and connects directly with the Liver, Lungs, Heart, and other organs.

Fig. 24 Bladder Meridian

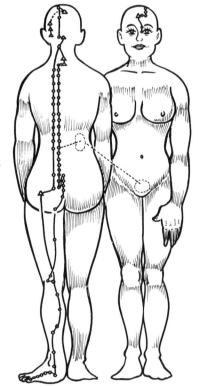

● *Symptoms and signs:*
External—Meridian: back pain, lumbago, cold feeling in the feet, weakness of the feet, thirst, sore throat, and pain in the back of the leg and thigh.

Internal—Organ: dizziness, facial edema, ashen complexion, blurred vision, shortness of breath, drowsiness, irritability, loose stool, chronic diarrhea or constipation, abdominal distension, vomiting, and impotence.

Bladder
The bladder is located in the lower abdomen behind and below the pubic bone. The main functions of the bladder are to receive, temporarily store, and excrete urine from the body. Urine is made by the filtering action of the kidneys. The Bladder function is accomplished with the help of Kidney Ki. All urinary problems are caused by dysfunction of the Kidneys and Bladder.

The Bladder Meridian of the Foot (Yang Meridian)
There are sixty-seven points on this meridian. The Bladder meridian pertains to the Bladder connecting with the Kidneys and has some direct connections with the brain and Heart.

● *Symptoms and signs:*
External—Meridian: alternating chills and fever, headache, stiff neck, lumbago, sinus trouble, frequent tearing, and pain of the eye, thigh, back of the knees, leg, and feet.

    Internal—Organ: lower abdominal pain, dysuria (painful urination), retention of urine, enuresis (bed-wetting), and mental disorders.

HEART GOVERNOR AND TRIPLE HEATER

Heart Governor
The Heart Governor or Pericardium is considered the outer layer of the heart. The function of the Heart Governor is to protect the Heart from outside disease causing factors. When invasions come it is the Heart Governor that is first affected. The Heart Governor and Triple Heater combined are said to correspond to the "Ministerial Fire" while the Heart and Small Intestine are considered "Sovereign Fire." One common problem of Heart Governor energy is the difficulty in the Heart housing the mind. When this occurs there is loss of consciousness and delirium.

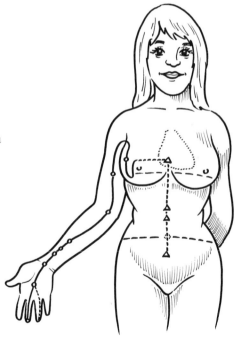

Fig. 25 Heart Governor Meridian

The Heart Governor Meridian of the Hand (Yin Meridian)
There are nine points on the Heart Governor meridian. The Heart Governor meridian pertains to the Heart Governor and connects with the Triple Heater, communicating with the Heart and Lung meridians.

● *Symptoms and signs:*
External—Meridian: stiff neck, spasms in the arm or leg, flushed face, pain in the eyes, underarm swelling, and hot palms.
    Internal—Organ: impaired speech, fainting, irritability, fullness in the chest, palpitations, chest pain, immobility of tongue, and mental disorders.

Triple Heater
The Triple Heater was described as "having a name but no form" in a third century classic. It is regarded as the function that coordinates all the functions of water metabolism. Its responsibility is to govern all the internal organs in their function to separate the

useful from the waste. It also provides water passage for water metabolism. At various times in written literature the "three burners or spaces" were but three regions of the body that were used to group the organs. The Upper Heater extends from the pharanx to diaphragm and includes the chest, neck, head, and the functions of the Heart and Lungs. The Middle Heater spans the region between the chest and the navel, and includes the functions of the Stomach and Spleen. The Lower Heater contains the lower abdomen and the functions of the Kidneys, Bladder, Large and Small Intestines (and usually the Liver which, however, is sometimes placed in the Middle Heater). As such, the upper portion has been compared to a mist that spreads the blood and Ki, the Middle Heater is like a foam that churns up food in the process of digestion, and the Lower Heater is likened to a swamp where all the impure substances are excreted. This description can be used in diagnosis. Symptoms associated with poor function include swelling (edema), bed-wetting (enuresis), excessive urination, and water trapped in the chest (pleural infusion).

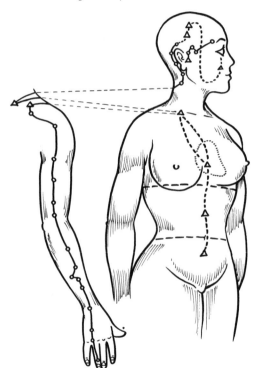

Fig. 26 Triple Heater Meridian

The Triple Heater Meridian of the Hand (Yang Meridian)
There are twenty-three points on the Triple Heater meridian. The Triple Heater meridian pertains to the Triple Heater and connects with the Heart Governor.

● *Symptoms and signs:*
External—Meridian: swelling and pain in the throat, pain in the cheek and jaw, redness in the eyes, deafness, and pain behind the ear or along the outside of the shoulder and upper arm.

Internal—Organ: abdominal distension, hardness and fullness in the lower abdomen, bed-wetting (enuresis), frequent or excessive urination, painful or impaired passing of urine (dysuria), and edema.

Fig. 27

Organs	Triple Heater	Location
Heart and Lungs	Upper Space	Pharanx to Diaphragm
Spleen and Stomach (Liver)	Middle Space	Diaphragm to Belly Button
Kidneys and Bladder Large and Small Intestines (Liver)	Lower Space	Below Belly Button

LIVER AND GALLBLADDER

Liver

The Liver corresponds to the wood phase, the direction of east, the season of spring, the climatic condition of wind, the color of green, the emotion of anger, the sour taste, the goatish odor, and the sound of shouting. Its point of entry is the eyes. It controls the sinews (muscles, joints), and its health is reflected in the nails.

The Liver is responsible for spreading and regulating the Ki throughout the body. Its character is flowing and free. Thus, depression or frustration can disturb its function. It is also responsible for storing blood when the body is at rest. This characteristic, combined with its control over the lower abdomen, makes it the most important organ with regard to women's menstrual cycle and sexuality.

Depression or long-term frustration can upset the Liver's spreading function and result in continuing depression, a bad temper, and a painful, swollen feeling in the chest and sides. If it worsens, it may lead to disharmony between the Liver and the Stomach and/or Spleen. This disorder is marked by the "rebellion" of Ki in the latter two organs, whereby the Ki moves in the opposite direction than it is normally proper. In the case of

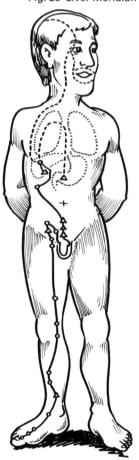

Fig. 28 Liver Meridian

the Stomach, whose Ki normally descends, rebellious Ki means hiccoughing, vomiting, and so on. The Ki of the Spleen, on the other hand, is ordinarily directed upward; rebellious Ki in this Organ means diarrhea.

1. The Liver stores blood: One of the Liver's most important functions is storage of blood, with the emphasis on nourishing and moistening. It regulates the volume of circulating blood. During activity the Liver will release more blood for circulation to be sent around the body while during rest, blood is stored in the Liver. The Liver dominates the Sea of Blood—acu-point SP10, a location that affects blood purity and skin troubles.

Deficient Liver blood: dry, painful eyes with blurred or weak vision, lack of suppleness or pain in moving the joints, dry skin, dizziness (lack of blood in the head), and infrequent or spotty menstruation.

2. The Liver maintains an unrestricted condition for free flowing Ki: The Liver makes Ki flow without obstructions both within the Liver and the other Zang-Fu organs. The Liver function is like a tree in spring that grows unobstructed. If restriction occurs so can Rising Liver Fire with symptoms of ill temper, restlessness, headache, vertigo, red face and eyes, and a parched mouth.

3. The Liver dominates the tendons: This also includes the ligaments and fingernails. Deficiency of Liver energy produces undernourishment of the tendons, spasms, numbness, difficulty in contraction, and tremor. If it becomes more serious then it becomes an interior movement of Liver

Wind with symptoms of sudden onset of dizziness while moving about, spasms, paralysis, difficulty in movement, or severe vertigo.

4. The Liver opens into the eyes: All five pairs of Zang-Fu organs flow through the eye but the Liver, Heart, and Kidney organs have the greater influence.

The Liver Meridian of the Foot (Yin Meridian)
There are fourteen points on the Liver meridian. This channel pertains to the Liver, communicating with the Gallbladder and connects directly with the Lungs, Stomach, and brain.

● *Symptoms and signs:*
External—Meridian: headache, dizziness, blurred vision, tinnitus (ringing in the ears), and fever. Spasms of the foot and the hand also may appear in severe cases.

Internal—Organ: fullness and pain in the lower chest, hard lumps in the upper abdomen, abdominal pain, vomiting, jaundice, loose stool, pain in the lower abdomen, hernia, enuresis (bed-wetting), retention of urine, and dark urine.

Gallbladder
The gallbladder is attached to the lower portion of the liver. Its main function is to store bile produced by the liver and excrete it into the large intestine when fats enter the digestive system. The excretion of bile is controlled by the liver. Problems of the liver will effect the flow of bile. Eating rich foods high in fat such as meats, eggs, oils, and dairy products stimulate bile production. These foods, as well as overeating, promote damp and heat to be produced.

For some people bile fluid concentrates and forms stones. If the passage from the gallbladder to the duodenum becomes obstructed or blocked, this usually happens from the presence of cholesterol-rich gallstones, the bile goes directly into the blood. This gives the skin a yellowish-green color and the feces become white from lack of bile pigmentation. Other symptoms include an oppressive sensation of fullness in the abdomen and yellow coloring in the eye whites.

The Gallbladder is sometimes considered an extra Fu organ because food does not actually pass through it. It is also a hollow organ (Fu) but it has a function similar to Zang organs. The Gallbladder and Liver together are responsible for the movement of unrestrained vital energy.

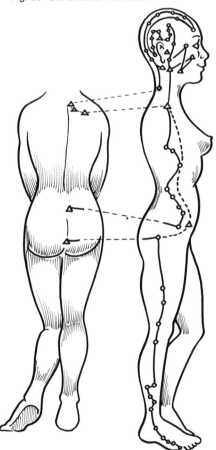

Fig. 29 Gallbladder Meridian

The Gallbladder Meridian of the Foot (Yang Meridian)
There are forty-four points on this meridian. The Gallbladder meridian pertains to the Gallbladder and communicates with the Liver, and it has some direct connections with the Heart.

● Symptoms and signs:
External—Meridian: chill and fever, headache, malaria, gray facial appearance, eye pain, redness in the eyes, pain in the jaw, underarm swelling of lymph nodes (scrofula), pain along the channel in the hip region, leg, and foot, and deafness.

Internal—Organ: pain in the ribs, vomiting, bitter taste in the mouth, and chest pain.

The Gallbladder stores and excretes bile, which is produced by the Liver. Together with the Heart, the Gallbladder is responsible for decision making. The principal disease associated with the Gallbladder is a disorder affecting the flow of bile, caused by dampness and heat. This is manifested by pain in the region of the Liver, an oppressive sensation of fullness in the abdomen, and yellowish eyes, skin, urine, and tongue.

GOVERNING AND CONCEPTION VESSELS

Governing Vessel (Yang Meridian)
The Governing Vessel flows from the anus area up the center of the back over the neck and head to inside the upper lip. There are twenty-eight points on this meridian. This regulates all the yang meridians.

● *Symptoms and signs:*
Tetanus, shaking, convulsion, apoplexy (stroke), aphasia (inability to speak after stroke), epilepsy, headache, redness and swelling of the eye, excessive tearing, lumbago, pain in the leg, knee, and the back, febrile disease, sore throat, toothache, swelling in the gums, numbness of foot and hand, and night sweating.

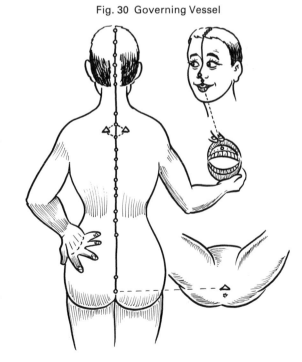

Fig. 30 Governing Vessel

The Governing Vessel acu-points located on the head and the neck, are usually indicated for disorders of head and brain, and febrile diseases. The points on the back are indicated for the diseases of the lungs, the heart, the pericardium, the liver, gallbladder, spleen, stomach, and diseases of the back, loin, and lower extremities while those on the lumbosacral region are indicated for diseases of the kidneys, bladder, and large and small intestines.

Conception Vessel (Yin Meridian)
There are twenty-four points on this channel. It regulates the functions of all yin meridians and nourishes the fetus. Its function is closely related with pregnancy and therefore
has intimate links with the Kidneys and uterus.

Fig. 31 Conception Vessel

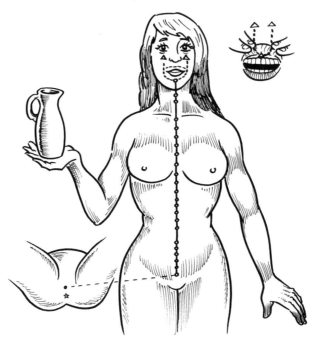

● *Symptoms and signs:*
Hemorrhoids, diarrhea, dysentery, malaria, cough, hemoptysis (coughing up blood),
toothache, swelling of pharynx, dysuria (painful urination), pain in the abdomen,
difficulty swallowing, post obstetrical palsy, lumbago, cold sensation in the umbilical
region, vomiting, hiccup, and pain in the breast. It also affects the throat, chest, abdomen, umbilical region, diseases of the digestive and urogenital systems, and cold diseases.

Summary of Meridian Pathology

The Three Arm Yin Meridians
   1. Arm Greater Yin Lung meridian is indicated for diseases of the chest, throat, trachea, nose, and Lungs.
   2. Arm Absolute Yin Heart Governor meridian is indicated for diseases of the chest,
Stomach, and Heart, as well as mental disorder generally.
   3. Arm Lesser Yin Heart meridian is indicated for diseases of the chest, tongue, and
Heart, as well as mental disorders generally.

The Three Arm Yang Meridians
   1. Arm Yang Brightness Large Intestine meridian is indicated for diseases of the

face, eyes, ears, nose, gums, throat, and Large Intestine, as well as febrile diseases generally.

2. Arm Lesser Yang Triple Heater meridian is indicated for diseases of the temporal region, eyes, ears, throat and ribs, as well as febrile diseases generally.

3. Arm Greater Yang Small Intestine meridian is indicated for diseases of the vertex, eyes, ears, throat, as well as mental disorders generally.

The Three Leg Yin Meridians

1. Leg Greater Yin Spleen meridian is indicated for diseases of the upper abdomen, Stomach, Intestines, and urogenital system.

2. Leg Absolute Yin Liver meridian is indicated for diseases affecting the hypochondriac region, lower abdomen, urogenital system, and head.

3. Leg Lesser Yin Kidney meridian is indicated for diseases affecting the waist, urogenital system, throat, and mental disorders generally.

The Three Leg Yang Meridians

1. Leg Yang Brightness Stomach meridian is indicated for diseases of the face, nose, gums, throat, Stomach and Intestines as well as mental and febrile diseases generally.

2. Leg Lesser Yang Gallbladder meridian is indicated for diseases of the temporal region, nose, eyes, throat, and ribs, as well as febrile diseases generally.

3. Leg Greater Yang Bladder meridian is indicated for diseases affecting the vertex, nose, eyes, and lumbar region, as well as febrile and mental diseases generally.

Circulating Direction of the Meridians

Downward Movement	Upward Movement
Lungs	Large Intestine
Stomach	Spleen
Heart	Small Intestine
Bladder	Kidneys
Heart Governor	Triple Heater
Gallbladder	Liver

Special Acu-points

Many individual acu-points (*tsubo*), as well as groups of acu-points have been known to bring about remarkable changes in the body. They have controlling, stimulating, sedating, and strengthening effects. The most useful acu-points in practice are the Front and Back points. The Front—*Bo* (*Mu* in Chinese) points and Back—*Yu* (*Shu* in Chinese) points give special diagnostic information as well as therapeutic results when stimulated.

Front Points

The Japanese *Bo* and Chinese *Mu* meaning for Front points is connection and accumulation. This meaning comes from the Ki of the Zang-Fu (solid and hollow) organs accumulating in the chest and abdomen. They are distributed according to anatomical location. Front points are on both sides except those on the midline. They are often

Fig. 32 Front Points

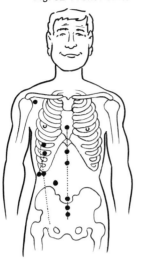

Organ	Point Number
Lungs	LU 1
Heart Govemor	CV 17
Heart	CV 14
Liver	LV 14
Gallbladder	GB 24
Spleen	LV 13
Stomach	CV 12
Triple Heater	CV 5
Kidneys	GB 25
Large Intestine	ST 25
Bladder	CV 3
Small Intestine	CV 4

called alarm points and are used to treat the disorders of the Zang-Fu organs. Tenderness on or near a Front point is a useful diagnostic indicator of disease in the organ associated with that point. Because the Front points are located near the organs, they are sensitive to imbalances. When there is trouble in the lungs, treat their Front point—LU l; and when there is trouble with nausea and the stomach, treat the Stomach Front point—CV 12. In practice the Front points are almost always used in combination with the Back points.

Back Points

This is the site where the infusion of Ki from the Zang-Fu organs occurs. This group is distributed on the first line closest to the spine on the Bladder meridian of the back

Fig. 33 Back Points

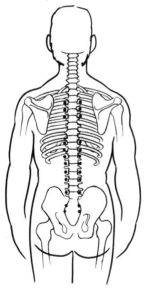

Organ	Point Number
Lungs	BL 13
Heart Governor	BL 14
Heart	BL 15
Liver	BL 18
Gallbladder	BL 19
Spleen	BL 20
Stomach	BL 21
Triple Heater	BL 22
Kidneys	BL 23
Large Intestine	BL 25
Bladder	BL 27
Small Intestine	BL 28

(called *Yu* in Japanese and *Shu* in Chinese). They are in close proximity to their related organs. When an internal organ malfunctions, an abnormal reaction such as tenderness will occur at the corresponding Back point. Besides the organ bearing its name, such as Liver point, the Back points can be used to treat their related organs. For example liver disturbances (such as vertigo, flushed face, or migraine headaches), as well as optic neuritis (because the Liver opens into the eye) are both treated with Liver Back point—BL 18. Gradual difficulty of hearing that comes with age (because the Kidneys open into the ear) can be treated by stimulating Kidney Back point—BL 23. Following this reasoning and studying the relationships presented in the Five Transformations Theory as well as the previously discussed Zang-Fu organ functions, you can see the depth of use possible with each of the Back points.

Strengths of Traditional Wisdom

The use of anesthetics in surgery was first introduced in the West in the mid-1800s. The Chinese were using "narcotic soups" for minor surgery some 700 years ago. For centuries, the Chinese treated "ulcer of the lung," what we know to be streptococcal diseases, with the fermented brine of salted vegetables—a process and remedy similar to modern penicillin. The use of the plant ephedra (*Ma Huang*) for the treatment of asthma became standard practice in Chinese medicine as long ago as the second century. They knew of its bronchi dilating effects. It has been a Western and worldwide practice only since 1887. Sea vegetable which contains iodine was used by the Chinese at least 1,000 years ago to treat enlarged thyroids; its essence iodine is now a common remedy in Western medicine used in the treatment of goiter.

External Traditional Applications

The first line of defense against ill-health is diet. Simultaneously traditional wisdom developed supplemental forms of treatment to enhance and strengthen the effects of good nutrition. Internal and external treatments go hand-in-hand, despite the type of ailment.

External treatments include: acupuncture, massage, moxibustion, tapping, scraping, cupping, bloodletting, compresses, poultices, liniments, and ointments. Sites for treatment are chosen among the vital acu-points along the meridians associated with the diseased organ. To get the full impact of the long-term development of ancient traditional medicine I thought you could appreciate the diversity of treatment plans that have been practiced. The following are brief get-acquainted description of some other unusual traditional applications. These are still in use today. We can use these methods when appropriate.

Moxibustion
Moxibustion uses a burning herb held or placed either directly on or over the skin at specific acu-points. *Moxa* is derived from Japanese and means "burning herb." It is a soft, downy material obtained from the common mugwort plant (*Artemisia vulgaris*). It

can be rolled tightly in paper to form a tube that looks like a cigar, or on rare occasions it can be placed directly on top of another substance such as ginger, miso, or garlic. One end is ignited until it glows evenly, then it is held about an inch from the skin over the acu-point and rotated slowly. Its healing effects radiate directly through the skin to influence the meridian below. It is used whenever cold has invaded the organism or when increased circulation and stimulation is needed.

Human blood has liquid plasma and solid red blood cells and white blood cells. White blood cells destroy bacteria when it penetrates into the human body, and thus prevent bacterial infections. Therefore, as long as the white blood cells are strong and balanced, our bodies will fight any infectious disease. In ancient times, people practiced moxibustion for such diverse conditions as tumors and bacterial infections such as venereal disease, intestinal or lung disorders.

When moxibustion is administered, the body protein below the surface of the skin is transformed into histotoxin by heat, and this chemical substance and the essential oil that moxa contains help to increase the number of white blood cells, and alkalize the blood. At the same time, white blood cells help to prevent infections and the alkalized blood helps to maintain health. According to studies, the number of white blood cells in the body is multiplied several times after moxibustion. Thus moxibustion really helps keep your body healthy.

Tapping

Tapping is also known as "Seven Star" needle therapy, but most often poetically referred to as "Plum-blossom" therapy. The term *plum blossom* produces much less anxiety with patients than the name *seven star needles.* Patients appreciate the not so subtle difference.

The art of tapping consists of using a special needle (the plum blossom or homemade variety) on an area to be treated. The patient is positioned in a comfortable posture and the tapper is used in a pounding or tapping manner on the troubled area (the same motion as a hammer). The area is tapped until it becomes pink or until small drops of blood begin to appear on the surface of the skin. Although the treatment may sound somewhat gruesome and torturous it usually is only slightly more uncomfortable than the sensation from sore points during finger pressure.

Information concerning Plum-blossom therapy in China goes back over one thousand years. The earliest Chinese medical classic *Ling Shui Jing* (part of the *Huang Di Nei Jing,* compiled from 475 B.C. to A.D. 23) describes its use. The ancients gave the name of plum-blossom needle to five needles bound in a bundle like a plum blossom, and of seven star needle to the seven needles bound in a bundle.

When to Use Tapping

The tapping method can be used on all conditions of heat or excess: muscle soreness, skin irritations, hypertension, stiff neck, painful lower back, and tension between the shoulder blades.

Getting the Instrument

The instrument can be purchased from acupuncture supply houses through mail order and from Chinese medical herbal shops in China towns around the world. The needle also can be made at home.

Holding the Needle

Holding the needle needs a certain amount of skill. It should be neither too tightly nor too loosely gripped. If it is too tight, this will cause muscular tension of the wrist joint, and affect the flexibility of movement. If it is too loose, it will shake the needle and tend to cause bleeding. The correct method of holding the needle is to have the handle in the center of the palm, held in place with the ring and little fingers. The index finger is extended with the tip resting on the handle of the needle. The thumb also braces the needle. The most important part is to keep the wrist flexible. From this position you can make use of the elastic force of your wrist.

Methods

The manipulation of the plum-blossom needle consists of tapping with the force of the wrist. Tapping must be stable and accurate. The tip of the needle should vertically touch the skin, lifting quickly after each tap. You will hear a short, clear, and crisp "tah" sound. Wrist force must be elastic and even. Slow, pressing, oblique or dragging styles are incorrect techniques and should not be used. The frequency is neither too quick nor too slow, generally seventy to ninety times a minute. The intensity of stimulation is divided into three kinds.

1. *Light tapping:* The wrist force is light and the force of impact is also small. Tap the local skin till it becomes pink.
2. *Heavy tapping:* The wrist force and the force of impact are heavy. Tap the local skin till it becomes very red and a slight bleeding occurs.
3. *Moderate tapping:* The force is between light and heavy tapping. Tapping is applied on the local skin till it becomes red and purple but not bleeding.

The force of tapping depends on the illness, the age and strength of the patient, and the area to which the tapping is applied. In children, in patients in poor health, or nervous patients treated for the first time, a light stimulation should be used. In the middle-aged person or a patient with acute or hot diseases, generally a heavy stimulation is applied. Yet according to the condition of disease as well as his sensitivity and tolerance of needling, you can apply light stimulation at first time then gradually change it to moderate or heavy stimulation.

Position for Treatment

Depending on the area of treatment the receiver can be arranged in either a sitting or lying (prone or supine) positions. It is important for the receiver to remain comfortable during the treatment.

How Often?

In chronic diseases, treat once daily or every other day. Four to seven treatments to the first series (short course), afterward treat once every other day, seven to eight treatments may be considered a long course. After a long course of treatment, it may take a rest for ten to twenty days, then continue the treatment as before.

In treating acute diseases, there are no fixed courses, you may treat once in every several hours successively till the condition is improving, then once daily or every other day. These are general guidelines. You should use common sense when applying this, or any other, technique.

Caring for the Instrument
After being used the needle should be kept dry. If the needle is found not even, loose or rusted, it should be repaired or replaced by a new one. Sterilization of the needle is generally done by soaking the needle in alcohol for thirty minutes or so.

If the patient has hepatitis or AIDS, the needle used on them should be put aside and reserved for their use only. It should not be used on other patients to avoid infection. In the last few years, disposable tapping needles have become available.

Scraping

Scraping is a simple technique and is used for fever, heat stroke, colds, headache, painful joints, and indigestion. A coin is lubricated with salted water and scraped over the surface of the skin in gentle strokes with moderate pressure. Another way to scrape is to use the index and middle fingers and pinch the area to be treated. Once pinched the skin is let go and repeated several times. Common sites for scraping are the back of the neck, both sides of the neck, both sides of the throat, the bridge of the nose, the space between the eyebrows, the upper chest, and along both sides of the spine. This technique relieves symptoms of hot and full ailments by drawing excess heat and energy to the scraped area, releasing it. Usually the treated area becomes red.

Cupping

Suction cups have been used for a variety of complaints. Using traditional terms, cups are good when the problem is caused by wind-chills, damp-excess, and such common problems as arthritis, rheumatism, abdominal pain, bruises, and abscesses. Cupping is often preceded by tapping. This combination is very effective. The cups are made of bamboo or glass and vary in size from a shot glass to a water glass. A couple of matches are lit or a piece of cotton held in forceps is dipped in alcohol and ignited. The cup is held mouth down near the patient and the inside briefly flamed with the burning material. This burns the oxygen in the air thus reducing air pressure inside the cup. The cup is then immediately pressed against the treatment site, to which it adheres firmly by suction. After fifteen to twenty minutes, the cup is released by pressing down on the skin around it and allowing air to enter and equalize the air pressure. It may leave a red circle on the skin, and the treated surface will be beaded with droplets of moisture and, sometimes, blood. This method literally sucks out excess moisture, chills, dampness, and leaked blood from the areas treated.

Bloodletting

Unlike the complexity of Transylvanian Count Dracula's vampire methods, bloodletting is a rather simple procedure. A sharp triangular needle is used to prick open the site of treatment. Sites can be either specific acu-points or areas of trouble such as an injury. A small amount of blood is released. Bloodletting is commonly used for heat stroke, fever, colic, vomiting, diarrhea, abscesses and swelling, strokes, and traumatic injuries. After the site has been selected it is sterilized with alcohol and pricked. The release of blood induces excess "evil energy" and excess heat energy to escape.

Compresses

The most common compress is the ginger compress. It is heated water to which fresh grated gingerroot has been added. Towels are dipped into the steaming brew, wrung out, and placed on the area to be treated. The compress heats muscles and tendons while it relaxes and expands them. It also increases blood and lymphatic circulation in the area treated. For aches, pains, and strains it is applied directly on the painful area, for internal organ strengthening, it is placed directly on the affected organ, such as the lower back for the kidneys or the abdomen in the case of the intestines. Treatment time is approximately from ten to twenty minutes. For cancer, compresses should not be used directly on a tumor area.

Herbal Poultices

Herbs are ground to a very fine powder and mixed dry for storage. Just before use, some powder is mixed with a little water until a sticky texture is achieved. This is spread thickly over a piece of cloth or wax paper, stuck tightly over the injured area, and taped in place for eight to twelve hours. The combination of moisture and body heat activates the herbal mix that draws out excess "evil energy" and radiates in healing vapors. Herbal poultices are used for arthritic and rheumatic conditions, strained backs, sprained joints and tendons, blocked meridians, nervous disorders, bruising, swelling, and abscesses. They are usually applied after shiatsu. Taro potato mixed with gingerroot is an example.

The Value of Traditional Wisdom

Universal truth prevails throughout the field of traditional Chinese medicine. The same ideas and terminology that define the traditional Chinese view of the universe are also used to describe the phenomena of health and disease. The Chinese regard the human body and all its functions as a microcosm of the grand cosmic order. They believe that the same forces that permeate the universe and animate nature in all its variety are also at work in man. The principles of Chinese medicine are drawn from traditional Taoist philosophy, China's most ancient and pervasive school of thought.

The depth of traditional wisdom is fathomless. Its principles are observations of the workings of the universe and are timeless. So much so that the present-day text books used in the classrooms of traditional Chinese medicine universities are excerpted from the classics of pre 500 B.C. times. The principles remain valuable.

Taoist thought stresses fluctuation and mutability and explains all natural phenomena in terms of the constant ebb and flow of cosmic forces. Many modern people tend to prefer to deal with structured ideas, fixed qualities, and absolute laws and reasoning. For these people the principles of Chinese medicine, especially the concepts and terms used to explain them, are difficult to absorb at first glance. Closer observation reveals the soundness, sense, and profundity of this system. It draws its symbols directly from nature. When dealing with the traditional system remind yourself that the descriptions are always symbolic of natural phenomena.

Shiatsu and macrobiotic theory and practice have borrowed liberally from these ancient traditional sources of wisdom. In the past before sophisticated electronic equipment existed, venerable wise ones were able to detect a bioenergetic field in the human body that only recently has been scientifically confirmed. The sensitivity and depth of thought expressed in literature left behind by past sages concerning the order of the universe, evokes a sense of wonder in modern man. With such comprehensive teachings, it is no wonder that there is the temptation to borrow the essence of their discoveries and insight. They are truly a universal gift. In the realm of the eternal, things change slowly. Natural truth that was accurate 5,000 years ago remains true today. For the benefit of humanity this information has valuable practical and theoretical applications.

Chapter 4

Whole Health Diagnosis

The human body is endowed with the ability to resist the invasion of various kinds of disease causing factors. This defensive action is what keeps us healthy and alive. When factors adversely affect the body imbalances may develop. To accurately deal with these health-threatening conditions knowledge is necessary. How do we get this information? In other words, how do we diagnose or assess the body's condition?

Diagnosis is the art of discovering the nature of the patient's illness and the underlying cause. I have to stress the importance of remembering the part about underlying cause. Diagnostic techniques have developed according to an eras prevalent belief system and available technology. Modern diagnostic techniques include traditional visual as well as invasive methods to gain greater information about a patient's condition. Because of the arrival of the microscope, the electron microscope, and other useful technologies, diagnosis has advanced greatly. The drawing of blood, spinal fluid, and other body secretions are routinely done. Often examination of urine and stool specimens are requested by doctors. The injection of radioactive dyes and photographing the results gives specialists information concerning size and function of internal organs. From these methods, information is gained on how the body is functioning. These can give strong clues when the body is not functioning properly. Modern use of technology in diagnosis is relatively new. It has not always been used.

I once had an elderly female patient over ninety years of age who recalled when she would visit her doctor as problems arose. Her doctor would sit next to her quietly for up to fifteen minutes. He would not speak a word. He merely sat quietly, listened, and thought. After his meditation on her condition he would recommend his treatment. She compares the older doctor's methods with his son who also became a physician. Years later when she would visit the younger doctor he would send her for a battery of tests never looking at her nor sitting with her. She felt without the tests the younger man would know nothing about her. She told me she wonders why medicine has progressed backward. Her older doctor always knew what her problems were and now the younger doctor does not. Sometimes he did not know even after a host of expensive tests.

French bacteriologist Louis Pasteur (1822–1895) championed a theory of disease that described nonchangeable microbes as the primary cause of disease. Pasteur's view that all diseases are caused by microbes that invade the body from the outer environment and come from preexisting microbes is the basis of modern microbiology. With techniques based on Pasteur's theory, it is easy to see why the development of diagnosis and treatment seek to explain the involvement of the outer world as extremely important.

At a much earlier time in history a noninvasive assessment system had developed. Observation of what is generally considered to be normal and correct, compared against current symptoms, gave traditional practitioners information necessary to prescribe adjustments appropriate to balance an imbalanced condition. This is the foundation of traditional diagnosis.

Getting an Accurate Picture

The art of assessment or diagnosis has ancient beginnings. My purpose for diagnosis is somewhat unconventional. I am not interested in only discovering the name of the ailment that is causing the patient's discomfort. The naming of a disease does nothing to change it. My purpose is to understand the imbalances that cause the body to create the symptoms that we name. To be accurate in diagnosis, we must find out the imbalance in the realms of body, mind, and even spirit. Every problem is complex and interrelated to other parts, nonetheless there are symptoms or disturbances that affect one aspect of the body-mind-spirit combination more than another. In order to balance you must sense which of these three parts are most affected. For example, a woman with breast cancer has first and foremost a body imbalance. Therefore the physical body must be adjusted. Yet, she always has concern, worry, and even fear. These strong emotions may create imbalance and must also be addressed. How do you know which segment is of primary importance? This is a difficult question to answer. The body and mind are not separate. The world is not only black nor white. The solution to this dilemma comes from your intuition and experience. However, the beauty of this treatment style is that all three areas are corrected with proper diet and shiatsu. Until you gather many direct experiences you need not be overly preoccupied with such concerns. Do your best and keep your eyes and ears open and alert.

The majority of patients who come to macrobiotic shiatsu practitioners bring a medical diagnosis with them. Their problems have sent them to their regular doctor who after tests, has given them a diagnosis and usually information about the eventual outcome of their problem. Others may come to you just for a checkup. They ask, "Am I O.K.?… am I developing any serious problems?" A growing number of others are bypassing conventional medicine and coming directly to alternative practitioners. While this is a wonderful gesture of confidence in alternative therapies it also exerts greater pressure on the practitioner to be accurate. Students in my classes continually ask for information on how to diagnose. They are feeling the pressure of primary health-care providers.

There are three observations that enhance your ability to assess accurately. These lay the foundation for the specific types of traditional diagnosis that follow.

1. All parts are connected: No matter where the major area of complaint is located you can be sure there are other areas of trouble. While the primary complaint area is usually the source of the problem there are other parts that cause the problem yet they display no symptoms. For example, a patient may complain of pain in the mid-back area, the right shoulder, and the rims of the eyes when the gallbladder is inflamed. Ironically, the gallbladder is located below the right ribs. A child may wet the bed every night. Initially it appears that kidney and bladder imbalance is present. Yet it may be the child is emotionally disturbed and releases his frustration nightly. In both cases by treating the whole person you are being complete.

There are front and back connections, left side and right side connections, top and bottom connections, inside and outside connections, and physical and emotional connections.

2. *The inside shows itself on the outside:* The interior of the body is visible with a trained eye by observing the surface. This includes the face, skin, hair, and nails. The muscle-bone relationship gives information about relative yin-yang balance useful to reestablish harmony. The internal organs' function creates an energy field that surrounds the body. This force field can be sensed. Viewing the eye in its complexity can explain many telltale clues about a person including emotional states.

3. *Energy must flow:* Life is movement. Troubles arise when energy slows down and stagnates. Commonly seen as sinus congestion, constipation, or asthma, various sites in the body display symptoms as energy flow diminishes.

Diagnosis at a Glance

I have compiled several types of diagnosis that I have found to be valuable and relatively easy to learn. For our purposes, diagnosis or assessment is a method to get to know an individual better. This includes the physical, emotional, and even the spiritual levels. Each of the major assessments will be explained in detail. There are lifestyle categories that should be looked into when someone comes to see you. These are the preliminary categories that will lead us into a greater investigation. The following signs begin to paint a picture of the individual's current condition.

Chills and Fever: Intermittent fever and chills usually indicate an ailment which affects both the internal and external parts, or is moving from one to the other. Fever and thirst with no chills indicates an internal ailment, chills without fever reflects yang deficiency, and fever without chills indicates an overabundance of yang energy. Other factors, such as what time of day chills and fever occur, further refine the reading of this indicator.

Perspiration: The amount and thickness of perspiration, when it occurs and on what parts of the body it appears, are the main questions regarding this sign.

Stool and Urine: Constipation accompanied by hard stools is a sign of "hot" and "full" disease. Loose stools containing partially digested food indicates a "cold" and "empty" ailment. The presence of blood or mucus in the stool must also be reported. Scanty, dark urine reflects "heat excess," while profuse, clear urine is a sign of "cold" and "empty" disease. Cloudy urine indicates "moist heat excess."

Food, Drink, and Taste: An inclination for hot drinks reflects a "cold" disease, while a preference for cold drinks and food indicates a "hot" type disease. A revulsion toward drinking water is a sign of "moist" disease. The presence of a flat, bitter, sweet, or other dominant taste in the mouth has significance. A strong desire for spicy, deep-fried foods or strange materials (such as dirt, candle wax, coffee grounds, and so on) usually indicates the presence of parasites in the system.

Sleep: Excessive sleep indicates yang deficiency (a yin state), while insomnia is a sign of poor circulation, excessive worry, or spleen deficiency. Fitful sleep indicates emotional disturbance or overindulgence in food and drink. Unusually early rising often indicates an overactive heart.

Sex, Menstruation, and Pregnancy: For men, the vital questions in this area involve sexual vitality, impotence, incontinence, nocturnal emissions, and spermatorrhea, and frequency of intercourse. For women, frequency of menstruation, its color and texture, other vaginal discharges such as leukorrhea, past pregnancies and/or abortions, childbirths, and frequency of intercourse are vital indicators of the nature of disease in the body. In addition to the history of the specific disease based on the above indicators, a brief past history of the patient is also taken.

Besides stressing past illnesses, living habits, environmental surroundings, allergies, and so forth, the general health history of the patient's family is also covered. In cases involving infants, the deaf and mute, and others who are unable to conduct the interview for themselves, the relevant information is provided by the patient's spouse, parent, close family member, or friend.

Adjustments to a Healthier Lifestyle

When beginning the practice of a healthier way of living, you may experience some physical and mental reactions during a short transition period. The times vary but can last from three to ten days, and sometimes for up to four months. Such physical and mental reactions have various symptoms, but none of them have any harmful or lasting influence. Usually such reactions are almost negligible, if our native constitution is strong and well-structured, due to strong genes and our family's way of life. The transition symptoms are of short duration especially if the condition of our digestive system has not been affected by any sickness and we have not had unhealthy dietary habits in the past. More pronounced reactions, physical and emotional, are experienced by people who have had the following conditions:

1. Chaotic dietary habits, especially as a child.
2. Used drugs or medications, including eating artificial and chemicalized foods.
3. Have received surgery and had organs removed, such as tonsils, appendix, ovaries, gallbladder, and spleen. Abortions physically weaken women.

The healing crisis or discharge is known as "Jarisch-Herxheimer reaction." It is similar to an allergic reaction. It is a basic phenomenon that occurs whenever there is any substantial die-off of microbiotic pathogens such as the yeast cell fungal infections associated with systemic candidiasis, or the amoebic-type manifestations often found in severe cases of rheumatism and arthritis in adults.

Do not worry if you experience these reactions. They are usually desirable, since most of them are either symptomatic displays of the recovery process, or the elimination of accumulated toxins from the body. These reactions may be generally classed as follows:

1. General fatigue
2. Aches and pains
3. Fevers, chills, and coughing
4. Abnormal sweating and frequent urination
5. Skin discharge and unusual body odors
6. Diarrhea or constipation
7. Decrease in sexual desire and vitality
8. Temporary cessation of menstruation
9. Mental irritability
10. Disturbed sleep

These symptoms vary from person to person, depending on individual constitution and condition, and usually require no special treatment, naturally ceasing as the body makes functional adjustments and begins to work better. In the event that the symptoms are severe, modify your diet to include 10 to 30 percent of your previous foods. This may mean including one to two pieces of fruit each day if you were a big fruit eater, or two to four ounces of milk if you were a heavy milk drinker. This will slow the discharge process. When you are stable and feel better, kick out these recent additions and clean up the diet again.

Summary

Historically there are four principal methods of diagnosis. They are observation, which includes seeing an individual's body, face, and vibration; listening to body sounds and smelling its odors; inquiry, asking questions and noting responses and how the patient responds; and palpation, touching the body, abdomen, and pulses.

Observation: The practitioner observes and notes the overall external appearance of the patient. If the patient has a robust physique and good nutrition, he has a firm confirmation; whereas if the patient has a delicate and slender physique, pale complexion, frail and thin skeleton, and little strength, he has a weak confirmation. Diagnosis is made by observing the physique, complexion, and condition and color of the nails, lips, and eyes.

Listening and Smelling: The practitioner listens for coughs, gasping, and length and frequency of respiration and by noting odors from the mouth and body.

Inquiry: The practitioner questions the patient about complaints like pain sites, chills, fever, perspiration, thirst, dry throat, headache, dizziness, ringing in the ears, bowel and urine routines, vomiting, appetite, swelling, and any other category that will give useful information to determine the causes for their problem.

Palpation: The practitioner feels the body by giving a shiatsu treatment. He also feels the abdomen and pulse. In pulse taking, the practitioner presses his fingers on the radial artery's pulse and from the bounce, speed, length, and tension determines whether the patient's confirmation is superficial or deep, weak or firm, cold or hot. In abdominal touching the practitioner presses the patient's abdomen to test the elasticity and reaction of the skin and internal organs.

These four methods of diagnosis have been used for a very long time to determine the correct treatment that a patient requires. With practice and experience, you can make these methods become useful in your shiatsu practice. In every treatment that you give spend some time trying to decide the confirmation of your patient. In the long run this time will be well spent.

Vibration

All living creatures move, that is the nature of being alive. Each human also has subtle internal and external movements that are their particular vibrational and energy fields. As human beings we should have an even, clear, and consistent vibration. When you look at a magnificent giant redwood tree, you feel calm. You feel calm because this tree has a good, calming vibration. It is the same with people. Vibrations that are rough or irregular are disturbing. People who are prone to violence, drug use, or seizures are examples of disharmonious energy fields. Vibrations are like television waves that are always beaming a message outward. Human vibrations are made up from the combination of energy from the internal organ functions, emotions, education, and dreams of a person. It is not easy but if you practice you can see vibrations. They are similar to an aura. We have all seen pictures or drawings of angels or saints with halos above their head. This is an artists view of what vibrations look like.

When we meet someone it is our Ki or energy fields that meet first. The vibration of one person meets the vibration of the other person. If you have a good conversation with someone, your Ki met well. If conversation is difficult, your Ki is not blending smoothly. When you feel faint, your vibration is low, when a baby cries, their vibration is high.

In a shiatsu treatment session there are several types of vibrations that we exchange. The first is talk. The second is through touch. Depending on the receiver, there will be a need for more of one or the other. You as the practitioner must decide how to spend the session time. This will depend on your instinct, experience, and judgment. Your consciousness along with your technical treatment skills meet the receiver's consciousness. Your attitude and personal condition affect the receiver very much. Try to train yourself to be sensitive to the world of vibration. If the receiver picks up some strange feeling and has no trust in you, you cannot be a good treater. The treatment will be ineffective. This initial introduction to another's vibration is instinctive. We also can study vibration and energy movement and its effects by reviewing traditional diagnostic information. The following rules and descriptions are based on energy and vibration.

Fig. 34 Two People with Energy Fields

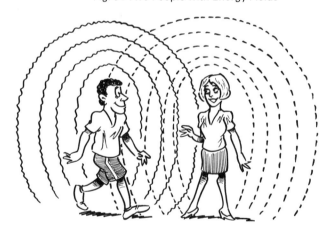

Yin-Yang and the Four Diagnostic Methods

Yin and yang are vibrations. After careful study, I normally reduce all four methods into the singular yin-yang analysis. This makes it easy for me. However, in your study you should acquaint yourself with a fuller range of assessments because these four reflect distinct sets of symptoms that can lead us to understand an individual's problem more clearly. The following are practical guidelines to distinguish yin or yang vibration.

Yang diagnosis: Excess body heat and desire for coolness; great thirst and desire for fluids; constipation and hard stools; scanty, hot, dark urine.

Yin diagnosis: Cold feeling and desire for warmth; lack of thirst and preference for hot drinks; loose stools; profuse, clear urine; flat taste in mouth; poor appetite.

The Eight Diagnostic Principles

These provide a systematic framework for the assessment of the quality, nature, and depth of the patient's disorder.

- Yin and yang
- Cold and hot
- Emptiness and fullness
- Internal and external

These features of the patient's ailments allow you to distinguish the severity and depth of their problem. Because of the many possible combinations of the four categories there may be at times apparently contradictory qualities. For example, emptiness of yang in chronic diarrhea adds up to be a yin condition. When assessing the four categories feel intuitively for overall, general tendencies. In this way you will not lose sight of the major problem. Someone with fever (a yang, hot symptom) may be suffering from internal, empty, deficient causes (yin causes) such as asthma. While apparent contradictions exist, the majority of signs point to one or the other side of the coin—yin or yang. Study, practice, and allow your intuition to guide you. Do full shiatsu treatments and recommend a whole foods diet and you can trust that nature will give the appropriate treatment.

Yin and Yang

These are the two main principles which distinguish the different groups of disorders. They are very broad categories which embrace the other six diagnostic principles. Assessment of yin-yang quality helps to determine the development of the illness and its localization.

Ailments that are localized in the surface tissues and principal meridians are generally yang (such as fever and perspiration), while those involving the organs and insides are yin (creating an underfunctioning state). Yang active organs may frequently have yang (heat) diseases for which ginger compresses or moxibustion would be ill advised, for example a condition of dry heat in the liver in the case of cancer or cirrhosis from excessive alcohol consumption.

The main distinguishing features of yin disorders are as follows: symptoms tend to move inward (sore throat turns into a cough that leads to difficulty breathing, and so forth. The person becomes weaker and sicker as the disease moves deeper into the body); tendency to withdraw, little talking, lying curled up; respiration is feeble; limbs are cold; seeks warmth, no thirst, urine is clear; pulse deep and slow; tongue pale, moist, and indented (teeth marks).

Yang qualities are movement of warmth to the surface, and upper part of the body (often producing fever). This motivates the person to desire coldness and crave for cold drinks. The pulse is full, hard, or bounding. The tongue is dry and coated. These symptoms are generally seen in a yang condition.

Let me explain about yin and yang. There are many instances that may be confusing for those without a great deal of clinical experience. The first thing to remember is that rules about yin and yang are guidelines. There are plenty of circumstances where classification is not clear cut. Depending on the interpretation of the practitioner, the condition can be explained one way or another. I consider the upper body location as yin. This is the standard macrobiotic interpretation. This makes the head region susceptible to influences such as heat and fever, which are yang symptoms. But remember that most of these yang symptoms are caused by yin foods and drinks like sugar, fruits and juices, fats, oils, alcohol, spices, and drugs. This is an example of the contradictory nature of illness. The yin (expansive) foods dilate the blood vessels allowing the excessive heat and irritation they produce to be expelled. This expelling movement creates heat—a yang symptom (a glass of red wine makes your face hot). So the symptoms are yang, but the cause is yin. Unfortunately not all yang symptoms are caused by yin or vice versa. You must look at each case to determine the individual truth of the situation. If you are not completely confused, let me add one more set of tendencies. External yang (like hot weather) causes yin response (skin pores dilate and heat escapes the body and you cool down). Internal yang (infection or foods like beef, bacon, and eggs) causes yang response (you eat hot foods and you become hot).

Cold and Hot

This indicates the state of the disease. If the patient fears the cold and craves warmth, and the body is cold, a disorder is classed as a cold, yin type, deficiency disease. The converse is true of yang disorders.

There are frequently manifestations of both hot and cold in the body, or parts of it, and before deciding treatment it is necessary to determine whether one is faced with combinations of hot and cold, or local heat or coolness in the upper or lower parts of the body. Many people experience hot face and head with cold hands and feet.

Clinical signs of cold disorders may include: no thirst, cold limbs, pale skin, abundant and clear urine, whitish tongue, and slow pulse.

Clinical signs of coldness in the upper part of the body are: breathlessness, indigestion, and vomiting.

Coldness in the lower part of the body manifests as: hard and dry stools, abdominal pain, herniation, and cold limbs.

Some complex combinations can occur, for example, in the *Nei Jing* it states, "Cold, with fullness, moves down and transforms to heat; the heat, with fullness, moves upward and transforms to cold." There are also such conditions as "false yang" that include restlessness, constipation, breathing difficulty (dyspnea), painful throat, and thirst without desire to drink. The point here is to be attentive to variations in confirmations. Do not be confused when opposing diagnostic signs present themselves. Overall the patient will be either yin or yang. Give a full shiatsu treatment and adjust the diet to match the overall condition.

In the presence of signs of general weakness, quiet voice, pale clear urine, tongue flabby and coated at the center, pulse deep, fine, and feeble, the disorder may be due to the presence of cold energy calling for a heat treatment such as moxibustion and hot salt baths.

Emptiness and Fullness

In general, "fullness" and "emptiness" can be distinguished by touching the affected areas. In emptiness (deficiency of energy) firm pressure is comforting and gives relief (by increasing the compressive qualities of yang). In fullness (excess of energy) pressure aggravates the discomfort (by adding to the excess).

In assessing the requirements of the patient it is necessary to discover the cause of the fullness or emptiness. Fullness feels hard (excess, yang condition), but the hardness may come from expansion (yin) as in the case of a swollen liver like a balloon that has been blown up. Normally, during a shiatsu session, if you allow your hands to guide you you will apply appropriate treatment.

The signs of emptiness are: fine pulse, cold skin, weakness, diarrhea, and abundant urine.

In general the constitution of the patient is a good indication of fullness and emptiness. Those of slender and feeble constitution tend to suffer from the disorders of emptiness which require reinforcement.

Fullness of the muscle-tendon group, for example the legs, will manifest as spasms and contractions along with acute sensitivity of surface acu-points. Pulse diagnosis may reveal a relative deficiency of the principal meridian that passes through this area. In this situation you can work vigorously on the muscle group directly (a dispersing technique) while you tonify the corresponding meridian with moxibustion or foods that strengthen that particular organ. For example, if someone gets leg cramps in the calf muscle you can vigorously press the calf muscle directly at first (a dispersing technique) followed by sustained holding pressure on the kidney points (BL 23) on the low back. The calf muscle has the Bladder meridian pass through it therefore tonifying the low back area will strengthen the calf.

Emptiness of a muscle-tendon group may be seen by weakness, numbness, and flaccidity. There will be tenderness on deep palpation, though not a sharp sensitivity to superficial touch.

Internal and External

These qualities designate the locality of the malady and overlap aspects of the other diagnostic principles. The external area is made up of the skin (epidermis) and principal meridians. The internal area is made from organs and other inside materials.

Symptoms from external disorders, due to the invasion of cold, include: headaches, radiating from the neck, fear of cold, pains in the joints, thin and whitish tongue, and superficial and fast pulse. The pulse of external disorders due to emptiness of yang is superficial and slow.

Internal disorders due to cold manifest as symptoms including: cold limbs; lack of perspiration; abdominal pains; nausea and vomiting; coated and moist tongue; deep and rapid pulse.

Emptiness of functional energy internally gives rise to feeble respiration, poor appetite, cold limbs, racing heartbeat (tachycardia), whitish tongue, and deep and very fine pulse.

Symptom Summary of the Eight Rules of Diagnosis

	Major Symptoms	*Tongue and Coating*	*Pulse*	*Treatment*
YIN	Pale complexion; fatigue; shortness of breath; weak voice; loose stools; profuse, clear urine	Pale, tender; white, slippery coating	Sunken; weak; slow	Warming; tonifying
YANG	Flushed, red complexion; restlessness; loud voice; rapid, hard breathing; scant, dark urine; constipation and hard stools	Bright red; thick, yellow coating	Floating; heavy; fast	Cooling; sedating
COLD	Aversion to cold; cold hands and feet; pale, white complexion; no thirst and preference for hot drinks; profuse, clear urine; loose stools	Pale; white, slippery coating	Slow	Warming, dispelling cold
HOT	Aversion to heat; hot hands and feet; great thirst with preference for cold drinks; nervousness; scant, dark urine; hard stools	Red; dry, yellow coating	Rapid; bounding	Cooling; sedating
EMPTY	Weakness and fatigue; shortness of breath; low resistance; poor appetite; weight loss	Thick; tender; little or no coating	Weak; slow	Tonifying
FULL	Overactive body functions; restlessness; loud voice; coarse breathing; abdominal distension; scant, dark urine; constipation	Hard; thick coating	Bounding	Scattering, expelling, and purging
INTERNAL	No independent symptoms; depends on hot-cold and full-empty indicators	Changing	Sunken	Depending on hot-cold and full-empty indicators
EXTERNAL	Fever and/or chills	Normal color; white, thin coating	Floating	Expelling; inducing perspiration

Perverse Energy

The term *perverse energy* is applied to any otherwise normal external or internal phenomenon that creates a disturbance because of disequilibrium in the body's function. There are six normal factors that when they become excessive or abnormal are then called *pathogenic* (disease causing). Ailments most commonly arise from failure to adjust to climatic factors which create disturbances in the external area, and initially in the Small Intestine and Bladder meridians. Normal weather changes can be pathogenic for weak people. When interior resistance (a disharmony of interior yin and yang) is low it is easy for external pathogenic factors to invade. Shiatsu and moxibustion can be used to reinforce the defensive energy.

The external perverse energies, or "external evils or devils" are wind, cold, heat, humidity, dryness, and fire. It is wind, cold, and humidity, or their combined effects, that are most likely to call for warmth and tonification, while heat and dryness like dispersing movements.

The perverse energies that originate from the inside, such as fear, anger, depression, and so forth, may create disturbances when the equilibrium of the meridians, by which they are controlled, is disturbed.

External Evils

Killing germs eliminates the immediate symptoms but does nothing to restore the original energy of the diseased organ and tissues. It is only a matter of time before it is attacked again. Ancient China did not have the technological means to observe and identify minute germs. But even modern practitioners of the ancient art consider the presence of germs to be more a manifestation rather than a cause of disease. Why do germs attack some people and not others? Why do common bacterial infections invade the lungs of one patient, the knees of another, and the bowels of a third? The reason according to Oriental theory, is that germs gather and thrive only in weakened parts of the body of patients with low resistance. The true cause of disease are those conditions that lower a patient's resistance, weaken certain parts of his body, and expose him to attack by germs. Similarly, the true cure of disease is not simply to kill germs. It is to counteract those conditions which permit disease to develop in the first place; to reestablish the body's optimum relative balance or energies and tonify the primordial energies of the weakened organs. Germs simply cannot attack strong healthy organs.

The study of the cause of disease is important because long-term treatment is based on cause. Balance is everything. In the interior of the body the movement of yin and yang, Ki, and blood must be kept in a relative balance. This is extremely important for normal life activities. The body has an autoregulation system. With this ability it can adapt to the environment. Once this balance is destroyed, disease will occur. There is the balance with the interior and a balance with the external environment. The factors that destroy this balance are the pathogenic or disease causing factors.

The body constantly has to adjust its internal function to adapt to the variations in the six factors of the natural environment. If these factors change abnormally or overtax the adaptability of the human body, or the body's anti-pathogenic factor is weak and the vital function is impaired beyond its ability to adapt itself to the changes in weather, the occurrence of disease may be caused by such factors as wind, cold, and so on.

Wind

In spring the body is accustomed to the warm temperatures and the pores dilate easily, making it easier for "evil wind" excess to enter the body. The main characteristics of wind troubles are acute onset with quick development. Symptoms can include tremor, convulsions, vertigo, moving pain, shaking head, and itch. Wind usually affects the head, Lungs, and Spleen. Other symptoms include coughing, stuffy or runny nose, headache, dizziness, and sneezing. Wind often combines with heat, damp, or cold, depending on the weather, and such winds induce symptoms of both excesses. There is also an "inner wind" unrelated to weather, which originates in the heart, liver, or kidneys due to energy imbalances. Symptoms of "inner wind injury" are fainting, weakness, nervous spasms, blurry vision, and stiffness in the muscles and joints.

Cold
Cold is a "yin evil" which usually injures the body's yang energy. If cold enters the exterior surface of the body, it produces symptoms of fever, aversion to cold, headache, and body pains. It is easy for cold to cause Ki and blood to stagnate resulting in severe pain. If it reaches the meridians, it produces muscle cramps and pains in the bones and joints. If it enters as far as the internal organs, cold excess causes diarrhea, vomiting, abdominal pains, and internal noises. "Inner cold," again unrelated to weather, is usually caused by deficiency of yang energy in the Stomach and Spleen, inducing the internal cold symptoms of nausea, diarrhea, coldness in the limbs, and a pallid complexion. Excessive consumption of cold foods ("cold" in the sense of energy, as well as in temperature) can also induce inner cold.

Summer Heat
Major symptoms of summer heat, which occurs in summertime, are excess body heat, profuse sweating, parched mouth and throat, constipation, and heart palpitations. When summer heat combines with dampness, it produces abdominal pains, vomiting, and intestinal spasms. Iced drinks taken in the heat of midsummer sometimes cause "yin summer heat." The two excesses combine in the stomach and induce symptoms of unpleasant chills, dull headache, abdominal pains, and profuse perspiration.

Dampness
Ailments of damp excess can be induced by sudden exposure to fog or mists, immersion in water or exposure to rain, and living in excessively damp locations or climates. The characteristic symptom is that dampness lingers. It is not easily cured. The symptoms—lethargy, aching joints, and oppressive sensations in the chest—are characteristically heavy and sluggish in nature and tend to block the flow of energy throughout the body. "Inner dampness" is caused by excess consumption of liquor, tea, cold melons, and sweet and oily or greasy foods. These impede Spleen functions and cause symptoms of abdominal swelling, edema, eczema, vomiting, and diarrhea. It is easy to remember that external causes come from exposure to water, wearing damp clothing, and so on, while internal causes of dampness come from a deficiency of Spleen energy. Dampness can be associated with wind, cold, and heat.

Dryness
There are two types of dryness—hot and cold. Dryness easily injures the Lungs, causing symptoms of heavy coughing, blood in the sputum, dry nose and throat, and pains in the chest. Dry excess is also harmful to the body's fluid balance. "Inner dryness" is caused by excessive loss of fluids due to too much sweating, vomiting, bleeding, or diarrhea. Characteristic symptoms are dry, wrinkled, or withered skin, dry hair and scalp, dry mouth and cracked lips, dry stomach, and hard, dry stools.

Heat (Fire)

When any of the five excesses as described above become too extreme, they often transform to fire excess. The symptoms are usually more intense forms of those associated with the original excess, plus symptoms of extreme heat excess. "Inner fire" is caused by excess emotional activity or by overindulgence in food, drink, and sex. Violent anger, for example, often causes a sensation of heat rising from the upper abdomen, where liver fire is raging. Too much strong food and drink causes fire to collect in the stomach; deep grief or passion will often cause it to rise in the Lungs.

With heat it is easy to exhaust the yin body fluids, therefore you will find dry skin with thirst and constipation. It also can impair the blood vessels causing hemorrhage. If heat is caused from internal sources there will be no fever, if the cause is external there will be high fever. If other pathogenic factors like cold, damp, or wind are not eliminated immediately they stay in the interior and become fire.

Internal Evils

There are seven principal emotional factors that when excessive are considered "internal evils." They are: joy, anger, anxiety, excessive thinking, grief, fear, and being surprised. Under normal conditions these are called "emotional factors." It is normal for people to experience these emotions from time to time. However if the emotions are intense and persistent or the individual is hypersensitive to the stimulation, they may result in drastic and long-standing change in emotion that leads to disease. Sudden, drastic, or prolonged stimulation can give rise to disorder in Ki, blood, and yin-yang balance. This directly influences the internal organ function. The internal evils can be viewed as "paralyzing" states while the opposite positive emotional aspects can be seen as "enabling" states. In the *Nei Jing* it states, "Anger injures the Liver, Joy injures the Heart, Anxiety injuries the Spleen, Deep Sorrow injures the Lung, and Fear injures the Kidney."

The external excesses that occur during the four seasons do not affect every person in the same way. Nor do the internal excesses. Healthy people are not adversely affected by any of them. An "evil excess" will attack the body only when and where it is weak and only when the protecting Ki is deficient somewhere along the surface of the body. One of the purposes of preventive medicine is to keep the body strong and resistant to such outside attacks.

Areas of Accumulated Evil Influence

Imbalanced energy can accumulate in different parts of the body. When this happens there will be pain and hypersensitivity (yang, excess Ki) or numbness and a dull feeling (yin, deficient Ki) in a corresponding area. At times there may be blemishes, pimples, or discoloration in these areas. Using this diagnostic information and treating the affected part will enhance your shiatsu session.

Organ	Display Area
Lungs and Heart	Forearms
Spleen/Pancreas	Inside the thighs
Kidneys	Back of the knees
Liver	Armpits

Seeing

One of the first features that we notice when we meet someone is their face and expression. On the face we observe color and individual characteristics such as the size and shape of the eyes, mouth, lips, nose, and so forth. If you remember one important rule, "The inside shows itself on the outside," you will appreciate the beauty each face displays.

To identify the various diagnostic confirmations, Oriental medicine employs four methods of diagnosis: observation, listening and smelling, inquiry, and palpation. Observation includes inspection of expression and general appearance, body type, color of complexion, and a look at the tongue proper and its coating.

Preliminary facial observations can be reduced to either yang or yin analysis. Simply stated a yang face is flushed and red, while a yin face is pale and of light complexion. But realistically we cannot leave facial diagnosis at such a basic level. There are a great number of hues that like an artist's palette, color our facial landscape, each with significance.

Constitution and Condition

When we look at the person who has come for a Whole Health Macrobiotic Shiatsu session we are struck with two main concerns: what is their constitution? and what is their condition? Understanding their constitution and condition points out tendencies why they have developed problems and it points to a direction to appropriate treatment.

Constitution is the structured makeup that you inherit at birth. It is your ancestral influence. It includes those family traits that have been passed down from parent to child. Constitution can be divided into two varieties: yin and yang. Yang, gathering energy forms a yang constitution, yin, dispersing energy produces a yin constitution. In giving treatment it is important to estimate how the patient will survive and carry on. For those with serious health problems, if their constitution is strong they have a good chance of survival.

Yang Constitution
The following are attributes contributing to the physical structure of someone with a yang constitution: broad shoulders; the person tends to be shorter with a square, wide body; an angular face with nose, eyes and mouth being small and close together; the

Fig. 35 Energy Movement Develops Constitution

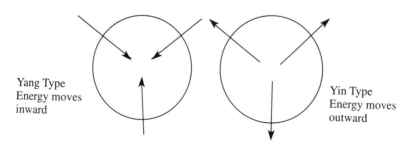

Yang Type
Energy moves
inward

Yin Type
Energy moves
outward

speech and voice are strong and loud, the person speaks clearly; the eyes move more and the iris is centered in the eye.

Yin Constitution

A person with a yin constitution has narrow shoulders, small bones, soft exterior, an oval face with eyes, nose, and mouth larger and further apart on the face. The voice is weaker than normal.

Condition is a reflection of our current state of health. Yin and yang factors affect the condition in an immediate way. Whereas the constitution is your biological foundation, a gift from your parents, condition is a result of how you have lived your life day-to-day. If you eat excessively yin foods and live in a chaotic way, you will acquire a yin condition. The opposite is true, if you consume excess yang foods and are overactive you will develop a yang condition.

Facial Colors and How They Affect Condition

The five colors correspond to the the five paired organs. Each is a reflection of the function of an organ. Disorders in the five paired organ systems create your condition. All facial colors, when disorders are present, have a stronger than normal coloration. To spot when color is out of sorts you must study what is normal, healthy color. First look at the color and determine if it is yin or yang, then decide what is the source of the problem. Color also is related to pain, heat, and cold symptoms. If there are disorders in the Liver and Kidney systems there will be a tendency for pain to be present. When the Spleen and Heart are affected, the patient will feel hot and there may be fever. When the Lungs are affected the patient will display cold symptoms.

Fig. 36 Facial Color and Symptoms

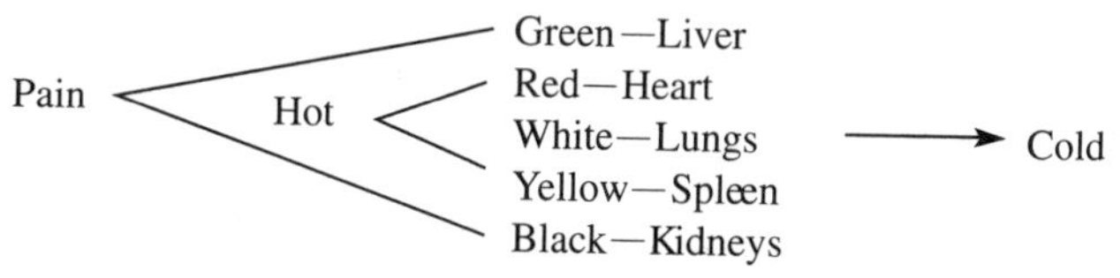

Pain < Hot < Green—Liver / Red—Heart / White—Lungs → Cold / Yellow—Spleen / Black—Kidneys

1. White: The pale, transparent, washed-out, whiter than normal color reflects the condition of the Lung and Large Intestine systems. Usually the posture displays rounded, drooped shoulders with a hollow chest. Often constipation (a yang symptom) or diarrhea (a yin symptom) is present. The soft tissue of the body has contraction or expansion power. Trouble occurs when the system is weak. With contraction the intestines are stuffed. While not necessarily smaller, they do not function well. When they are expanded, they are soft and weak and their function is slower than normal. Overall, the Lung energy is yin.

2. Yellow: The sallow, yellowish green tinge to the skin reflects the condition of the Spleen/Pancreas and Stomach systems. When the stomach is overly contracted (a yang condition) from excessive amounts of eggs and meat, the body is thin. Stomach expansion can be caused by fruits, pastries, sugars, and excessive liquid consumption. The stomach can not contract and may even drop from its normal position. In the case of the Spleen/Pancreas system, diabetes (excessive sugar in the blood) is yin caused and hypoglycemia (lower than normal sugar level) is yang caused. The overall energy of the Spleen is yin.

3. Red: The flushed, bright complexion reflects the condition of the Heart and Small Intestine systems. Always check additional diagnostic methods to confirm heart trouble because the heart is so important you must be accurate when recommending diet. For example there can be redness caused by contraction (a yang condition) that comes from meat, chicken, eggs, salt, and so on or redness created by expansion (a yin condition) caused from sugars, fruit, and juices. The flushed condition does not have only one source. Overall the energy of the Heart is yang.

4. Black: The dark, dirty facial color comes from an inadequate function of the Kidney and Bladder systems. The body's filters, the kidneys, are not doing their job. They cannot throw off the toxins that have accumulated. The kidneys can become hard (a yang condition) usually from excessive protein and fat deposits, or they can become swollen and soft (a yin condition from improper mineral balance and fluids, especially fruit juices). The bladder also can become either expanded or contracted. The overall energy of the Kidneys is yin.

5. Green: The grayish green, or yellow, jaundiced color reflects the condition of the Liver and Gallbladder systems. Bile produced by the liver is greenish in color and taints the skin. Additionally, if there is a blockage in the common bile duct the eyes and skin will take on a yellow pigment. Excessive eating, as well as excessive amounts of meat, eggs, sugar, and chemicals adversely affect the liver, the body's main defense system. The overall energy of the Liver is yang.

Expression

An individual's expression can be seen in the complexion, eyes, speech, movement, and breathing patterns. Expression has a lot to do in deciding at what rate someone will heal themselves. If the patient has a good spirit, natural facial expression, bright eyes, distinct speech, clear mind, and quick responses, we view these signs favorably. If on the other hand they have low spirit, indifferent facial expression, dull, cloudy eyesight, slow response, feeble voice, shortness of breath, and profuse sweating, these indicate serious disease and does not bring optimism. Expression is an indicator of the patient's life-force.

Relationship between Internal Organ and Facial Diagnosis

One of the most popular facial diagnostic methods used in macrobiotics is face reading. The internal organs and their functions are reflected on specific parts of the face. From observing abnormal or distinguishing characteristics on the face, details relating to the workings of the internal organs can be discovered. Figures 37 through 41 show the five paired organs and their display on the face. A more detailed analysis of this method can be found in my book, *Barefoot Shiatsu* (Tokyo and New York: Japan Publications, Inc., 1979).

Fig.37 Lungs and Large Intestine

Fig. 38 Spleen / Pancreas and Stomach

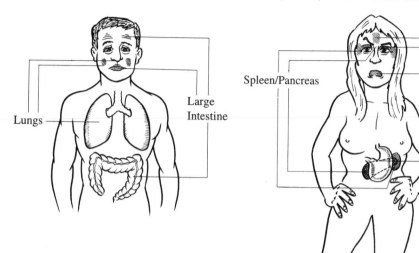

Lungs

Large
Intestine

Spleen/Pancreas

Stomach

Fig.39 Heart and Small Intestine

Fig.40 Kidneys and Bladder

Small Intestine

Heart

Kidneys

Bladder

Fig.41 Liver and Gallbladder

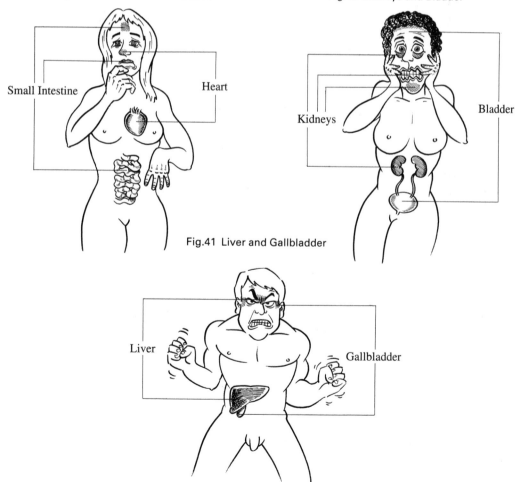

Liver

Gallbladder

The Tongue

Fig. 42 Tongue

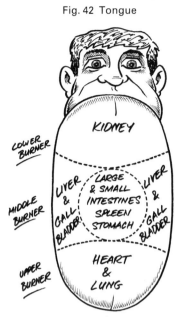

Observation of the tongue including the tongue proper and its coating is an important procedure in diagnosis. There is a close connection between the tongue and the internal organs, meridians, Ki, blood, and body fluid. Any disorder of these may result in a corresponding manifestation on the tongue. Indications of the nature of the disease can be learned by observing the color, form, and condition of dryness or moisture of both the tongue proper and its coating, and the movement of the tongue.

A normal tongue is of proper size, light red in color, free in motion and with a thin layer of white coating over the surface which is neither dry nor over moist.

Tongue Abnormalities

Pale Tongue: A less than normally red tongue indicates syndromes of deficiency or cold type caused by weakness of yang Ki and insufficiency of Ki and blood or due to invasion by outside disease causing cold.

Red Tongue: An abnormally bright red tongue indicates various heat syndromes of the excess type due to invasion by pathogenic heat and various heat syndromes of the deficiency resulting from consumption of yin fluid.

Deep Red Tongue: A deep red color of the tongue occurs in the severe stage of a fever disease in which pathogenic heat has been transmitted from the exterior to the interior of the body. It can also be seen in those patients suffering from prolonged illness in which yin fluid has been exhausted and internal fire, which is of the deficiency type, is hyperactive.

Purplish Tongue: A tongue purplish in color, or with purple spots indicates stagnation of Ki and blood. It also indicates preponderance of internal cold due to deficiency of yang.

Flabby Tongue: A tongue larger than normal, flabby, and whitish in color, sometimes with teeth prints on the border, indicates deficiency of both Ki and yang and retention of phlegm-damp in the interior. Flabby tongue, deep red in color, indicates preponderance of pathogenic heat in the interior and hyperactivity of fire due to deficiency of yin.

Cracked Tongue: Irregular streaks or cracks on the tongue indicate consumption of body fluid by excessive heat, loss of the essence of the Kidneys and hyperactivity of fire due to deficiency of yin. Congenital cracked tongue and cracked tongue without any morbid signs are considered normal.

Thorny Tongue: The papillary buds over the surface of the tongue swelling up like thorn, and usually red in color, indicates hyperactivity of pathogenic heat.

Rigid and Tremulous Tongue: A tongue that is rigid and difficult to protrude, retract, or roll leads to stuttering and indicates invasion of outside heat and disturbance of the mind by phlegm-heat. It also indicates damage of the yin of the Liver by strong heat which stirs up the wind, or obstruction by wind-phlegm. The tremulous tongue seen in protracted illness often indicates deficiency of both Ki and yin.

Tongue Coating

White Coating: The tongue's whitish coating may be thin or thick, sticky or dry. A thin white coating is normal, but when it is seen in a disease state, it usually indicates invasion of the Lungs by wind-cold. Thick white coating usually indicates digestive trouble and retention of food. White sticky coating usually indicates invasion by the outside cold-damp or retention of phlegm-damp in the interior. Dry white coating usually indicates invasion by external sources.

Yellow Coating: A yellow coating on the tongue may be thin or thick, sticky or dry. A thin yellow coating usually indicates invasion of the Lungs by wind-heat, while a thick yellow coating usually indicates persistent accumulation of food in the stomach and intestines. Yellow sticky coating usually denotes accumulation of damp-heat in the interior or blockage of the Lungs by phlegm-heat. Dry yellow coating usually indicates accumulation of heat in the Stomach and Intestines which results in damage to the yin.

Grayish Black Coating: A grayish black coating in the tongue may be moist or dry. Grayish black moist coating usually denotes retention of cold-damp in the interior or too much internal cold due to deficiency of yang. Grayish black dry coating usually indicates consumption of body fluid by excessive heat or hyperactivity of fire due to deficiency of yin.

Peeled Coating: The tongue with its coating peeling off is known as "geographic tongue." If the entire coating peels off leaving the surface mirror smooth, the condition is known as "glossy tongue." Both manifestations indicate the crisis in a long-term ill

Summary of Diagnosis Based on Examination of the Tongue and Tongue Coating

Tongue	Tongue Coating	Diagnosis
Pale white and weak	White, thin	Ki and blood empty
Pale white; swollen with teeth prints	White, thin	Yang empty
Pale white, swollen, tender	Grayish black, slip, moist	Yang weak; internal organs cold
Pale red; tender and jagged	No coating	Ki empty; yin weak
Pale red	White, thin, slippery	External wind-cold
Pale red	White, thick, oily	Indigestion; internal heat
Pale red, moving	White with yellow traces	External evil Ki inward
Pale red already	Yellow, thick; white edges	Interior heat
Bright red	White, very thin	Yin empty; heat excess
Red, deep and jagged wrinkles	No fur	Yin weak; fluid deficient
Red	Yellow, thin	Heat excess rising
Red	Yellow, oily	Moist, heat excess
Red	Yellow, thick and dry	Heat excess, deep inside
Red	Black, dry	Heat excess, injuring yin
Crimson	Dark yellow	Heat excess, injuring Ki
Dark purple	Dark yellow, thin, dry	Heat excess, penetrating to blood
Light purple and blood	White, slippery	Internal cold; Ki blocked

ness in which the anti-pathogenic factor is severely damaged and the yin is grossly deficient.

The abnormal changes of the tongue proper and coating suggest the nature and changes of disease from different aspects. Generally speaking, observation of the changes in the tongue proper is mainly to differentiate whether the condition of the internal organs, Ki, blood, and body fluid is in a deficient or excess state, while observation of the tongue coating is for judging the condition of disease causing factors. Analyzing the changes in both the tongue proper and its coating is therefore necessary when diagnosis is made by observation of the tongue. Observation should be done in daylight.

Asking, Listening, and Smelling

Asking and Listening

When someone comes for Whole Health Shiatsu normally they have symptoms and troubles that bother them. Their main concern is to rid themselves of these problems. Asking questions and listening to their complaints have been noted as two of the four diagnostic methods used traditionally. Besides the actual complaint we listen to the patterns of speech. A strong, high tone of voice shows sufficient vital energy. A feeble, low voice indicates just the opposite—weakness. As they explain their situation to us we also listen to breathing. Weak breathing or shortness of breath after light exertion suggests a deficiency of energy in the Lung and often the Heart systems. If the breathing is coarse, with wheezing and mucus, the Lungs may have excessive or stagnant energy. If there is a cough, we listen to its sounds discovering if it is dull, heavy, crisp, or clear.

As a practitioner you should listen to the chief complaint of the patient, and then ask about onset and duration of the illness and the past history. Based on the patient's complaint and with the view of regarding the body as an integrated whole, several general questions regarding body temperature, sweating, urine and stool abnormalities, diet and cravings, thirst, sleep, and pain locations, are asked in order to get to the bottom of their problem. For women ask questions concerning menstruation and any abnormal bleeding or discharges.

After listening to the patient's story and assessing the speech, breathing, and cough sounds, it is important to make sure they have expressed themselves as completely as possible. We would like to resolve any frustrations that may contribute to their condition. Encouraging the patient to freely tell their story helps in this process.

Each of the five primary organs has a sound or tone that demonstrates an abnormal state if it is persistent. They are:

Organ	Tone
Lungs	Crying
Spleen	Singing
Heart	Talking
Kidneys	Groaning
Liver	Shouting

Smelling

Another of the four diagnostic methods is based on the sense of smell. A healthy body does not have much odor. Foul or sour smelling odors coming from the mouth may show Stomach heat or stagnation from overeating. The stools and urine also should not have offensive odors. If the smell is heavy and foul there is heat in the interior and digestion is not processing smoothly.

Each of the five primary organs has an odor or smell that demonstrates an abnormal state if it is persistent. They are:

Organ	Tone
Lungs	Fishy
Spleen	Sweet/Fragrant
Heart	Burned
Kidneys	Putrid
Liver	Oily/Greasy

Summary

Inquiry or asking, listening, and smelling provide useful information in making judgments for treatment direction. They can be reduced to the following diagnoses.

Yang diagnosis: Talkative and loudmouthed; rapid, coarse breathing; heavy, foul-smelling secretions, body fluids, and discharges.

Yin diagnosis: Soft, low voice; few words; shortness of breath; shallow breathing; light, raw-smelling secretions, body fluids, and discharges.

Making Contact

The Body Surface—Skin, Hair, and Nails

The sense of touch is familiar to all of us. It is the skin that allows such sensitivity. The skin is the barrier that keeps the outside world out and the inside world in. All living cells in the body are in a watery environment and the substances that enter and leave the cells are either dissolved or suspended in water. The skin and the mucous membrane lining the passages that open to the surface of the body provide a barrier between the dry external environment of the body and the watery environment of the body cells.

The surface layer of skin consists of dead cells that are constantly being rubbed off and replaced from below. This lower level provides the living cells that make up the surface. Sweat glands and pores are located in this material.

Hair grows from follicles found in the skin. Hair is not living material. It is formed by cell growth at the base and as they are pushed upward, away from their source of nutrition, the

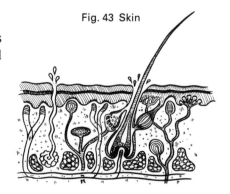
Fig. 43 Skin

cells die and are converted to keratin. The color of the hair depends on the amount of melanin present. White hair is the result of the replacement of melanin by tiny air bubbles. The skin also provides oil glands that keep it soft, pliable, and to a large extent waterproof. Sebum (the secretion from the oil glands) and tears contain chemical substances that kill microbes. These contribute to the body's defensive energy.

Nails are derived from the same cells as skin and hair and consist of a hard, horny type of dead cell. Fingernails grow more quickly than toenails and growth is quicker when the environmental temperature is high.

In addition to the sense of touch, the skin is one of the main protective organs of the body. It protects the deeper and more delicate organs and acts as the main barrier against the invasion of microbes and other harmful agents. Pain receptors found in the skin protect the body from further injury by making pain serve as a stimulus to avoid the source of pain. The skin manufactures vitamin D_3 from exposure to sunlight and uses this substance in the maintenance of bone. The skin also regulates body temperature. This temperature balance is maintained by regulation of the pores. The nervous system activates the skin to match heat produced in the body and heat lost to the environment.

What to Look for in Touch
The characteristics of texture, suppleness, blemishes, moisture, and temperature serve as indicators to give feedback to the patient's condition. A healthy skin is smooth, clean, and compact. It is not rough, nor is it loose. If it is too loose there has been an overconsumption of sugar and fat in the diet. There can be precancerous cysts that are not visible to the eyes but can be felt when you treat the skin. You can feel lots of fatty dots under the skin.

There normally should not be much body hair except on the head, pubic, and underarm regions. This becomes a diagnostic indicator in the case of women, especially when hair is found in more than normal amounts on the upper lip and chin, and to a lesser degree on the arms and legs. How much hair is normal? This depends on ethnic background. Orientals tend to have less hair while southern Europeans tend to have more. Therefore it is more significant if a Chinese or Japanese woman has more hair on her legs than a Greek or Sicilian woman. The cause is excess animal protein consumption. Animal protein and its accompanying fat content clogs the pores so the skin cannot sweat. The fatty layer below the skin does not separate from the skin, the pores do not adjust and open, and toxins are trapped inside the body.

Skin to Skin Test: You should be able to pinch and pick up with your thumb and index finger a small amount of skin without much fat between the skin layers. When you release the skin it should return back to a normal position.

Muscle Quality: The muscle should be firm and lean. When you press the muscle it should not have a spongy texture to it. If you were to take a look at a cross section of the arm it should not look like marbled meat. It should be fat-free. If it looks like salami or sausage, the fat content interferes with the circulation of energy. This creates stagnation.

Touch the muscle lightly with your fingertips, then press more deeply with your thumb into the large muscles of the arm. Determine the quality of the muscle.

Bone Quality: The density of the bone should be hard and solid yet it should feel resilient. This is the quality of bones produced with mother's milk. It matches the muscle, not too big nor too small. In my opinion, cow's milk produces bones that are too big and excessively hard without resiliency. They have a greater tendency to break. The bone does not match with the muscle.

Touch the bones of the arm with thumb on top and fingers beneath. Press thumb and other fingers together feeling for bone quality.

Skin Surface: Because of its discharging ability, the skin can be considered a third kidney or lung. It is a major excretory organ and helps the body rid itself of unwanted waste. When the body is filled to excess with material it will discharge this excess to the surface of the body. There are many forms of discharge. The following are many of the most common and their causes:

Skin Conditions	*Cause*
Pimples	Sugar and fat
Freckles	Sugar
Warts	Sugar and protein
Mole	Sugar and fat
Tiny, pin-sized red dots	Excess protein
Beauty marks	Chemicals, sugar, and chocolate
Age spots	Toxins, sugar, and fats
Keratosis (excess skin thickening)	Protein and toxins
Nail Conditions	*Cause*
Showing white with stretched fingers	Anemia
Brown dots	Protein
White dots	Sugar
Breaking easily	Lack of minerals, sugar
Having moons	Sugar
Slow growth	Slow metabolism
Fast growth	Eating too much
Having ridges	Excess sodium, animal food
Thick cuticle	Excess eating
Cracking skin around base and red	Excess eating

Checking the Internal Organs

This is a subjective test that takes many years to develop, but there is only one way to develop this skill, it is to do it. During a treatment session include time to assess and treat the abdominal area. This area, which can be sensitive to some, houses the internal organs. Check charts to learn the correct locations of the five paired organ sets. When you palpate the abdomen, imagine what a good condition of each organ would be like. If an organ is in good condition you do not feel much. The area does not feel strange to you. If it feels like it is full of material or hard, you know that it is not in good shape. Your fingers are supposed to be able to

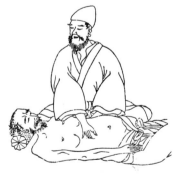

Fig.44 Chinese Doctor and Abdomen

go into it without much tenderness or resistance. If the patient complains, fidgets, or you find hardness, things are not right. When we press a part of the body we look to discover if it is hot or cold, soft or hard, and are there pain on pressure, swellings, nodes, cysts, or tumors. Here are some clues concerning each organ.

Lungs: When tapping them in clavicle area (LU 1) there should be a clear, firm, healthy sound. There is trouble if the area is spongy and fatty and if the sound is dull or strange.

Large Intestine: It should feel flexible and empty. There is trouble if there is pain and your fingers cannot go in. It also can feel watery and swollen. It is easy to get irritated and produce lots of mucus, like in the case of colitis, allergies, or environmental reactions.

Stomach: It should feel firm and happy. There is trouble if it feels hard, heavy, or hollow, without energy.

Spleen: This organ is located under the left ribs therefore you should not be able to feel anything. There is trouble if it has enlarged and comes out under the ribs and is soft and watery.

Pancreas: It should not feel much and a bit firm is O.K. There is trouble if it feels tight, hard, or spongy.

Heart: When you tap and press over the heart at the center of the chest it feels alive and balanced. There is trouble if when you tap there is pain, swelling, or a strange feeling. Also if the muscles around the chest area are too tight heart circulation is probably impaired.

Small Intestine: It should feel flexible and empty. There is trouble if there is pain and your fingers cannot go all the way to the bottom. There can be accumulated hardened fat and impacted feces. In time when this is discharged it appears in the stool like rabbit pellets. Pockets inside the villi are full of material.

Bladder: It should feel pleasant resistance. There is trouble if it is too hard (yang) or if your fingers can go in too far without resistance (yin).

Kidneys: Probed them from the back side, you should not feel much. There is trouble if when you push the patient screams. There may be kidney stones. You also may feel like rocks are there.

Gallbladder: It should not feel much. There is trouble if when you press the patient screams. It also may be hard with fat around the organ.

Liver: You should feel a lively, peaceful organ that has resiliency. There is trouble if you cannot get your fingers under the ribs, it is expanded and tight, or it is expanded with a soft layer of fat insulating it. You may have seen examples such as chicken liver in the market with fat attached to it.

Touching Specific Acu-points

There are variety of surface locations that reflect internal function. Point and meridian diagnosis has been used for thousands of years. Some of the most useful follow:

Trouble	Acu-point
Lungs, breathing	LU 1, BL 13
Liver, digestive, vision	BL 18, LV 14
Stomach, indigestion	BL 21, ST 36
Nausea	HG 6
Appendicitis	2 inches below ST 36

Trouble	Acu-point
Gallbladder, gallstones	1 inch below GB 34
Headache, intestines	LI 4
Low back pain	BL 57
Intestinal heat	LI 11
Menstrual trouble	SP 6, SP 9
Neck pain, vision, colds	GB 20
Kidneys, urinary organs	KI 1
Sinus	LI 20
Ear, hearing	Indention at base of ear

Touch Diagnosis and Pain

The nature of pain can be determined by its response to touch. When pain is aggravated by pressure we know this is a condition of excess (yang). There is blockage of the meridians and a stagnation of Ki and possibly blood. This can be caused by invasion of external factors such as flu microbes as well as wind, cold, damp, and so on. It also can be the result of intestinal parasites, food retention, or excessive mucus production and stagnation.

When pain is alleviated by pressure we know that it is a deficiency condition (yin). This area of the body lacks sufficient Ki and possibly nutrient substance also. Adjust the diet and apply tonifying treatments.

Oriental Pulse Diagnosis

The most subtle and difficult of diagnostic techniques is taking the pulse. If mastered it can be an important part of diagnosis. It is said that the pulse tells of the state of Ki and blood as well as the struggle between disease causing and health promoting factors. This diagnostic method was described in detail in the *Nei Jing*. It is the diagnostic technique that relates each of the strengths and weaknesses to give us a picture of the overall condition. Normal pulse signs are an even, smooth pulse, forceful with regular rhythm of sixty to eighty beats per minute. The pulse is judged by the throb, frequency, rhythm, width, location, smoothness, and whether it is tense or not. However, in practice this is easier said than done. For our purposes the pulse can give basic information that will confirm other more obvious signs to help complete the diagnostic picture.

Before taking the pulse it is important for both the patient and the practitioner to be rested and very quiet. While possible to take the pulse in a seated position, it is best with the patient lying on the back. This will allow the patient to feel rested and comfortable, and it will let proper breathing be established. You may want to take the pulses after abdominal palpation (*Hara* diagnosis). You should examine each side for between twenty-five and fifty pulse beats. Classically, the examiner observed the ratio of beats to number of breaths. Generally considered healthy people have one complete inhalation and exhalation to every four pulse beats. If the ratio is less than one breath to four beats this is a much better sign. This rhythm of breath and pulse is the first important diagnostic observation.

There are three essential elements of the pulse: position, depth, and quality.

Position: Position consists of placing three fingers above the wrist where the radial

Fig. 45 Fingers on Pulse Positions

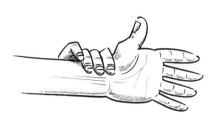

artery throbs. The middle finger is placed on the styloid process (the bump) of the radius. Finger pressure is exerted first lightly, then moderately, and finally heavily to get a general idea of the depth, frequency, rhythm, strength, and form of the pulse. Abnormal changes in any region of the pulse should be determined by exerting an even force on the three regions, then by feeling the three regions separately and making comparisons in order to have a correct impression of the pulse as a whole.

Depth: The first level of depth is lightly touching and registering the qualities of the pulse at the superficial level. The second level is pressure applied deeply, pressing against the radius.

Quality: A normal pulse is of medium frequency, and regular rhythm. It is even and forceful.

Abnormal Pulses

Superficial (Floating) Pulse: The pulse responds to pressure when pressed lightly and becomes weak on heavy pressure. This often occurs in the early stage of a disease from the outside, that is an exterior syndrome. It may also be seen in those suffering from prolonged illness and who are in a state of general weakness.

Deep (Submerged) Pulse: Superficial palpation reveals no clear pulse, which is felt only upon heavy pressure. This often occurs in interior syndromes.

Slow Pulse: The rate is very slow. This often occurs in cold syndromes. This is different from an athletic pulse which also is slow. It also signifies deficient yang. Symptoms include pronounced sensitivity to cold, poor circulation, loose bowels, white coating on the tongue, and general weakness.

Rapid Pulse: The pulse is very quick. This often indicates a situation of heat caused by heat excess or deficient yin.

Deficient (Weak) Pulse: The pulse is weak and forceless and disappears on heavy pressure. Deficiency is in Ki and/or blood or in the organ corresponding to the specific pulse location.

Excess (Strong) Pulse: The pulse is forceful and is felt even on deep pressure. It signifies the presence of an excess in a sick person, but a good condition among the healthy.

Wiry Pulse: The pulse feels taut and forceful, as though pressing on the string of a drawn bow. It often occurs where this is insufficiency of yin energy and hyperactivity of yang in the Liver. A wiry pulse appears in Liver diseases and accompanies pain.

Rolling Pulse: The pulse feels smooth (like pearls rolling on silk), flowing and forceful, and often occurs when there is excessive phlegm or retention of food. Rolling pulse may be seen in healthy people with ample Ki and blood, and during pregnancy in women. Symptoms include mucus, sluggish digestion, difficulty in moving the joints, and heavy coating on the tongue.

Thready Pulse: The pulse is fine and thin. It often occurs in the cases of deficiency of both Ki and blood. Symptoms include thirst, irritability, low grade fever, and a tongue with a red tip.

Fig. 46

Pulse Internal Organ Locations			

	Forearm		Wrist	
Superficial	Cubit	Bar	Inch	
Deep	Bladder Kidneys	Gallbladder Liver	Small Intestine Heart	Left
Superficial	Cubit	Bar	Inch	
Deep	Triple Heater Heart Governor	Stomach Spleen	Large Intestine Lungs	Right

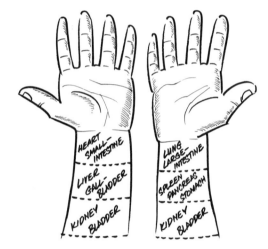

Fig. 47 Organs and Pulse Locations

HEART SMALL INTESTINE
LIVER GALL BLADDER
KIDNEY BLADDER

LUNG LARGE INTESTINE
SPLEEN PANCREAS STOMACH
KIDNEY BLADDER

The quality of a pulse may vary according to such factors as body-build, activity, and general constitution of the individual, and weather.

Summary

Yang diagnosis: Fast, floating, heavy, slippery pulse; warm hands and feet; abdominal pain with aversion to applied pressure.

Yin diagnosis: Slow, sunken, weak pulse; cold hands and feet; abdominal pain with desire for applied pressure to relieve cramps.

Learning from the Body—Structure and Function

We are made from nature. Humans are not man-made. While not perfectly nor symmetrically constructed, the human body is both simple and complex. Simplicity and diversity fuse in the production of cells, tissues, organs, and systems working in combination to create an entity much more valuable than any machine. There is no comparison between the human body and machines as no machine can repair itself. Within the animal world, humans make up in ingenuity and intelligence what they lack in muscle or teeth strength. The complexity of the human nervous system and its thinking capacity has set man apart from all animals. Even those who may be critical of such statements are using the very capacity of intellect that makes mankind the highest animal. Let us investigate the physical body, viewing it from both the Western explanations and traditional Oriental medical and biological understandings. Keep in mind that information should help you develop a clearer picture of what is going on inside the body and how you can use this information to formulate more effective treatments. Your explanations to patients should help them understand their condition and inform them what they can do about it.

Formation of the Body

Before we investigate the specifics of structure and function of the major parts of the body, let me briefly explain how the body is formed. As you have learned, the physical body is the result of the interaction of yin and yang. These energies mix. As yin and yang energies move within the developing embryo the internal organs, as well as the skeletal, circulatory, and nervous systems grow. Simultaneously, the appendages, in the forms of arms and legs also develop. As all internal energy is governed by the result of these two opposing energies, spirals are formed. These spirals unwind and straighten out, yet their original folds remain. We see the unwound spiral as the bending places or articulations of the arms and legs. If an outstretched arm is marked at half point, and the remaining segment is marked at half point (approximately), and the remaining part marked off at half point, and again and again, we will see a marked arm, now straight, that was formerly rolled up in a spiral. The first bend down from the shoulder is the elbow, then at the wrist and three places on the fingers.

Fig. 48 Bisected Spiral Marked and Unwound   Fig. 49 Segmented Arm and Unfolded Spiral

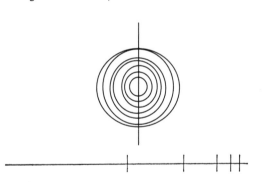

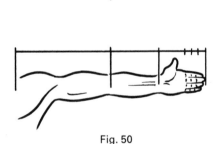

Fig. 50

Body Structure
The body is as tall as is the length of the outstretched arms. This ratio is considered balanced.

Height and arm length are equal.

The Body Systems
For convenience and also to acquaint you with the traditional view of looking at the body in three distinct segments, I have classified the structure and function of the body parts according to the Oriental Triple Heater system. This system divides the main body segments into three distinct areas. It is within these areas that all major structures as well as functions are performed and located.

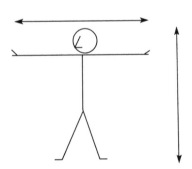

Upper Section—The upper section consists of respiratory, circulatory, and nervous systems.

Middle Section—The middle section consists of digestive, immune, and nervous systems.

Lower Section—The lower section consists of reproductive, excretory, urinary, and nervous systems.

Triple Heater Controls the Three Principal Body Sections

The Triple Heater function is one of the most important in the Oriental medical system. When disorders occur in the body, including major life-threatening problems, they can often be corrected by an adjustment of this system. These adjustments take place with treatment but also through diet, exercise, and breathing techniques.

Unfortunately many people have limited their understanding of this system as having to do with circulation. Because it has no tangible organ, such as the Lung system with its lungs and large intestine, many westerners have not grasped its significance. In an attempt to understand its physical nature some people have correlated the Triple Heater to the omentum. This is the fatty, apron-like membrane hanging down from the small and large intestines. It is rich in blood vessels. The omentum along with the lymphatics are believed to be responsible for the Triple Heater function.

Classically the Triple Heater has dealt with the production and movement of fluids and with energy. It is the function that coordinates the entire body. This is a major function indeed. At the core of this function is the ability to separate the useful material from the waste. The useful material and energy is processed on to the vital systems while the waste is processed out of the body. This essential metabolic process is controlled by the Triple Heater.

Main Components of the Three Body Sections

Upper Section:
- The respiratory system consists of the lungs, larynx, and the windpipe.
- The blood system is made up of the lymph vessels, heart, and blood vessels.
- The nervous system consists of the brain, spinal cord, and several nervous systems.

Middle Section:
- The digestive system is the alimentary canal and organs, teeth, tongue, and salivary glands.
- The skeletal system consists of the bones.
- The articulatory system consists of joints and ligaments.
- The muscular system are the muscles.
- The integumentary system includes the skin, hair, and nails.

Lower Section:
- The urogenital system consists of the urinary and reproductive organs.

Upper Section

Respiratory System: This is the system through which oxygen is taken into the body from the external environment and carbon dioxide, a waste product of cell metabolism, is excreted. The respiratory passages are the nose, pharynx, larynx (voice box), trachea, two bronchi (one for each lung), and a large number of bronchial tubes that subdivide and lead to millions of tiny air sacs called *alveoli*. The hundreds of millions of alveoli make the total surface area of the lungs very large, so that a maximum amount of oxygen can be passed to the blood. The oxygen travels in the blood to each cell in the body where it is used for respiration. Air also may enter the pharynx through the mouth.

The two lungs are located one on each side of the heart in the chest cavity. They consist of bronchial tubes, alveoli, blood and lymph vessels, and nerves, all which are supported by connective tissue. Each alveolus is surrounded by a dense network of blood capillaries.

Air containing oxygen and carbon dioxide is breathed into the lungs, filling the tiny alveoli air sacks. It is then separated from the blood in the capillaries by two semipermeable membranes. Because the wall of each alveolus is only one cell thick, oxygen can easily seep through and pass into the tiny capillaries covering its surface. The oxygen combines with hemoglobin in the red blood cells and is carried around the body. While oxygen is leaving the alveolus, carbon dioxide—produced during respiration in the body's cells—is entering, ready to be breathed out. Oxygen is in higher concentration in the alveoli so it passes from the alveoli to the blood. Carbon dioxide is in higher concentration in blood so it passes in the opposite direction, from the blood to the alveoli. The cells throughout the body get their oxygen and rid themselves of carbon dioxide by the reverse process. Oxygen is in higher concentration in the blood than in the cells and the interstitial fluid around the cells, so it diffuses down the concentration gradient from the capillaries to the cells. Carbon dioxide is in higher concentration in the cells and interstitial fluid and diffuses down the concentration gradient from the cells to the blood. Breathing maintains a steady movement of these gases in the lungs and alveoli.

The lungs have no muscles of their own. It is the muscles in the chest that control breathing. The diaphragm is a sheet of muscle tissue that forms the floor of your chest. There are other muscles between your ribs that can contract to move the ribs.

Breathing occurs when the diaphragm contracts and moves down. The rib muscles contract and the ribs move up and out. This increases the space inside your chest. The lungs themselves are in their own airtight space called the *pleural cavity*. When the space inside the chest increases, the air pressure in the lungs is less than the air pressure outside the body. Air rushes into the lungs to make the pressure equal. You breathe out when the diaphragm relaxes and moves up. The muscles between the ribs relax so air pressure in the lungs is greater than outside the body. Air rushes out to make the pressure equal.

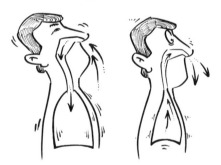

Fig. 51 Breathing

Adults' lungs hold about five pints of air. In quiet breathing the diaphragm moves up and down less than 1/2 inch and about one pint of air is breathed in and out, roughly fifteen times every minute. During vigorous exercise, the breathing rate increases and breathing is much deeper, because the diaphragm can move as much as two inches.

The area of the lungs is 753 square feet, about forty times greater than the area covered by your skin. This is because of the enormous number of tiny alveoli and means that you can take in the amount of air that you need.

Outside air may be too cold or hot, too dirty or too dry for the lungs. To protect the lungs, air is warmed and filtered. Dry air is moistened inside the nose and cold air is heated by the blood vessels in the nasal cavity. The nose contains hairs that trap large particles of dust and dirt. Smaller particles are trapped by sticky mucus in the nose, throat, and air passages. Tiny hair-like cilia move the mucus which contains these particles away from your lungs and back up to your nose or mouth to be sneezed or blown out, or swallowed. When irritation is present, for example with a cold or allergies, more mucus is produced. Coughing forces a gust of air up from the lungs and carries with it harmful particles that irritate the lining of the bronchi, trachea, or throat.

Problems related to respiration are: bronchitis, asthma, emphysema, pneumonia, infections, collapse of the lungs, tuberculosis, and cancer.

Circulatory System: The blood system is the main transportation system in the body. The red and white blood cells and blood platelets are pumped by the heart. The heart pushes blood to the lungs where oxygen is absorbed from the air in the lungs and at the same time carbon dioxide is excreted from the blood into the air and to the cells in all parts of the body.

Fig. 52 General Circulation

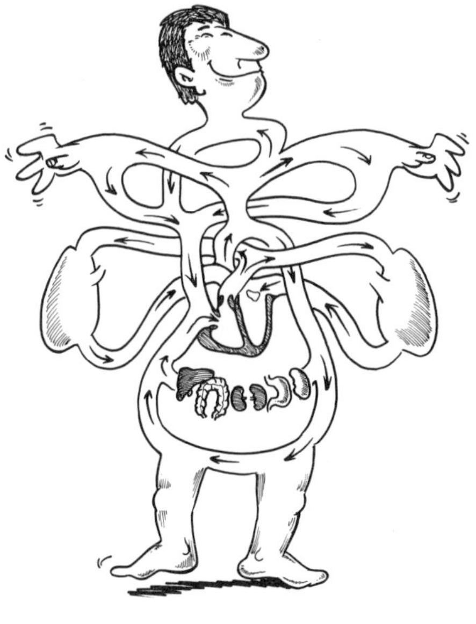

Circulation consists of deoxygenated (without oxygen) blood moving from the right ventricle of the heart to the lungs and back to the left atrium. In the lungs, carbon dioxide is excreted and oxygen is absorbed. From the left atrium oxygenated blood flows to the left ventricle. From here blood is carried by the branches of the aorta around the body and is returned to the heart by the superior and inferior vena cava.

Problems related to heart and vessels in-

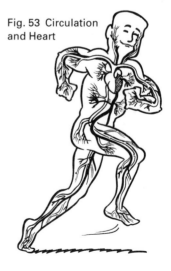

Fig. 53 Circulation and Heart

clude: arteriosclerosis, plaque deposits in vessels, inflammation of the heart and vessels, aneurysms (balloon-like swelling in vessels), clots, varicose veins, hemorrhoids, angioma (benign tumors of vessels), hypertension, kidney disease, hypotension, congestive heart failure, angina pectoris, heart attack (myocardial infarction), and arrhythmia.

Nervous System: This system receives communications from outside as well as inside the body through the five sense organs and nervous impulses and chemical substances circulating in the bloodstream. The nerve endings related to the five senses of vision (eyes), hearing (ears), smell (nose), taste (tongue), and touch (skin)

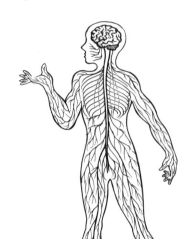

Fig. 54 General Nervous System

Fig. 55 Brain with Five Senses

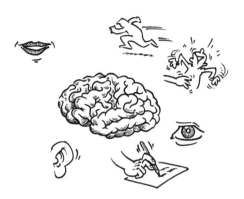

are stimulated by sensations outside the body and transmit this information to the brain for interpretation. The brain processes this material with information obtained from previous information stored in the memory to make sense out of the perceptions. In a similar way, information from inside the body is processed. This regulates and coordinates the activities of organs and systems. The major parts are the brain and spinal cord, central and autonomic nervous (with sympathetic and parasympathetic branches) and peripheral systems.

Problems related with the nervous system: headaches, nerve damage, meningitis, multiple sclerosis, herpes, mental disorders, Alzheimer's disease, epilepsy, pain, Bell's palsy (facial paralysis), Parkinson's disease, growth and hormonal imbalances, and nerve and brain tumors.

Specifics about Pain

Pain is nature's warning sign to alter activities. If your finger becomes hot while touching a hot pan you drop the pan protecting the finger from severe damage. The skin is sensitive to these types of stimuli. Normally the internal organs are insensitive to generally considered pain stimuli like cutting, and so on. However, a sensation of dull, poorly located pain is experienced when organ nerves are stretched or circulation has been disrupted by increased waste products or when the threshold of pain has been lowered because of disease. Inflammatory pain is usually easy to locate. This is because the peripheral nerves supplying the superficial tissues also supply the area in trouble. Appendicitis is an example of this type of pain. Initially it is dull and vaguely located around the midline of the abdomen. As the condition progresses the area near the appendix becomes involved and acute pain is clearly located in the lower right abdominal area.

However, in some cases of internal disease pain may be perceived to occur in superficial tissues remote from the source. We call this *referred pain*. The following list pinpoints the source and referred pain sites.

Origin of Pain	Site of Referred Pain
Heart	Shoulder
Liver and Gallbladder	Right shoulder
Kidneys and Ureter	Loin and groin
Uterus	Low back
Male genitalia	Low abdomen
Prolapsed intervertebral disc	Leg

Specifics about Headaches

According to the National Headache Foundation, over forty-five million Americans suffer from chronic, recurring headaches. Of these, sixteen to eighteen million people annually are plagued by migraine headaches. And headaches are big business. More than 400 million dollars is spent annually on over-the-counter pain relievers for headaches, not to mention eight million doctor's office visits that are made each year by headache sufferers.

This situation is a big headache for business! Companies that employ chronic headache victims can attest to that. The National Headache Foundation estimates that American industry has lost fifty billion dollars due to absenteeism and medical expenses caused by headaches. Migraine sufferers lose more than sixty-four million workdays each year.

There are three different types of headaches. Organically caused, or secondary headaches, occur because of an underlying disease or condition. Pain in the head can be caused by infections and flu. Headaches also can be traced from toothache or improper jaw alignment (TMJ). The pain also can be associated with vision problems, signaling a needed eye examination. When sinuses become infected, a gnawing pain also may develop in the nasal area and cause a headache. However, some experts say sinus disease is present only in a small number of people, and the victim is actually a migraine sufferer.

Fig. 56 Brain

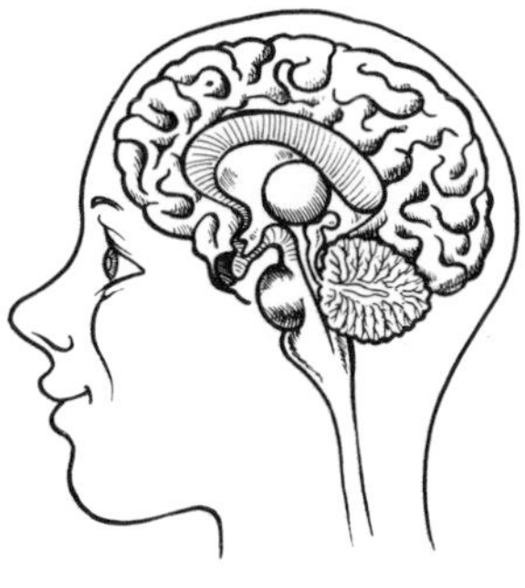

In very few cases, less than one-tenth of 1 percent, the headache is caused by serious illness such as a brain tumor. Even though most headaches are not from immediately life-threatening illnesses, they occur for a reason. Frequent headaches are your body's way of telling you there is a problem somewhere.

Muscle contraction headaches are often referred to as tension headaches. These types of headaches are usually dull, non-throbbing pain, frequently bilateral and associated with tightness of the scalp or neck.

Tension headaches signal emotional stress, fatigue or hidden depression. The tightening of muscles is a body's protective defense against stress. When life seems threatening, people tense muscles. The regular medical recommendation is rest, aspirin, ice packs, and muscle relaxants. However, drug therapy is unnecessary if the problem of headaches is approached from a whole health point of view.

Many hospitals, clinics, and specialists offer classes that teach how to deal with tension, including relaxation techniques that can be lifesavers for the chronically stressed-out individual.

Vascular headaches are a very real problem for many people. They have been around for a long time, with famous sufferers including Julius Caesar, Saint Paul, Thomas Jefferson, Chopin, Charles Darwin, and Sigmund Freud.

Vascular headaches include migraine and cluster headaches. The National Headache Foundation says that 70 percent of migraine sufferers are women. These sufferers often share many common characteristics. There are highly energetic, ambitious people who strive for perfection. The length of an attack can last from several minutes to several days, sometimes totally incapacitating the sufferer.

There are different types of migraines. Common migraines account for about 75 percent of vascular headaches. The victim has severe, one-sided throbbing pain, often accompanied by such symptoms as nausea, vomiting, cold hands, tremors, dizziness, and sensitivity to sound and light.

Recent research has proven that migraines have physical causes. Stress, like tension headaches, can trigger migraines as well as diet. Certain foods such as ripened cheeses, peanut butter, and pizza can be associated with migraines. Also foods that contain caffeine or preservatives such as monosodium glutamate (MSG) are popular culprits. Changes in environment, such as a difference in altitude or weather, excessive light, noise or pollution also can cause migraine pain.

Classic migraines are the same as common, except the victim develops warning symptoms such as visual disturbances, numbness in arms or legs, and in some cases, hallucinations. Symptoms usually subside in a half-hour and then the head pain will occur.

Ninety percent of cluster headaches sufferers are male. Victims have excruciating pain around or behind an eye. The pain frequently develops during sleep. Alcoholic beverages and excessive smoking can be the cause; however, the cluster headache should not be associated with a hangover headache. These headaches are clustered into a few weeks, during which the headaches may occur every day or several times a day. Standard treatment includes oxygen inhalation or medication. Whole Health Shiatsu has extremely beneficial effects on all headache types.

Middle Section

The principal area of congestion and trouble for most people is the central area of the torso. It is in this portion of the trunk where the most active organs are located.

Digestive System: This system takes solid material and breaks it down and extracts the locked-in energy and makes it useful. Food is one of the sources of the raw materials that cells must obtain from the external environment, but it is not always in a form that cells can use. A specialized system has developed to modify or digest food to make it usable.

The alimentary tract is the long tube through which food passes. In an adult it is up to 29 1/2 feet (9 meters) long. Its parts are the mouth, throat (pharynx), esophagus, stomach, duodenum, small intestine, large intestine, and rectum. Two forms of digestion take place. The mechanical breakdown of food is accomplished by the teeth and the eating process. The chemical breakdown is accomplished by enzymes secreted by various glands. They are: saliva from the salivary glands, gastric juice from the stomach, intestinal juice from the small intestine, pancreatic juice from the pancreas, and bile from the liver.

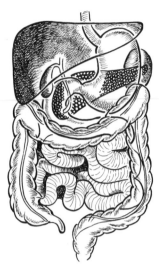

Fig. 57 General Digestive System

Digestion starts with the first bite. In the mouth, food is chopped up by the teeth and mixed with saliva, a digestive juice from the salivary glands that begins breaking carbohydrates down into glucose. The tongue rolls the food into a ball, which is pushed into the food pipe, the esophagus, and moved down to the stomach by a process called *peristalsis*. When you swallow food, a lid, the epiglottis, usually comes right down over your windpipe so that food does not go down there instead of down the esophagus.

Food stays in the stomach for about three hours. The rate at which the stomach empties, depends to a large extent on the type of food eaten and how well it was chewed. A carbohydrate meal leaves the stomach in two to three hours, a protein meal remains longer and a fatty meal remains in the stomach longest. Here it is mixed with more digestive juices containing enzymes and acid, which are produced in the walls of the stomach. Enzymes are special proteins that work throughout your body to speed up the chemical changes that are constantly taking place. Digestive juices contain several different enzymes that help to break down food. The acid in your stomach allows the enzymes to work and helps to kill any bacteria in the food.

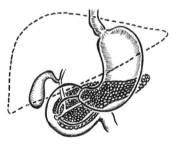

Fig. 58 Liver and Pancreas Close-up

By this stage the food is like a creamy soup. It leaves the stomach a little at a time and goes into the small intestine. This is the longest part of the digestive system, up to thirteen feet (four meters) long, and is neatly coiled in the abdomen. In the first part of the small intestine, the duodenum, alkaline digestive juices (pH 8) from the pancreas, gallbladder, and small intestine walls are added. The acid contents from the stomach move here where the contents become alkaline. Food gradually moves along, being digested as it goes. After food is ingested and digested, it must be absorbed.

Absorption takes place in the small intestine. The surface area through which absorption takes place in the small intestine is greatly increased by the circular folds of mucous membrane and by the very large number of villi present. It has been calculated that the surface area of the small intestine is about five times of the whole body. Carbohydrates, proteins, vitamins, mineral salts, and water are absorbed from the small intestine into the capillaries and into the bloodstream. Fats pass through the villi into the

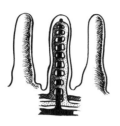
Fig. 59 Small Intestine Villi

lymph system. In the large intestine remaining water and useful vitamins and mineral are absorbed before the waste is passed out of the body. Feces consist of a semi-solid brown mass. Even though absorption of water takes place in the large intestine it still makes up about 60 to 70 percent of the weight of the feces. The remainder has undigestible material like roughage, dead and live microbes, old cells, some fatty acids, and mucus secreted by the lining of the large intestine. Feces are stored temporarily in the rectum before evacuation.

Metabolism

Carbohydrate: Absorbed into the blood capillaries of the villi of the small intestine, carbohydrate is transported by the portal circulation to the liver, where it is processed.

Carbohydrates in our food supply us with energy. The main types of carbohydrates are sugars and a substance called *starch*. Whole grains and their products such as bread and pasta contain starch. Table sugar is a sugar called *sucrose*, and fruit and jam contain a sugar called *glucose*. Only glucose can be used by the body for energy, so all other forms of carbohydrates have to be broken down and turned into glucose inside the body by the digestive process. It is important to remember that the rate of breakdown controls the rate at which sugar reaches the blood. Refined sugar enters the bloodstream fast. This elevates the blood sugar level producing dangerous symptoms. Complex sugars such as whole grains and vegetables are best for maintaining sustained energy. Oxygen is needed to obtain all the energy carbohydrates contain and the waste products are carbon dioxide and water. Some of the excess is converted to glycogen in the presence of insulin and stored in the liver and in the muscle. The amount of energy that can be produced from different foods is measured in calories. The number of calories a person needs each day depends on how active he is. For example, swimming uses up about 600 calories an hour, but sleeping uses only 70 calories an hour. On average, man needs about 3,000 calories each day, a woman needs around 2,200 calories, and a child of four years old needs about 1,600. If you eat more carbohydrates than your body needs, the extra amount is stored as fat. The body can convert this fat store into energy if it has to, but eating refined carbohydrates over a long period can make you put on weight. This can put a strain on your heart and is a common cause of heart disease. Any remaining glucose is converted into fat and stored in the fat depots like the hips, breasts, thighs, and abdomen.

Protein: Digestion breaks down the protein of the diet to its constituent amino acids in preparation for transfer into the blood capillaries of the villi in the wall of the small intestine. In the portal circulation amino acids are transported to the liver then into the general circulation, making them available to all the cells and tissues of the body.

Amino acids are used in the liver to form various substances. These are used by cells of the body for cell replacement, cell repair, and the production of hormones, enzymes, and antibodies. Amino acids not used by the body are further broken down by the liver with the nitrogen part converted into urea and excreted in the urine. Urea is a powerful diuretic. When urea and amino acids enter the kidneys on the way to elimination in urine, they cause not only the loss of excess water but also the excretion of large amounts of minerals. One of the most important minerals lost in this way is calcium.

The more proteins that are consumed, the greater is the loss of calcium. Researchers estimate that doubling the amount of proteins in the diet will increase by 50 percent the amount of calcium lost in the urine. For adults protein requirements are rather low. The World Health Organization suggests a protein level of twenty-nine grams for women and thirty-seven grams for men per day. The minimum daily requirement established by the Food and Nutrition Board of the United States is forty-seven grams for women and fifty-six grams for men. Both recommendations include safety margins to satisfy the protein needs and actually are requirements set higher than the need for most healthy adults. Most Americans consume 105 to 120 grams each day with some consuming even higher amounts. The remainder is used to provide energy and heat or deposited as fat in your body's favorite fat depots.

Fat: Absorbed into the lacteals of the small intestine then fat is transported into the lymph system. From here it gets into the bloodstream and eventually to the liver.

Fatty acids are utilized in the presence of oxygen to provide energy and heat, the waste products carbon dioxide and water being produced. Fat stored under the skin provides a store of energy and a layer of insulation. For many people who have too much insulation, extra fat is stored in the fat depots. When stored fat is required for oxidation it must first be desaturated by the liver. Fat is harder to digest than carbohydrates but produces twice as much energy as the same amount of carbohydrates. The average person consumes about 25 to 40 percent of their daily calories from the fats they eat. This is thought to be far more than what is required by the body. United States government dietary recommendations warn of the excessive use of fats as leading to heart disease as well as some types of cancer, notably cancer of the breast and colon. Lowering the dietary intake of fats decrease the likelihood of developing these diseases. Within the macrobiotic dietary approach 10 percent fat is considered adequate.

Mineral Salts: Small amounts of chemicals called *minerals* are vital for the smooth running of your body. Calcium and phosphorus, found in many vegetable, non-dairy sources, help to build healthy bones and teeth. Your red blood cells need iron. Sodium and potassium are needed by your nerves. We get sodium from good quality sea salt, sea vegetables, and organic produce. Small amounts of fluoride help to prevent tooth decay and iodine, found in sea vegetables and fish, is essential for growth.

Vitamins: You need small amounts of fifteen different vitamins to keep the chemical processes in your body going. Your body cannot make any vitamins except vitamin D, so you must eat foods that contain them to stay healthy.

Water: About 70 percent of your body is made of water. Although you might be able to live for two to three weeks without food, without water, you could die in two or three days. An adult loses about half a gallon everyday in sweat, urine, and through breathing. About half of this is replaced by drinking, and the rest comes from foods.

Cooking Food: Cooking makes food easier to chew and digest and makes many foods look and taste better. High temperatures kill many bacteria in food and so make it safe to eat. However, if green vegetable are overcooked, more than 50 percent of the vitamin C they contain can be destroyed.

Fiber: Roughage is the part of your food that cannot be broken down and passes out of your body. It comes from fruit, vegetables, and whole grains. Because it is bulky, it helps the colon muscles to work properly and so prevents you from becoming constipated.

Cholesterol: Cholesterol is a type of fat found only in animal foods, for example, in eggs and shellfish. Too much of it can increase the risk of a heart attack.

Problems related to the disorders in the digestive system are: gastritis, ulcers, pancreatitis, hepatitis, cirrhosis, liver failure, gallstones, jaundice, flatulence, constipation, diarrhea, hemorrhoids, nausea, obesity, anorexia, hypoglycemia, diabetes, dizziness, allergy, malabsorption, Crohn's disease, colitis, diverticular disease, hernia, and cancer.

Specifics about Ulcers

As many as 10 percent of all Americans can expect to suffer from an ulcer at some time. Men are still twice as likely as women to develop the disorder, but the gap is narrowing rapidly, and experts point to one reason: smoking, which is now believed to be the biggest factor in putting people at risk. In addition, smokers take longer to heal and run three times the risk of a recurrence.

Many medical researchers believe that heredity plays a significant role in the development of ulcers. The child of an ulcer patient is three times more likely to develop an ulcer than the average person. However experts do not know exactly what the genetic link is. To say that heredity has some influence may be partially true but is certainly not the whole picture. One major activity that is participated in by all members of a family is eating. Parents and children eat the same types of food and live under the same roof thus being exposed to the same types of environmental factors such as physical and emotional stresses. Poor eating habits are learned by the children. Problems created by such poor eating habits affect both parents and children alike.

Stress, while not the cause of an ulcer, will contribute to it. Allowing yourself to get too worked up can increase stomach acid production that in turn will eat away at the lining of the stomach. However it is safe to say, it is the person, not the environment, that creates the stress.

For most people, an ulcer makes its presence known with a heartburn type sensation, a burning or gnawing feeling in the mid- to upper abdomen that is often relieved by eating. Others experience nausea and vomiting. Still others—as many as one-third— have no symptoms at all. As up to 50 percent of ulcers are self-healing, many of these people do not even know they have ulcers.

More than 6,000 Americans die each year of ulcer complications. Left untreated, an ulcer can eat away at a critical blood vessel, causing bleeding that can result in anemia or, in extreme cases, death. Or the hole can penetrate through the stomach or intestinal wall, resulting in peritonitis, which also can be fatal. The public self-medicates with over-the-counter antacids such as Maalox or Mylanta. Doctors prescribe Tagamet (cimetidine) that was introduced a decade ago. In 1987, Tagamet became the biggest-selling prescription drug in history, not a particularly positive reflection on the state of American health. Studies show that up to 90 percent of ulcer patients have another ulcer attack in less than a year.

Specifics about Fat Distribution and Strokes

One of the reasons men have a higher risk than women for strokes and other cardiovascular diseases is because males accumulate more fat around the waist.

Fat tends to be concentrated in the hip, buttock, and thigh areas for women. If most fat is in the belly region, you are at much higher risk of hypertension, stroke, and diabetes than if it is in the hips and thighs.

Fat deposited around the abdominal area inhibits breakdown of insulin in the liver, which eventually could lead to adult-onset diabetes. Inhibition of insulin breakdown also increases the blood pressure.

Skeletal System: The bones of the skeleton provide the framework for the body. Movement is achieved when the muscles, lying between the skin and the bones, contract and move them at the joints. The skeleton system is living, supplied by blood and nerves. It can become weaker and thinner with disuse, or heavier and stronger with weight resistance exercises. The system also changes with transient illness and with malnutrition.

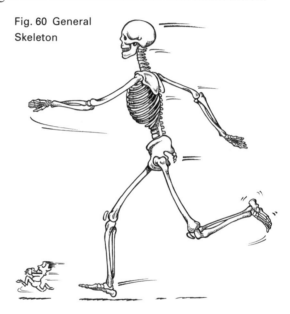

Fig. 60 General Skeleton

The skeleton is the framework of our bodies and the bones of it have specific functions that they do. The long bones of the arms and legs act as levers for the muscles so that both strong and delicate movements are possible. The flat bones that form the vault of the skull protect the brain. The cage of ribs protects the heart, lungs, and liver. The basin formed by the flat bones of the pelvis not only protects the abdominal viscera to some extent, but bears their weight. The bones of the wrist and arch of the foot are many and small, bound tightly together by fibrous structure called *ligaments* so that the force from impacts on the hands and feet can be dissipated through this flexible little network, without a fracture occurring.

Where muscles and tendons are attached to bone so that they can create movement, outgrowths of bone called *tubercles, tuberosities,* and *processes* can develop.

Although we have approximately the same number of bones (206), a few fuse together with age, and we can be born with extra or absent ones. But the main components of the skeleton are the same. We all have skulls, rib cages, and pelvises. However, these can vary greatly from person to person. A rib cage can be long and narrow, short and wide, rounded or flattened, and all the variations of these features. The skeleton contributes to the "build" of a person, regardless of the muscles and fat.

The vertebral column is made up of thirty-three vertebrae. The first twenty-four of these are separate bones that are capable of movement because there is a cushion or articular disc between each one. The next five vertebrae are fused in the adult into a composite bone and are then called the *sacrum*. The last four fuse in middle life and are called the *coccyx*. The first vertebra has a joint between it and the skull. This is called the *atlas*. The twenty-fourth vertebra has a disc between it and the sacrum.

The rib cage is formed by twelve pairs of ribs each of which has joints with one or two vertebrae. The upper ten pairs are joined in front to the sternum (breastbone) by pliable cartilage (gristle). This arrangement allows the sternum to swing up and the chest to expand during respiration. The lower two pairs of ribs are not joined to the sternum and are called *floating ribs* (though they are held firmly by muscles).

The pectoral girdle is made up of the clavicle that joins at the medial end with the sternum to make the sternoclavicular joint, and the scapula that is joined to the lateral end of the clavicle to make the acromioclavicular joint. The main function of the clavicle is to thrust the scapula back. The scapula has great freedom of movement to move up and down and rotate around the rib cage but is controlled by the clavicle and ligaments.

The pelvis is formed by the two hipbones that articulate with the vertebral column at the sacroiliac joint. They meet in the median plane in front to make a joint called the *pubic symphysis* (pubic bones).

There are twelve pairs of ribs all which articulate at the back with the vertebral column. At the front the ribs have a cartilaginous portion that is joined to the sternum except for the lower two pairs. The cartilage being flexible allows movement of the sternum and ribs during respiration. The upper seven ribs are joined directly to the sternum by cartilage. The cartilage of the eighth, ninth, and tenth ribs join with the cartilage above them. Those of the eleventh and twelfth ribs end in muscle.

All the ribs are joined together by the internal and external intercostal muscles that fill the spaces between the ribs. The muscle bundles of these two layers run diagonally to each other. They are muscles of respiration.

At birth the ribs are horizontal and the rib cage nearly circular in babies and young children. It is slightly more circular in the female than in the male. By the seventh year it is beginning to have anteroposterior flattening with more definite front, sides, and back and eventually becomes kidney-shaped in the adult.

The second most common joint injury occurs in the shoulder. The shoulder is made up of scapula (shoulder blades), clavicle, and humerus. The scapula are triangular flat bones slightly arched from top to bottom to fit against the rib cage. They are situated on the back of the thorax in its upper part, and with the two clavicles form the pectoral girdles.

Fig. 61 Types of Joints

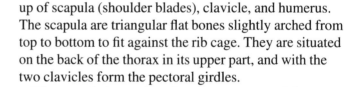
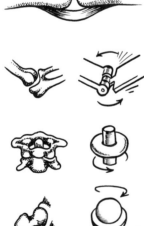

The scapula is capable of movements up and down on the rib cage, backward and forward, and rotation forward and up or backward and down, all depending on which muscles are contracting. It is this wide range of action that creates much of the changing form on the upper part of the back. The scapula vary in size and shape (short, long, wide, narrow) from person to person.

The two clavicles (collarbones) are classed as long bones because they have shafts and two ends. With the two scapula they form the two pectoral girdles.

A clavicle is S-shaped with the center part of the shaft curving forward and the side part curving backward. In males the bone usually lies horizontally or with the lateral end raised. In the female the lateral end is usually lower. This lateral end moves up and down and backward and forward. It joins with the scapula and is usually initiated by arm movement.

The clavicle holds the scapula back and out and provides surface for the attachment of neck, arm, and chest muscles. It has a thin sheet of muscle over it, lying between it and the skin that allows the skin to move more freely during the shoulder movements. It can be felt from end to end.

The Vertebral Column and the Vertebrae

The vertebral column is the central axis of the back of the trunk and in the adult it is made up of twenty-four separate vertebrae, five fused vertebrae called the *sacrum,* and three to five coccygeal bone's tail rudiments. The column is considered to have five regions: seven cervical vertebrae, twelve thoracic vertebrae, five lumbar vertebrae, the sacrum, and coccyx. Except for the first two cervical vertebrae all the separate ones have cushions between them of a fibrous-gelatinous substance called the *nucleus pulposus.* This is surrounded by a fibrous capsule that binds two vertebrae together. These are called *articular discs* and act as shock absorbers as well as allowing movement to take place at each vertebral level. The fibers of the capsule are arranged in layers of diagonal fibers of opposite direction to aid mobility of the joint. Each vertebrae is weight supporting so they increase in size down to the fifth lumbar. At this point weight is transferred to the sacrum and then out through the hipbones to the legs if one is standing or to the two places of the pelvis on which one sits. The discs are relatively more generous in the cervical (neck) and lumbar (waist) areas so the column has a little greater freedom of movement in these areas.

Fig. 62 Spine

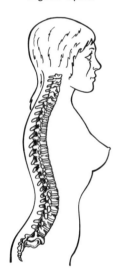

The vertebrae of each region vary, and each vertebra is different to some degree, but there is a common pattern. The weight bearing part is called the body and consists of a small cylindrical block of bone, one inch (twenty-five millimeters) or less high and a little greater in width. It is covered on its upper and lower surfaces by cartilage where it is involved in the joint. From the back of this solid cylinder an arch of bone projects that creates a hole through which the spinal cord runs and in which it is protected. When the vertebrae are placed on top of each other the holes form a continuous canal from the skull so the spinal cord is protected from the moment it leaves the brain and skull. A transverse process projects from either side of this arch of bone and a spinous process from the back. These serve as levers for muscle attachment so the column can be bent. There are four articular processes on each vertebrae for joints with the vertebrae above and below. These are mainly to restrict movement and to prevent forward displacement of one vertebra on the next. They are so placed as to allow for rotation and in the thoracic region the movement between vertebrae is mainly that.

The Curves of the Vertebral Column

The vertebral column has four curves that give a basic flow or rhythm to the body. The cervical curve is composed of the seven cervical vertebrae and their discs. It begins to develop late in uterine life and becomes more convex forward when the child starts to hold up its head and later when it is sitting upright. The thoracic curve is concave forward and is composed of the twelve thoracic vertebrae and their discs. It is already present at birth. The lumbar curve is convex forward and appears when the child begins to walk at about eighteen months. It becomes more prominent in the female than the male. This fact added to the forward tilt of the female pelvis create a more backward thrust of the buttocks. The pelvic curve, concave forward, is composed of the five sacral vertebrae and the coccyx and is already present before birth, though not fused as in the adult.

The pelvic girdle is composed of the two hipbones. These, with the addition of the sacrum and coccyx of the vertebral column, form the whole pelvis. The two hipbones articulate behind with the sacrum making the two sacroiliac joints. At the front they articulate the pubic symphysis. Both these joints allow limited movement. Each hipbone has three parts: ilium, ischium, and pubis. These three parts are fused by the sixteenth year and each contributes an element to the acetabulum that is the socket for the head of the femur. This is a deep socket in comparison with the socket for the head of the humerus.

Bone Landmarks on the Posterior Aspect of the Trunk
The central axis of the vertebral column can always be seen. The form of the spine of the seventh cervical vertebra is usually apparent. The deep indentation in the lumbar areas is where the lumbar vertebrae are curving forward and are more buried by the longitudinal back muscles.

The form of the scapula can be seen. Look for the vertebral border, the inferior angle and the change of plane at the spine of the scapula. The acromion (shoulder tip) creates the most lateral point on the shoulder.

The big form of the whole thorax, which is caused by the rib cage, is the main structure.

The thrust of the ilia (the upper parts of the hipbones) with their iliac crests is seen in the hip area. The two "dimples" are the posterior superior spines of the crests where tendons from the back and hip muscles are attaching to the bone, and the bone is close to the surface. The triangular area between them with its apex at the cleavage between the buttocks is the sacrum, covered by fibrous tendons and ligaments attaching to it.

Muscles
The two components of a skeletal muscle are the fleshy part (meat) composed of the muscle cells and a fibrous part that is called a *tendon* or *aponeurosis*. Tendons are usually round and cord-like or flat and band-like. They are built for strength, consisting mainly of strong tensile protein fibers called *collagen*, which are arranged longitudinally in the muscle axis and are plaited. There also are present a low percentage of elastic fibers that allow for about 4 percent contraction. It is now believed the tendons can store energy for the next muscle movement. When the tendon needs a wide area of attachment it assumes a sheet-like form and is then called an aponeurosis. The collagen fibers extend into the bone at their origins and insertions and it is this which results in the tubercles, tuberosities, and processes, as extra bone growth is stimulated in this area. It therefore makes an exceedingly strong union.

Muscles throughout the body have different arrangements for their muscle bundles and tendons according to the largeness of the movement and the weight involved. The bundles of cells are arranged in long parallels if the action is to be sustained through a great distance, and in short diagonal bundles with far more numerous cells, if great power is needed through a short distance.

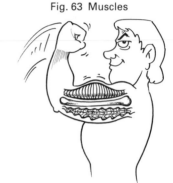

Fig. 63 Muscles

Muscles act on our skeleton to move it. This is possible for two reasons: first, because a muscle is attached at both ends (from one bone to another, from bone to muscle, or from bone to skin) and secondly, because muscle cells are specialized to perform one function, and that is to contract. It is the contraction of bundles of cells comprising the fleshy part of the muscles that brings its two ends together, and so the two points to which it is attached.

Nature created muscle cells long and slender, some being up to 1 1/2 inch (40 millimeters) in length, so that they can shorten. When they do so, they become plumper. They contain within their protoplasm tiny fiber-like structures called *myofilaments* (*myo*, Greek for muscle). It is thought that these myofilaments have charged sites along their lengths that make a potential attraction between them. When a nervous impulse is received, one myofilament slides along and lays against another to which it is attached. This process of "doubling up" occurs throughout the cell and it can shorten by approximately half. This is an extremely simplified explanation of the intricate mechanism of contraction. Thus a whole muscle that is composed of masses of these cells can contract by approximately half.

Each muscle cell is enclosed in a loose connective tissue that is a combination of fibers and cells imbedded in a jelly-like substance. These muscle cells line up end to end and side by side into bundles that are also surrounded by connective tissue that is then called a *muscle sheath*. The cells are always free to contract and relax within this loose covering.

One end of a muscle attachment is always more fixed than the other end and is called the *origin*. When a muscle contracts, the other end, called the *insertion*, is pulled toward the more stationary point.

All the cells in one muscle do not have to contract at one time. If the work demanded of it is for a small movement, a small number of cells will perform. But there is an "all or nothing" law for the cells. The cell itself must contract fully. When this happens with a group of cells in the muscle bundles the plumpness, because of them shortening, shows on the surface as a bulge under the skin. This also explains why a slow change of form can take place on the surface as more and more cells are brought into the contractive state.

Well-developed muscles indicate a yang physique. Undefined or weak muscles demonstrate a yin condition.

Hormone System

The endocrine system consists of glands widely separated from each other with no direct anatomical links. The glands are commonly referred to as the ductless glands because the hormones they secrete pass directly from the cells into the bloodstream.

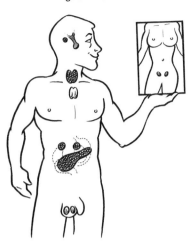

Fig. 64 Hormone Glands

Hormones are chemical substances that influence activity, growth, and nutrition of the organs and functions of the body. The internal environment is regulated partly by the autonomic nervous system and partly by hormones. The endocrine system consists of the following glands: pituitary, thyroid, parathyroid, adrenal, islets of Langerhans in the pancreas, pineal, and ovaries or testes.

The correct regulation of the endocrine system is essential for balance within the body. Imbalance can be corrected by adjusting the relative balance of yin and yang through shiatsu, diet, breathing, and exercise. Imbalance stimulates many diseases such as: gigantism, acromegaly (distortion of the bones of the face, skull, hands, and feet), dwarfism, diabetes, hypothyroidism (Hashimoto's disease), goiter, hyperthyroidism (Grave's disease), exophthalmos (protrusion of the eyeballs), adrenal exhaustion (Addison's disease), hyperfunction of adrenal glands (Cushing's syndrome, obesity, and high blood pressure), coma, cardiovascular disturbances, infection, and kidney failure.

Immune System

The body is endowed with a wonderful preservation system that protects itself from external and internal disease causing influences. Throughout all the tissues and organs of the body there are certain cells which ingest foreign particles and bacteria. They are particularly concentrated in the lymph glands, spleen, liver, and bone marrow. These cells have great powers of multiplication and are related both to lymphocytes and to the blood-forming organs. They are concerned in protecting the body from infection.

Bone Marrow: Tissue rich in fats, containing plenty of nourishment for the comprehensive production of the different blood cells; red blood cells for the transport of oxygen, blood platelets for clotting, and the various white blood cells for the immune system.

Spleen: Forms red blood cells during fetal life and may do so in adult life if the function of the bone marrow is impaired. It separates worn-out red blood cells from the circulation. It manufactures lymphocytes and antibodies.

Lymph Nodes: Normally there is more fluid leaving the capillaries than there is coming back into them. This excess is removed by the lymphatics. The lymphatics permeate tissue spaces. (Blood and fluid flows from heart to arteries, capillaries, veins, and again heart.) The lymphatics carry broken-down fat particles from the intestine to the circulation. Lymphatic glands filter out and destroy microbes in order to prevent infection spreading from the point where the organisms entered the tissues, to other parts of the body. Following an infection the lymphatic glands produce antibodies to protect the body against subsequent infection. Nodes are small oval or bean-like bodies which serve as the sites where filtration is done. The main groups lie in the neck, underarm, thorax, abdomen, and groin.

Thymus: Location of vital training of the different types of lymphocytes such as killer, helper, and suppressor cells.

Liver: Modifies waste products and toxic substances to make them suitable for excretion in the bile or the urine.

Intestines: Mucosa of the small intestine is lined with lymphatic tissue.

Stomach: Acids in stomach destroy microbes on entry into the body. The mucous membranes contain lymph tissue.

Internal and External Attack

Microbes are everywhere. In the air, in water, in foods, and in our body. They live on the surface of the skin always ready to attack us. Inside of our body is the battlefield of a never-ending war. It is said that four microbes enter the body everyday.

The body is covered by a strong barrier of skin. The body excretes sebum (oil) and sweat which contain a variety of chemical agents such as oleic acid, lactic acid, and salt that are capable of intercepting and destroying harmful microbes. Mucous membranes secrete fluids and are protected by saliva and mucus, which also contain a special enzyme, lysozyme, and other substances to kill microorganisms and wash them away. The blood and tissue fluids contain many kinds of protective substances such as spermine, properdin, and defensin to kill microbes.

Defense Forces

White blood cells, known as leucocytes, are the main defensive cells. They are classified into two categories: phagocytes and lymphocytes. The first group phagocytes are eating cells (scavenger cells). Examples are macrophages, microphages, and granulocytes. The second group, lymphocytes, are originally from the bone marrow but receive special training from different organs. The stem cells, immature cells from bone marrow, migrate to the thymus gland and become T-cells. They then go back into the bloodstream and many of them go into the lymphoid organs. Only about 5 percent of cells survive thymus training. They become helper T-cells, killer T-cells, and suppressor T-cells. In the case of AIDS, the number of helper T-cells is decreased significantly.

The stem cells which receive special training from intestinal mucous membrane tissue, lymph nodes, liver, or spleen become B-cells. Their special abilities are that they produce antibodies and that they are monoclonal, which means that they can multiply quickly from one to two, two to four, four to eight, and so on. These are plasma cells. Plasma cells produce antibodies.

Antibodies

The antibodies are very important weapons in the body's defense system, but their production is rather slow, taking from one to three months. If a virus settles inside the body cells, the antibodies, once produced, cannot find the virus and do not attack the body cells. But, before antibodies have been made or the white blood cells can react to a viral attack, the body produces antiviral substances called *interferons*. These inhibitors of viral multiplication are also anticancer substances and are most important in the early stages of viral diseases. A special material was discovered from an extract of shiitake mushroom which stimulates body cells to produce more interferons. This special material, called an *interferon inducer*, can be injected or given orally in liquid or capsule form.

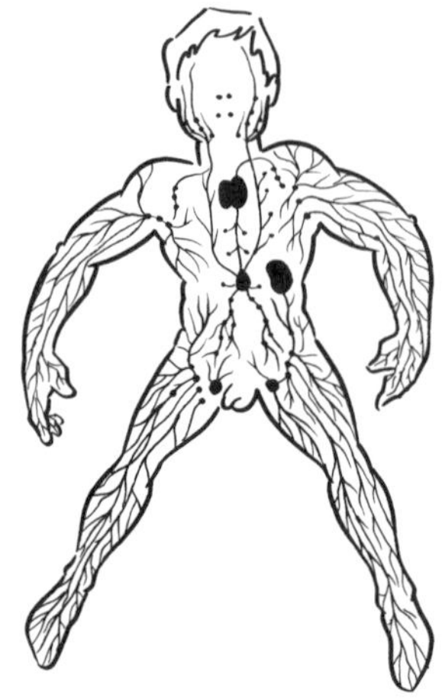

Lymphatic System: This system is a network of lymph vessels throughout the whole body. From this network small vessels emerge, pass to a neighboring branch, become larger and larger, and finally connect the thoracic duct with blood vessels. The prime purpose of this system is the draining of tissue fluid and returning protein to the bloodstream, but it is also very important for the transportation of the body's defenses. In the normal condition, red blood cells are not allowed to enter this system, probably because they would disturb the smooth flow of traffic. The entire system fills up with lymphatic fluid which is composed mainly of salt water and certain other components.

Fig. 65 Lymph System

The lymphatic system has many lymph nodes. Hundreds of them are strung along the lymph vessels and many are located at the intersections and joints of the branches. When a cut or other invasion occurs the normal cells which are destroyed release substances which enter the blood and lymph system. This is the chemical sign of alarm. Local blood cells permeate the broken site to repair it and to bring more white blood cells.

Macrophages start eating the invaders. Helper T-cells send a full-scale alarm to the various units of the body's defense system and also direct the immune response. With this, alarm cells are mobilized. Lots of blood comes to the entry site and the blood vessels swell up. The affected area becomes red and hot because blood brings heat from the interior of the body. Swollen tissues give pressure to sensory nerves and you feel pain. This is an inflammation, just a small local problem. If local forces are weak it could spread via the lymphatic system to other parts of the body. Generally the infection is controlled if the immune function is intact.

Lower Section

Urogenital System: This system consists of the urinary and reproductive organs. Many of the same organs and pathways are used for the functions of removing waste products in a liquid form and reproduction. The urinary system maintains the appropriate balance between water and substances dissolved in it, and between acids and alkalis. It also eliminates waste products that result from the processing of cell protein such as urea and uric acid. Reproduction of a species is essential if the species is going to continue. All of us are the products of successful reproduction. In its simplest form it is the union of the female ovum and the male sperm cell.

Urinary System: The kidneys, bladder, ureters (tubes from kidneys to bladder), urethra (tube from bladder out of the body), and the adrenal glands sitting on top of the kidneys make up the urinary system. The kidneys can be found on the back abdominal wall, one on each side of the vertebral column below the diaphragm. They extend from the level of the twelfth thoracic vertebra to the third lumbar vertebra. The right kidney is usually slightly lower than the left, probably because of the space occupied by the liver. Kidneys are bean-shaped organs, about 5 inches (12 centimeters) long, 2 1/2 inches (6 centimeters) wide and 1 1/2 inches (3 centimeters) thick. Each weighs about 5 ounces (140 grams). They are embedded in and held in place by a mass of fat. A sheath of fibrous capsule encloses the kidneys and the fat. Inside the kidneys is composed of over a million tiny filtering units called *nephrons*. Inside the nephron unit is the glomerulus (a filtering device) and collecting tubules.

Functions of the Kidneys

As the blood passes through the kidneys it is filtered. Filtration takes place through the semipermeable walls of the glomerulus. Water and a large number of small molecules pass through, some of which are reabsorbed later. Blood cells, plasma proteins and other large molecules are unable to filter through and remain in the capillaries. About 100 to 150 liters of dilute substance are formed each day by the two kidneys. Of these 1 to 1.5 liters are excreted as urine. The difference in volume and concentration is due to selective reabsorption and secretion in the tubules. The body reabsorbs materials needed by the body to maintain fluid and electrolyte balance (minerals dissolved in fluid) and blood alkalinity. Urine is an amber color that is due to the presence of uro-bilin, a bile pigment altered in the intestine, reabsorbed then excreted by the kidneys. Healthy urine is acidic, an average of pH 6. Urine is 96 percent water, 2 percent urea, and the remaining 2 percent comes from uric acid, creatinine, ammonia, sodium, potassium, chlorides, phosphates, sulfates, and oxalates.

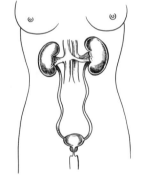

Fig. 66 Kidneys

The mineral balance of the body is maintained by the function of the kidneys. Sodium is the most common positively charged ion in extracellular (outside of cells) fluid, while potassium is the most common intracellular (inside the cell) positive ion. For body processes to run smoothly concentrations of minerals must be correct. Excess sodium is excreted from the body via urine and sweat, with sweat excreting an insignificant amount except when sweating excessively from high environmental temperature or during sustained physical exercise.

The bladder is a pear-shaped reservoir for urine. It lies in the pelvic cavity and its size and position vary, depending on the amount of urine it contains. When distended the bladder rises into the abdominal cavity. As the urine is formed in the kidneys it passes along the ureters into the bladder. The desire to urinate (micturate) is due to an increase of pressure in the bladder caused by the presence of urine there. This occurs when 6 to 8 ounces (170 to 230 milliliters) have accumulated. Urinating is a reflex act that can be controlled and inhibited by the higher centers in man. The act is brought about by the contraction of the muscular coat of the bladder, and relaxation of the sphincter muscles. It may be assisted by contraction of the abdominal muscles that increase pressure in the abdominal cavity. The organs pressing on the bladder assist in emptying it. The quantity averages 1 to 2 liters a day, but varies greatly with the amount of fluids taken. It also is increased when excess protein is taken, in order to provide the fluid necessary to carry the toxic residue—urea—out of the body.

Problems related to kidneys and bladder include: infections, inflammation, kidney stones, kidney failure, cysts, cancer, frequency of urination, bed-wetting, ureteritis, urethritis, cystitis, hypertension, and mineral loss.

Reproductive System: The reproductive organs of the male and the female differ anatomically and physiologically. Both males and females produce specialized reproductive cells containing genetic material (genes) and chromosomes. Other body cells contain 46 chromosomes arranged in pairs. The sex cells contain only one of each pair totaling 23 chromosomes. When an ovum is fertilized by a sperm cell, the resultant zygote contains the full complement of 23 pairs of chromosomes, half obtained from the mother and half from the father. The zygote embeds in the wall of the uterus where it grows and develops during the 40-week gestation period before birth. The function of the female reproductive system is to form the ovum and if it is fertilized, to nurture it until it is born then feed it with breast milk until it is able to take a mixed diet. The function of the male reproductive system is to form the sperm cells and transmit it to the female.

Females

The internal organs of the female reproductive system lie in the pelvic cavity and consist of the vagina, uterus, two uterine tubes, and two ovaries. The vagina's pH is maintained between 4.9 and 3.5. The acidity inhibits the growth of most microbes that may enter the vagina from the outside. After puberty the uterus goes through a regular cycle of change, the menstrual cycle, which prepares it to receive, nourish, and protect a fertilized ovum. It provides the environment for the growing fetus, during the 40-week gestation period, at the end of which the baby is born. The cycle is usually regular, lasting between 26 and 30 days. If the ovum is not fertilized the cycle ends with a short period of bleeding (menstruation).

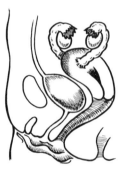

Fig. 67 Female Reproductive System

If the ovum is fertilized the zygote embeds in the uterine wall that relaxes to accommodate the growing fetus. At the end of the gestation period labor begins and is concluded when the baby is born and the placenta extruded. A women's reproductive cycle goes through 4 distinct parts. Beginning with change from childhood to puberty and menstruation, changes continue into menopause. Menopause usually occurs between the ages of 45 and 55, marking the end of the child bearing period. It may occur suddenly or over a period of years, sometimes as long as 10 years. It is caused by the changes in the concentration of the sex hormones. The ovaries gradually become less responsive to hormones and ovulation and the menstrual cycle become irregular, eventually ceasing. Common symptoms are short-term unpredictable vasodilation with flushing, sweating, and palpitations, causing discomfort and disturbance of normal sleep patterns. The breasts also shrink, pubic and underarm hair lessens, the sex organs atrophy, and there are episodes of uncharacteristic behavior.

Problems related to the female reproductive system include: infections like pelvic inflammatory disease, inflammation, venereal diseases, premenstrual syndrome, lack of menstruation, painful menstruation, irregular menstruation, vaginal candidiasis, cervical dysplasia, inflammation of the cervix, endometriosis, uterine fibroids, ectopic pregnancy (uterine tube pregnancy), and ovarian and uterine tumors.

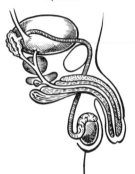

Fig. 68 Male Reproductive System

Males

The reproductive organs of the male are found outside the body. There is the penis, inside the scrotum are the testes, and below the bladder is the prostate gland. The testes are the reproductive glands of the male and are the equivalent of the ovaries in the female. They are about 1 3/4 inches (4.5 centimeters) long, 1 inch (2.5 centimeters) wide, and 1 1/2 inches (3.5 centimeters) thick and are suspended in the scrotum by the spermatic cords. The male hormone, testosterone, is produced in the testes. The prostate gland lies in the pelvic cavity in front of the rectum and behind the pubic bone, surrounding the first part of the urethra.

The male system produces semen. Semen is the fluid ejaculated from the urethra during sex. It is made up of sperm, a thick fluid, a thin lubricating fluid, and mucus. An ejaculation usually consists of 2 to 5 milliliters of semen containing 40 to 100 million sperm cells per 1 milliliter. If they are not ejaculated, sperm are reabsorbed by the body. Successful production depends on about 6 degrees F lower than normal body temperature. The testes in the scrotum outside the body keeps the temperature lower.

Problems related to the male reproductive system include: inflammation, venereal diseases, prostate enlargement, impotence, difficulty in urination, and testicle and prostate cancer.

Differences between Male and Female

Men and women, though equal, are clearly not the same. Men are more likely to hiccup. Boys sleepwalk more than girls. Women have only four-fifths as many red blood cells as men in each drop of their blood. Women suffer more from throbbing migraine headaches, while men more often get piercing cluster headaches.

Heat: A man's hands are usually warmer. At room temperature, healthy men have a larger flow of blood to their fingers than do healthy women. When a woman warms up, however, the flow of blood to her hands will exceed a man's because her blood vessels are more expandable. That is how her body can accept 40 percent more blood during pregnancy with no increase in blood pressure.

A women's forehead is more likely to feel warm, but it depends on the time of the month. The normal body temperature for a healthy adult of either sex is 98.6 degrees F. (Macrobiotic people have a slightly lower body temperature.) But each month at ovulation a woman's temperature rises about 1 degree F and stays there for twelve to fourteen days until just before menstruation.

Wrinkles: A woman's aging face is more likely to be wrinkled for a couple of reasons. The skin is made up of several layers of cells starting with the epidermis (the outer layer) and the dermis (the layer just underneath). As we get older the dermis thins, loses elasticity and sags, but a man's initially thicker dermis may hold elasticity longer. Also, women lose bone after menopause, which allows the skin to sag.

Color Vision: A man is more likely to be red-green color blind by a ratio of 10 to 1.

The gene for red-green color blindness is carried only on some X chromosomes. Women have two X chromosomes; men have an X and a Y. The woman who inherits just one X chromosome with the gene for red-green color blindness will not be color blind. A man whose one X carries the defective gene will be color blind.

Body Smell: A women's armpit will be smellier. Men perspire most heavily on the upper chest, from eccrine glands that secrete only salts and water. Women perspire most heavily under the arms, from apocrine glands that secrete fatty substances along with salts and water. Bacteria digest the fatty substances and their by-products make this sweat smelly.

Sense of Smell: A women has the ability to smell more keenly than a man. The ability to smell, taste, and hear is affected by a variety of hormones, particularly our daily secretion of adrenal hormones. At almost every point in the cycle a woman's senses are more acute. Also, her senses become even sharper as the monthly production of estrogen increases, peaking at ovulation.

Brain Recovery: A woman is more likely to recover after a stroke. The corpus callosum, the bundle of nerve fibers connecting the brain's two sides, is larger in women than in men. As a result, women have more left brain-right brain connections. If one side of the brain is damaged, women appear to recover more quickly and more fully than men do.

Long Life: The life expectancy of a women is 78.2 years and 71.2 years for men. Some attribute women's greater resistance to heart problems to estrogen.

Gout: Gout is a form of arthritis in which the body produces too much uric acid or excretes too little through the kidneys. In either case extra uric acid crystals may collect painfully in joints in the extremities. They also may form kidney stones. Ninety-five percent of those who suffer from gout are men.

Rheumatoid Arthritis: Women have rheumatoid arthritis 3 to 1. Women are also ten times more likely than men to suffer from systemic lupus erythematosus, the prime symptom of which is arthritis. In both these ailments the immune system is activated by female hormones and inactivated by male hormones.

Hay Fever: While both are affected in large numbers, men are more likely to be affected by hay fever than are women. The people most likely to be afflicted by airborne allergies are 18- to 24-year old men, 33 percent of who suffer when there is house dust or pollen in the air versus only 24 percent of woman that age.

Men (yang) of all ages are more likely than women to be allergic to plant pollen (yin); women (yin) are more likely to be allergic to cats and dogs (yang).

Skeletal System: The Hips and Spine
Many of the problems I encounter begin in the structural area of the body. The skeletal and muscular systems allow us to stand or move. These provide the framework for your body and protects delicate internal organs. Our bodies are similar to a building. It has the foundation, walls, and the roof. Needless to say, adequate groundwork is necessary for construction of the foundation. If the foundation is shaky, the walls and the roof will topple, no matter how pleasant looking the structure appears. The foundation of the body is the hip region and the walls are the backbones.

To understand the importance of body structure here is a little reminder about the skeletal foundation. The bones of your skull (29) form a very strong box, protecting your brain, the eyes, and the most important parts of the ears. Your heart and lungs are protected by the rigid cage formed by the breastbone and the ribs (24, 12 on each side) attached to the backbone. The spinal column, consisting of 26 vertebrae, protects the nerves of your spinal cord.

The thighbone accounts for 25 percent of your height. While your smallest bones, located in the middle ear, are less than a tenth of an inch long.

Much of bone consists of calcium, phosphorus, and other lifeless minerals. But about one third of bone is living tissue. Because living tissue needs a constant supply of nutrients and oxygen and waste removal, bones have their own blood vessels. Your bones are also supplied with nerves. The tough covering layer of a bone contains branching blood vessels that run through to canals within the bone. An adult has 206 bones: the skull has 29; spine has 26; ribs and breastbone have 25; shoulders, arms, and hands have 64; pelvis, legs, and feet have 62.

A variety of problems can arise with the hips and spine, a common one is spinal distortion. Spinal misalignment can be attributed to weight strain, habitual misuses of the body, and disease. Distortion is actually one of the body's means of protection. Since each vertebra corresponds to particular internal organs and the operation of the nervous system, spinal misalignment reveals internal malfunction. The autonomic nervous system originates at the base of the brain and travels the length of the spinal column. This system regulates the internal organ functions. The neck, serving as the communication center from the brain to the internal organs, is vital to life.

Spinal misalignment affects the spinal nerves, which originate in the vertebral canals. Irritated spinal nerves, in turn, give birth to various physiological problems. In an opposite way physiological problems irritate the spinal nerves causing spinal misalignment. The vertebrae, if displaced, bring pressure to the central nerves of the spine, and then to the base of the peripheral nerves. As a result, pains and malfunctions develop in the organs and intestines governed by the nerves involved. Additionally, vertebral displacement shrinks ligaments and muscles, resulting in blocked blood vessels and nerves.

Because spinal distortion as a protective device actually serves to maintain the yin-yang balance within the body, mere adjustment of the spine may not be enough. However, a specific exercise, consciously selected to give appropriate yin or yang stimulation, can be a proper means to gradual correction. Such exercise also strengthens the spinal muscles, connective tissue, internal organs, and most importantly, develops *Hara*—central to healthy operation of the mind and body. The exercises in this book serve this purpose.

Chapter 5

Creating Balance with Effective Treatment

The consumption of food and the volume of elimination must be in harmony or you will dehydrate (too much elimination) or swell (too little elimination); you will have diarrhea (too quick elimination) or be constipated (too slow elimination). If you become hot, the body pores open and you cool down. If you become cold, the pores contract, the body hair stands on end and you shiver. When you walk, one arm swings forward, while the other swings backward. Simultaneously, while the right arm swings forward (the top half of the body), so does the left leg (the bottom half). In each of these examples there is an action counteracted by another action. In a way they support each other. One complements the action of the other. Simply stated, you cannot have one without the other. The combination of the two create harmony or equilibrium. This is how nature works.

Fig. 69 Chakra

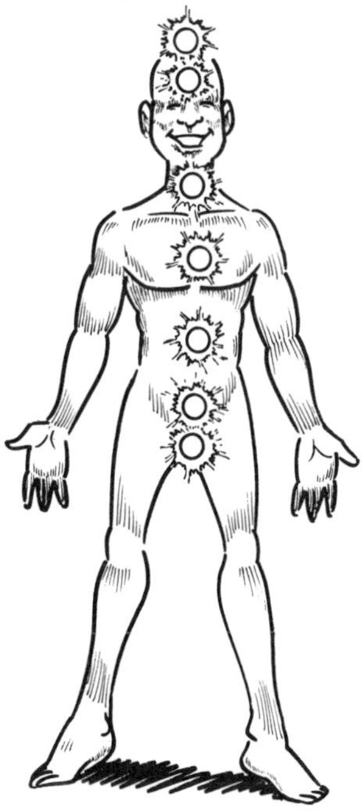

When we apply treatment methods we must always understand what are we trying to accomplish. Without understanding that all treatment is an attempt to follow nature's order and create balance we will fail to achieve our primary goal—to make humans whole. The earth exerts its gravitational pull on all creatures and objects that call this planet home. Gravity tends to draw all bodies in the earth's sphere toward the center of the earth. This natural force is constantly exerting its influence on the human body. Traditional Ayurvedic medicine (the 3,000 year old healing system of India) formulated a model of the human body that is influenced by internal energy fields called *chakras*. These "wheels of energy" line up geometrically with the earth. Each location has a relationship with all the others and with the earth. If your posture is good and these energy spirals line up correctly, you feel balanced. You can think of good posture as the combined effects of correct position and gravity. If you have correct posture you do not feel your body or organs much. You are stable. You feel balanced. This balance is reflected in the condition of the nerves and the spine. On the contrary, when imbalance exists the autonomic nervous system either over- or under-stimulates internal organs and you do not feel well. Unfortunately, many people are out of balance. When you are out of balance you feel uncomfortable.

The father of stress research, Dr. Hans Selye describes that various internal organs, especially the endocrine glands and the nervous system, help us adjust to the constant changes that occur in and around us. When imbalance exists a variety of symptoms are found. The following lists symptoms of autonomic nervous system or hormonal imbalances: general irritability; feeling of being keyed up; pounding of the heart; dryness of the throat and mouth; overpowering urge to cry or run and hide; inability to concentrate; trembling and nervous ticks; high-pitched, nervous laughter; grinding of the teeth; insomnia; sweating; frequent need to urinate; diarrhea and/or indigestion; migraine headache; premenstrual tension or missed menstrual periods; pain in the neck or lower back; loss of or excessive appetite; nightmares; and accident proneness. As you can see imbalance displays itself in many ways.

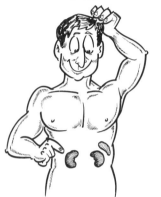

Fig. 70 Man Looking at Kidneys and Spleen

Little things add up to big things in the physical world. Small details, over time, can have major effects. Take for example how you use your body as you give shiatsu treatments or as you do exercises. If you are tense and hold your body improperly while doing shiatsu unfortunately you will be in need of a treatment at the end. When exercises are performed the hip, leg, and arm angles are of the greatest importance. Every degree change of the hip affects the spine and therefore the nerves that branch off the spine. This, in turn, affects the function of the internal organs such as the pancreas and kidneys.

Here are some pointers I would like to share with you. First, learn to feel the effects of posture. For example in the series of practical daily exercises that follow, how does the exercise change when you separate your legs or bring them closer together? Secondly, have the end result in mind before you start. Where does the influence of the twist, bend, or stretch affect the spine? Is this where you want to influence? Would moving the legs or arms closer together affect your target area? And lastly, learn to appreciate the power of breath. Are you or the receiver holding your breath, breathing too fast or too shallowly?

Helpful Hints:
• Learn to feel the effects of posture.
• Begin with the end result in mind.
• Learn to appreciate the power of breath.

Remember the main purpose of treatment is to create balance. More accurately, the purpose is to stimulate the body to correct internal and external imbalances so that it will stabilize itself. This goal is accomplished in many ways. I have presented a number of them in this chapter. You are in good condition if you feel like you are floating on clouds or on water. Your body feels light, you feel no tension. Treating the whole body from several positions; attending to dietary needs; addressing emotional and psychological concerns; and presenting daily and special exercise routines; make up my system. In the application of any exercise or technique, the practitioner should have a clear image of what you want to accomplish. With this vision you will supply the fine adjustments necessary to achieve mastery. When you understand, apply, and master the basics, your treatments will be effective.

Shape Up

In the search for solutions to the problems from hemorrhoids to heart disease, the development of effective treatment largely depends on underlying beliefs an individual or society holds. This may sound strange, but your perspective influences how you will see a problem. In developing health solutions, these treatments are limited by the quality of the developer's perceptions, thoughts, and experience. In short, if health care providers do not care for themselves and are out of shape and in poor condition what can be expected of their solutions?

The fact is people base their actions on perceptions and beliefs. All of us act how we believe we should or must. Actions repeated in daily life become your lifestyle or way of life. These consistent daily routines either support longevity and health or unfortunately, detract from it. The facts from numerous studies state most people are in terrible condition. Health levels are low. The high numbers of people suffering with obesity, lack of energy, sexual dysfunction, and depression point out that we are a people out of shape.

Health supportive day-to-day living forms the foundation of preventive health care. Exercise is the most physical challenge of these daily fundamentals. Many people have not cultivated good habits regarding exercise. Their exercise routines are sporadic at best and non-existent at worst. Yet, most people whom I have counselled have reported that every area of life from appetite, energy, personal confidence, and sex drive, have benefited from consistent training.

It is particularly important to share the pleasure and diversity exercise brings with children. Good lifestyle habits learned early may avoid much of the hardship and suffering experienced as adults. The human body declines steadily throughout your lifetime. It needs constant attention and care. Therefore it is important to stay in shape. At a minimum, training will slow down the aging process. Many people following my advice report friends are often surprised when they discover their age—an added bonus!

Actually, all life is training. Like the weather there are periods of calm, warmth, cold, and storm. Adaptability is essential to survival. If we are to survive, we must continually train and keep up.

The effort to practice my style of shiatsu can range from moderate to vigorous. To do the techniques in a correct way you must have a certain level of physical and emotional strength and particularly you must have endurance. These are the same requirements to survive on this planet. I have developed a series of physical and spiritual trainings for both patients and practitioners. My system of practical daily exercises can be used by everyone. It can be given as homework to clients. Practitioners should add the special training techniques for their development.

My treatment has been developed from many years of experience. But no treatment is any better than the person who provides it. These simple treatment methods may be ineffective if the practitioner does not continually train to discover their depths. I have given many treatments and each time I discover something new, interesting, and useful. I am sure if you apply yourself the same will be true for you.

Practical Daily Exercises

How to Do Exercises Properly

Breathing is especially important while exercising. The inhalation part of your breath makes the body contracted while the exhalation part makes the body relax. When doing these daily exercises always put attention in the exhalation half. Naturally to survive you automatically breathe in so it is not so important to pay attention to the inhalation. To breathe correctly, slightly open your mouth and breathe out when you are doing the strenuous part of the exercise. Inhale slowly and relax your body before repeating. Each exercise can be done 3 to 5 times.

Begin in standing position (Fig. 71).

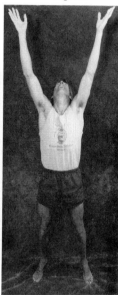

Fig. 73

1. Reaching Heaven

Bring hands up to shoulder height as you inhale (Fig. 72). Exhale lifting hands over head, stretching to reach heaven. Look up while you stretch your fingers out pointing to the sky (Fig. 73).

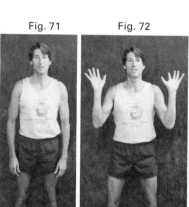

Fig. 71   Fig. 72

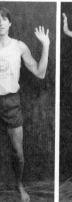

Fig. 74

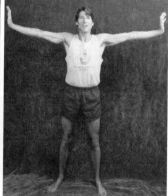

Fig. 75

2. Pushing Mountains

Bring hands up to shoulder height as you inhale (Fig. 74). Exhale pushing your outstretched arms away from you as if you were pushing back the surrounding mountains (Fig. 75). Bend your wrists back and look slightly up.

3. Upward Swing

Stand with arms at your sides (Fig. 76). Inhale and drop your upper body forward as you exhale (Fig. 77). Inhale and swing your hands and arms all the way around beginning on the right side (Fig. 78). Exhale midway through the circle (Fig. 79). Make a complete rotation (Fig. 80). Repeat this circle 3 times. Then swing to the left in the same way. Do both directions 3 times

Fig. 76   Fig. 77   Fig. 78   Fig. 79

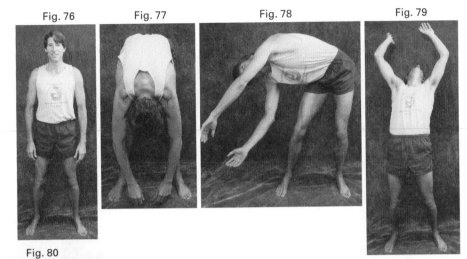

Fig. 80

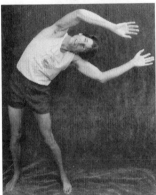

Fig. 81

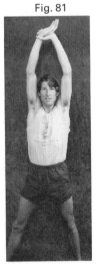

4. Bending with the Wind

Clasp your right wrist with your left hand. Holding them together straight over your head (Fig. 81). On an exhalation bend to the left side. Bend your right knee and move your hip slightly to the right side creating a stronger stretch (Fig. 82). Do this movement gracefully like bending with the wind. Do this 3 times with an exhalation. Repeat on other side (Figs. 83 and 84).

Fig. 82   Fig. 83   Fig. 84

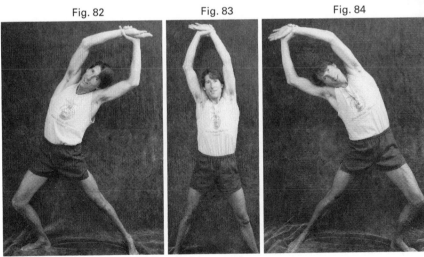

Fig. 85　　　　　　　Fig. 86

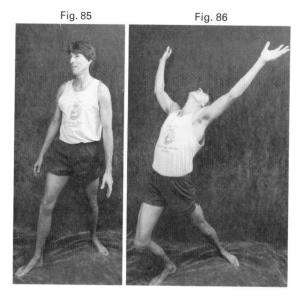

5. Pelvic Push

Step forward with right foot bending the knee (Fig. 85). While exhaling push hips forward as you look up, bring your outstretched arms over your head (Fig. 86). This opens and stretches the chest.

Fig. 87

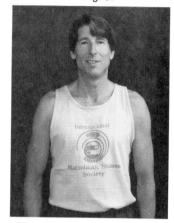

6. Shoulder Row

Drop your shoulders and roll them forward in a circular motion like rowing a boat, 3 to 5 times (Figs. 87–90).

Fig. 88　　　　　　Fig. 89　　　　　　Fig. 90

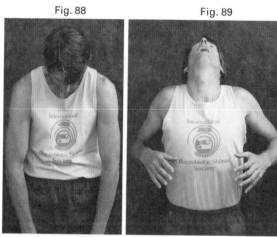
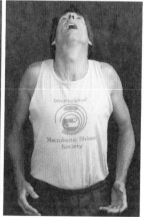

Fig. 91

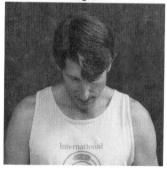

7. Neck Roll

Drop your head, open your mouth, and slowly roll your head in a clockwise direction (Figs. 91–93). Rotate 3 times. Reverse direction and repeat.

Fig. 92

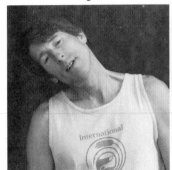

Fig. 93

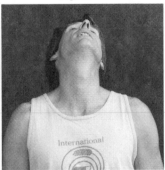

Fig. 94

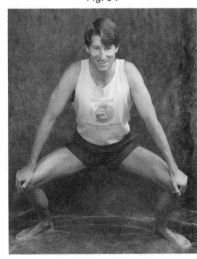

8. Sumo Squat

Separate feet as much as possible, feet parallel to each other. With your back as straight as possible lower your rear end. Your hands are supported on your knees. Move your center of gravity down (Fig. 94). Stretch the inner thighs holding this position for 5 to 10 seconds. Repeat up to 3 to 5 times.

Fig. 95

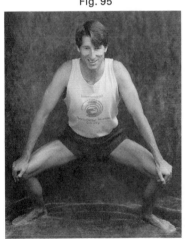

9. Kneeling Sumo

Assume Sumo squat position (Fig. 95). Lower your left knee and touch the floor (Fig. 96). Return to beginning position. Alternate and lower right knee to the floor (Fig. 97). Repeat each side 3 to 5 times.

Fig. 96

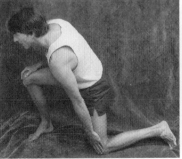

Fig. 97

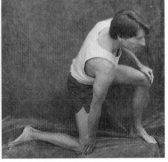

10. Full Spine Stretch

Stand with legs spread one and a half times waist width, feet parallel to each other. Slowly bend forward, keeping the knees straight. Place your hands on the floor, fingers spread apart, pointing forward. The arms should be straight and stretched out as far as possible in front of the shoulders (Figs. 98 and 99). Inhale and as you exhale, lower the hips near to the floor arching the head and upper torso up and back, keeping the arms straight (Figs. 100 and 101). Repeat this procedure 3 times.

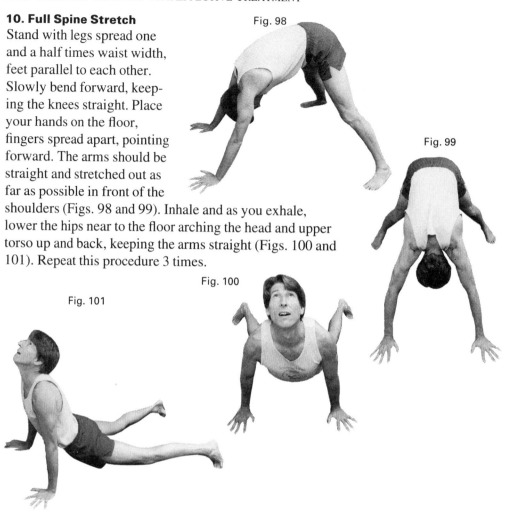

Fig. 98

Fig. 99

Fig. 100

Fig. 101

11. Modified Cobra with a Twist

Lying face down, forehead touching the floor, spread hands to about shoulder width in a push-up position. Bend your left knee which brings your left foot into your groin area. Stretch your right leg slightly out to the side (Fig. 102). Keep your abdomen on the floor. As you exhale raise your chest off the floor (Fig. 103), hold a few seconds, then

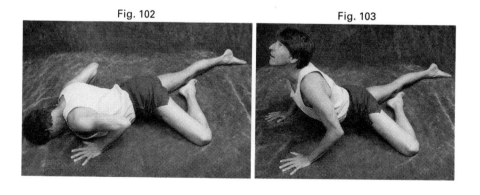

Fig. 102

Fig. 103

Fig. 104

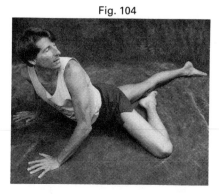

twist to left and look over your shoulder (Fig. 104). Inhale as you lower your upper torso. Repeat 3 to 5 times. Bend right knee and repeat on other side.

12. Sunrise to Sunset

Lie on your right side with outstretched hands together on the floor. Bend left knee up toward the chest (Fig. 105). Exhale as you move left arm over your body (Fig. 106) and place it on opposite side of your body with palm up on the floor (Fig. 107). Your face should be up following as if watching the sunrise and sunset. Look at the outstretched palm. Inhale returning left hand to right side. Repeat 3 to 5 times. Roll to left side with outstretched hands together on the floor. Repeat same movement 3 to 5 times. This twisting stretch affects the whole body.

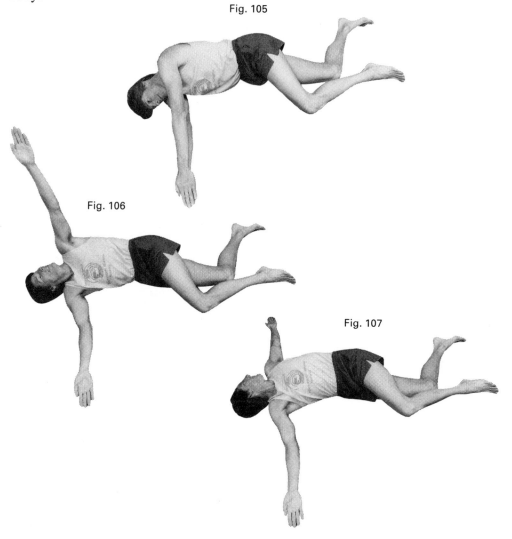

Fig. 105

Fig. 106

Fig. 107

Fig. 108

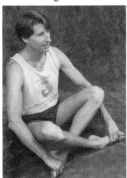

13. Back Roll

Hold the center of the soles of each foot with your thumb and other fingers (Fig. 108). Exhale and roll back on the spine throwing the legs overhead (Figs. 109 and 110). Inhale and roll upright. Repeat 3 to 5 times. Cross legs with other leg forward and repeat 3 to 5 times.

Fig. 109

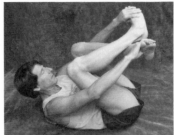

Fig. 110

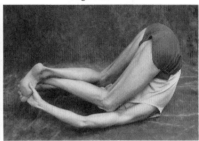

14. Hip Arch

Lying on your back, join the soles of your feet together and bring them up close to the buttocks. Clasp your hands together behind your head (Fig. 111). As you exhale arch up your hips raising them off the floor (Fig. 112). Hold for 3 to 5 seconds and repeat 3 to 5 times.

Fig. 111

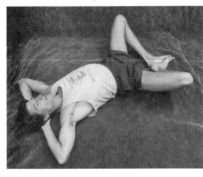

Fig. 112

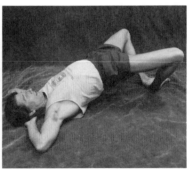

15. Equalizer (Side Stretch)

Lie on your back with hands clasped together behind your head. Extend your left leg, stretch out your heel by pulling your toes back. Bend your right knee and place your right foot near your groin area (Fig. 113). Exhale as you stretch your right knee up toward the head and you bend your head toward the knee trying to make the two meet (Fig. 114). Relax and repeat this side 3 to 5 times. Reverse body posture and do other side.

Fig. 113

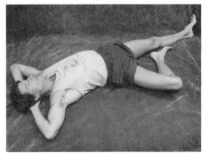

Fig. 114

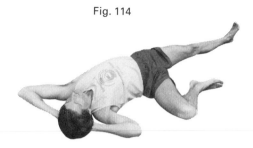

Fig. 115

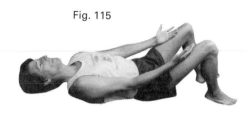

16. Abdominal Crunch

Lying on your back, bend your knees placing your feet flat on the floor (Fig. 115). Exhale and place your upturned palms on your knees (Fig. 116). Tighten your abdominal muscles by pulling your belly button toward your backbone and the floor. Hold for 5 to 10 seconds. Repeat 3 to 5 times.

Fig. 116

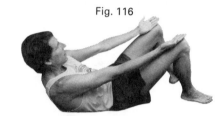

Fig. 117

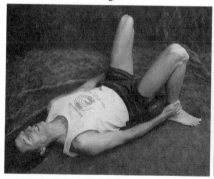

Fig. 118

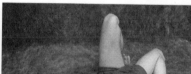

Fig. 119

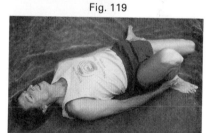

17. Hip Joint Stretch

Lying on your back grasp your ankles (Fig. 117). Bend right knee inward as you exhale (Fig. 118). Alternate with left knee (Fig. 119). Repeat 3 to 5 times.

Fig. 120

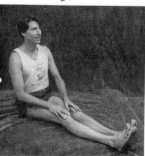

Fig. 121

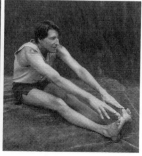

18. Forward Bend

Sit on the floor with both legs together (Fig. 120). Keeping the back as straight as possible, exhale and bend forward from your hip, trying to touch your toes (Fig. 121). Separate your legs to a 45 degree angle (Fig.

122). Try to touch your toes while exhaling. Open your legs as widely as possible and again exhale and try to touch your toes (Fig. 123). Hold each position for several seconds. Repeat 3 times.

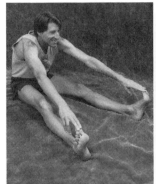
Fig. 122

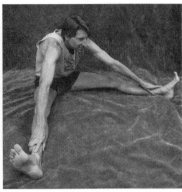
Fig. 123

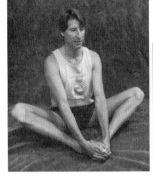
Fig. 124

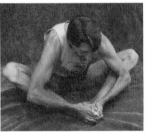
Fig. 125

19. Groin Stretch

Sit up with bottoms of soles joined together, knees outward (Fig. 124). Keeping your back straight, exhale and bend forward from your hip, trying to place your chest on the floor (Fig. 125). Repeat 3 to 5 times.

20. Lion's Roar

Sit on your heels with your knees open. Place your hands on your knees (Fig. 126). Open chest, look up, inhale and strongly exhale as you stick your tongue out. Stiffen your fingers and spread them wide. At the same time open both mouth and eyes wide, tensing the neck and throat (Fig. 127). Hold this posture for a few seconds, then relax. Repeat 3 to 5 times.

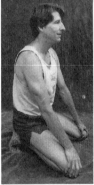
Fig. 126

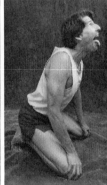
Fig. 127

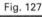

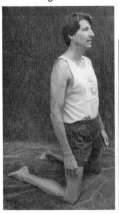
Fig. 128

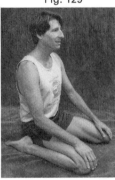
Fig. 129

21. *Seiza*

Kneel with legs separate (Fig. 128). Sit on the floor between your legs (Fig. 129). Hold this posture for 15 seconds to several minutes.

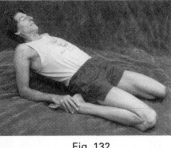

Fig. 130   Fig. 131

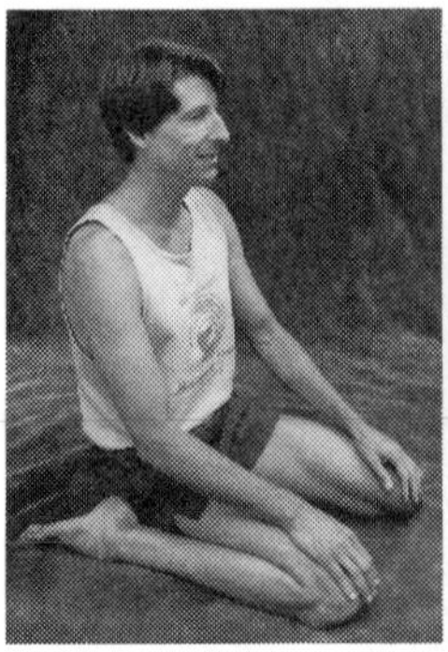

Fig. 132

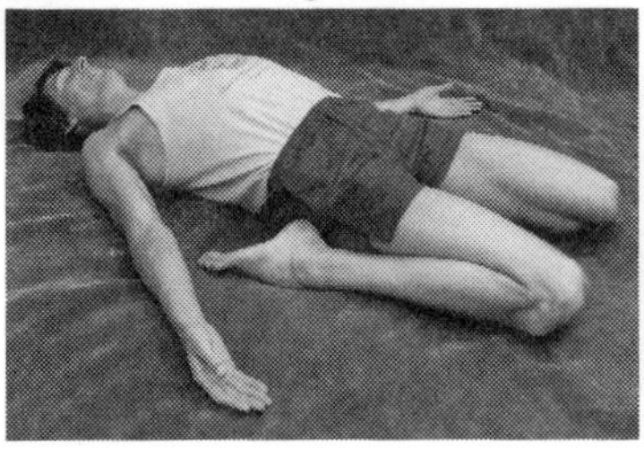

Fig. 133

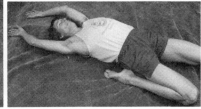

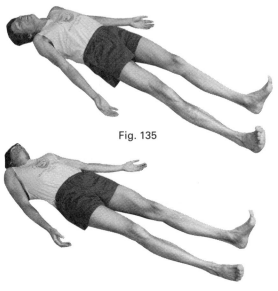

Fig. 134

Fig. 135

22. Leaning Back Stretch

Sit in *seiza* position (Fig. 130). Exhale and lean back, supporting yourself on your elbows (Fig. 131). If you can try to lower yourself all the way to the floor (Fig. 132). Stretch your arms overhead if possible (Fig. 133). Hold for 15 seconds to several minutes.

23. Shaking Body

Lying on your back, legs and arms are at your sides, palm up with hand open. Sway your hips up and down relaxing the whole body (Figs. 134 and 135).

24. Floating Pose

Lying on your back, legs and arms are spread out, palm up with hand open (Fig. 136). Imagine that you are floating on a cloud. Breathe 8 long, slow, and deep breaths. Relax the whole body completely. Maintain this posture for 3 to 5 minutes.

Fig. 136

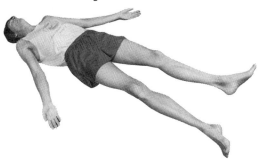

Training Exercises for Practitioners

Simple physical exercises that positively effect circulation and flexibility are useful for all practitioners. Ten of my favorites are:

1. Make fists and quickly stretch fingers open.
2. Rotate wrists in both directions.
3. Rotate ankles in both directions.
4. While standing, go up on toes and lower the heels up and down.
5. Stand on one leg and kick other leg out thereby stretching the knee.
6. Bend and straighten the elbow.
7. With arms outstretched to the side, twist in one direction and the other.
8. Rub the palms of the hands together vigorously.
9. Shake the hands overhead.
10. Clap the hands several times.

These simple routines warm the body and begin to circulate blood and Ki.

In preparation for treatment, practitioners should train the mind as well as the body. Some special time should be set aside to prepare yourself for the intensity of the work that comes with doing treatments. Treatments take a great deal of concentration. Your mind must have the ability to focus and not waver. And for the professional, you must be able to do this hour after hour—not an easy assignment.

I recommend you spend time regularly in various forms of meditation, visualization, or concentration practices. A brief meditation session at the beginning of the day, before the first treatment, helps you stay on track.

In their practices many practitioners forget the importance and effect of posture. Except for breathing, posture has the most influence on us. In order to have clear thoughts, the spine must be straight. Do not sit with legs crossed in the relaxed Indian style. This rolls the back, effecting the hips, and exerts pressure on the spine and nerves. This relaxed pose is fine for casual sitting such as talking with friends but I do not recommend it for meditation.

The important thing to remember concerning meditation is that the knees must be lower than the hips, preferably touching the floor. You can use a cushion to do this. The low back must be straight or the internal organs will drop and you will not be able to keep your center. The key point is the knees must touch the floor.

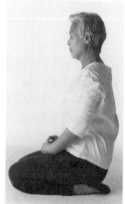

Fig. 137

I have developed a series of training exercises for the practitioners that helps to prepare the body and center the mind before treatment. Sit in *seiza* posture if possible. If this posture is not possible you may use a chair.

1. Straightening Spine
Sit with your spine straight. The big toes are crossed. Maintain a space of 1 to 2 fists between your knees for stability (Fig. 137).

2. Forward Bend

Bend upper body forward, push hips back, and place arms outstretched in front (Fig. 138).

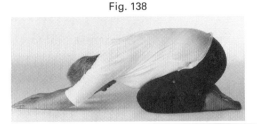

Fig. 138

Fig. 139

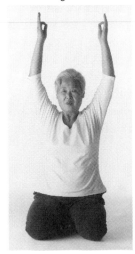

3. Thumbs Together Overhead

Place thumb and index finger together making a circle. Raise the arms overhead with palms facing each other (Fig. 139). Your eye focus is far away.

4. Thumbs Together at Side—Palm Down

Maintain same finger position and lower your arms to your sides. Palms are facing down (Fig. 140).

5. Thumbs Together at Side—Palm Up

Maintain same finger position and keep your arms to your sides. Turn palms to face up (Fig. 141).

Fig. 140

Fig. 141

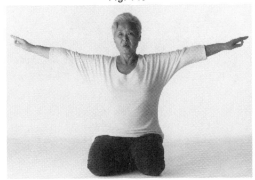

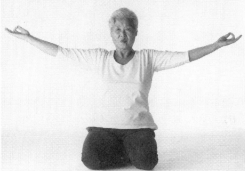

Fig. 142

6. Palm Up on Knee

Lower palms to rest on knees close to the body. Maintain the neck and head in a straight line. The eyes may focus far away in a half-closed position. Drop the shoulders. There should be a relaxed feeling of the arms like holding an egg in the armpit. Your thumb and index finger should form a circle with the other 3 fingers open and outstretched. Allow your body to float, like you are suspended between heaven and earth. Under your knees you are pressing the earth while you are holding heaven over your head.

Breathe deeply and maintain your center. The breath must

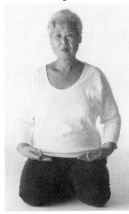

come from your *Hara*. Meditate in this posture for a while (Fig. 142). Allow yourself to empty, let everything go. Continue for 1 to 20 minutes, as long as you like.

You can arrange some special effects in the room if you like. Flowers, incense, bells, candles, and music have traditionally been used to set the mood. Experiment and discover what you enjoy.

After the quiet time you may reactivate your circulation with chanting, singing, shouting, and so on. Free yourself. It is your life. You may arrange it any way you feel is beneficial.

Fig. 143

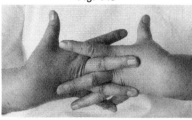

7. Finger Stretches
Interlace your fingers, holding at chest height, and stretch them inward toward you (Fig. 143). Repeat this 3 times. Turn palm out and straighten your elbow, stretching fingers (Fig.144).

| Fig. 144 | Fig. 145 | Fig. 146 |

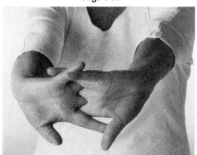 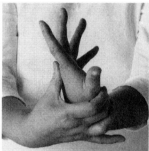 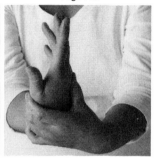

8. Wrist Bend—Palm In
Turn left hand out in clockwise direction. Your right hand holds inside wrist and thumb pushes at base of left ring finger. Pull palm down body's centerline toward waist (Fig. 145). Release and repeat 3 to 5 times. Repeat with other hand (Fig. 146).

Fig. 147

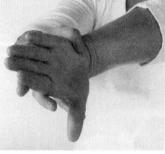

9. Wrist Bend—Palm Out
Extend left arm with palm out and thumb down. Your right hand holds top of hand (Fig. 147). Bend your elbow and bring hands to chest as you exhale (Fig. 148). Keep elbows level with horizons.

Fig. 148

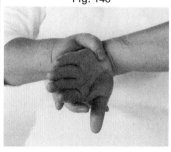

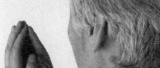

Fig. 149   Fig. 150   Fig. 151

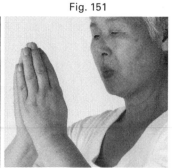

10. Prayer Breathing
Place palms together at nose level. Not too far, nor too close, hold at a comfortable position (Fig. 149). Make a hole between your thumbs (Fig. 150). Inhale and exhale from your *Hara*. As you exhale, blow into your palm through the hole (Fig. 151). Send your Ki. Continue breathing for 3 to 5 minutes.

Placing the palms together in a prayer position, immediately calms the mind and makes the nervous system more balanced. When you are breathing into your palm ask the question, "In the next treatment what am I to do?" Allow a clear picture to come to you. Now you are ready to work.

Fun with a Partner

Exercising with a friend can bring a new dimension to a familiar routine. With the added resistance that a friend exerts we use muscles and joints we cannot stimulate on our own. Exercising with a partner reminds us of our dependence on others. In a healthy way we discover some kinds of dependence free us. On all of the exercises that mention breathing, it should be understood that both partners breathe in and out together except for Inner Thigh Stretch (Number 8) when partners breathe in an opposite rhythm.

Fig. 152   Fig. 153

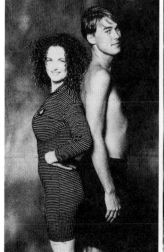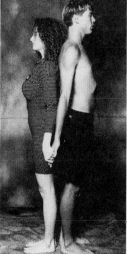

1. Side to Side Twist
Stand back to back (Fig. 152). Hold hands (Fig. 153). Twist to one side and the other (Figs. 154 and 155). Repeat 3 to 5 times.

Fig. 154

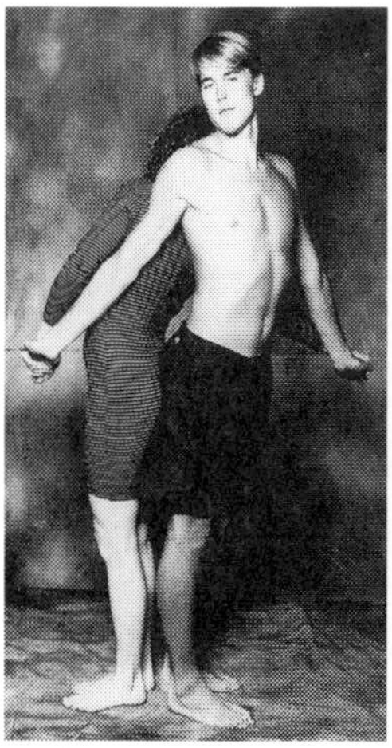

Fig. 155

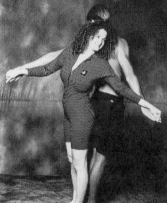

2. Side Stretch

Bend to one side while exhaling (Fig. 156) and to the other (Fig. 157). Repeat 3 to 5 times.

Fig. 156

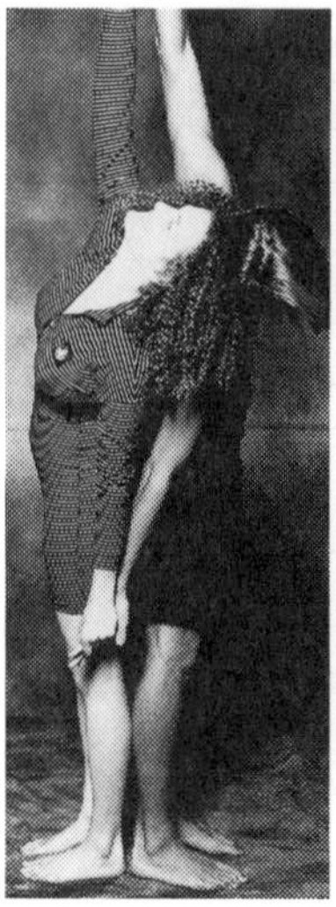

Fig. 157

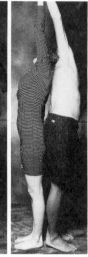

3. Back/Hip Stretch

Place hands on partner's shoulders. Step back and bend forward. Face each other and smile. Stretch by gently bouncing (Fig. 158). Continue for 10 to 30 seconds.

Fig. 158

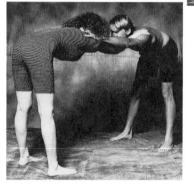

4. Leaning Back

Giver holds receiver's waist. Exhaling, receiver leans back allowing giver to support her (Fig. 159). Hold for 10 to 30 seconds.

Fig. 159

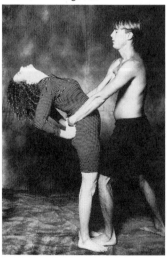

5. Back Lift Stretch

Giver puts receiver's buttocks, level with the small of his back. Exhaling, giver leans forward letting receiver

Fig. 160

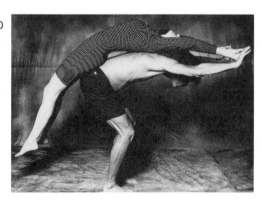

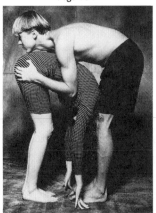
Fig. 161

go up onto his back (Fig. 160). This stretches and relaxes the spine.

6. Low Back Stretch

Receiver bends forward from waist, keeping knees straight and hands touching the floor. Giver leans over receiver's back and gently bounces helping her to stretch (Fig. 161).

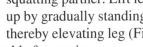
Fig. 162

7. Thigh Stretch

Place leg on shoulder of squatting partner. Lift leg up by gradually standing, thereby elevating leg (Fig. 162). Go up only as is comfortable for receiver.

8. Inner Thigh Stretch

Partners sit facing each other. Separate legs wide open and touch at ankles or feet. Hold hands. One person inhales and leans back while other partner exhales and leans forward (Fig. 163). After several rounds of back and forth, do same in circular movement (Fig. 164). Repeat in other directions.

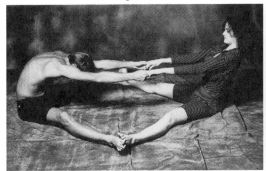
Fig. 163

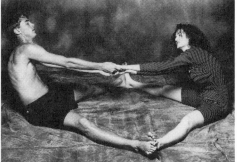
Fig. 164

Fig. 165

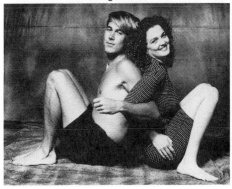

9. Full Body Forward Stretch

Sit back to back and interlock arms (Fig. 165). Receiver stretches legs out fully. The giver leans back onto receiver's back (Fig. 166). Hold for 5 to 15 second. Repeat 3 to 5 times.

Fig. 166

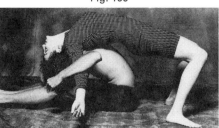

10. Standing up

Sit on floor back to back, arms interlocked (Fig. 167). Press against your partner and try to stand up (Figs. 168 and 169).

Fig. 169

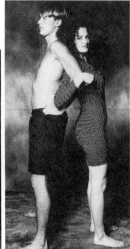

Fig. 168

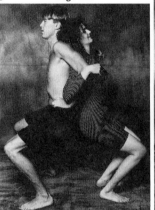

Fig. 167

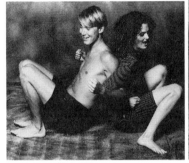

Fig. 170

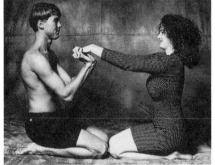

11. Forearm Strengthening

Sit facing each other. Interlock fingers (Fig. 170). One partner bends wrist forward while the other bends back. Resist each other (Fig. 171). Repeat 3 to 5 times.

12. Neck Resistance—Side

One partner sits. Standing partner places hand on side of head above ear. Exhale, the standing partner tries to push the head away while sitting partner resists (Fig. 172). Repeat 3 to 5 times. Do on other side.

Fig. 172

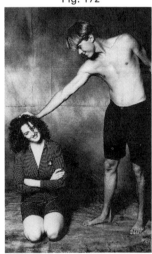

Fig. 171

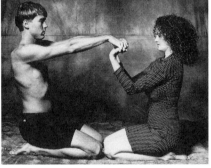

13. Neck Resistance—Front

Place hand on forehead of partner. Both people exhale as the standing partner pushes the head back. The sitting partner resists (Fig. 173). Repeat 3 to 5 times.

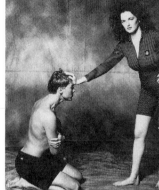

Fig. 173

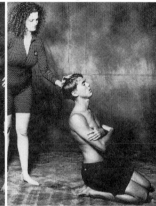

Fig. 174

14. Neck Resistance—Back

Place hand on back of partner's head. Exhale as the standing partner pushes the head forward. The sitting partner resists (Fig. 174). Repeat 3 to 5 times.

Fig. 175

15. Shoulder Resistance

Place both hands on one of partner's shoulders. Exhale as the sitting partner tries to lift one shoulder while standing partner pushes the shoulder down (Fig. 175). Repeat 3 to 5 times. Go to other side and do same technique on other shoulder.

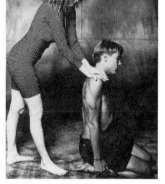

Fig. 176

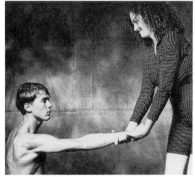

16. Arm Twist

Sitting partner extends arms to standing partner who holds hand. Exhale as sitting partner tries to twist the arm outward while receiving resistence from standing partner (Fig. 176). Repeat 3 to 5 times. Next twist the arm inward and resist. Grab other hand and repeat both techniques.

Fig. 177

17. Arm Lift

Sitting partner places hands up near head. Standing from behind other partner holds hands. Exhale as sitting partner tries to lift arms to outstretched position. Other partner exerts resistance (Fig. 177). Hold for 5 to 10 seconds. Repeat 3 to 5 times.

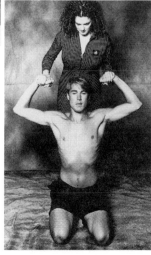

18. Leg Push

Lying partner bends one knee. Standing partner holds raised foot and braces herself. Exhale as lying partner tries to extend his leg. Standing partner resists (Fig. 178). Repeat 3 to 5 times. Do same technique on other leg.

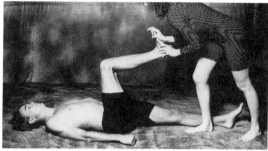

Fig. 178

Preparation for Treatment

While experts agree shiatsu brings comfort, it also is effective in dealing with specific problems, even serious medical ones. Shiatsu is suitable for everyone. From the very young to the very old, it helps to build a strong, resistant condition. For adults, it helps maintain a youthful appearance. For the elderly, it helps to keep the body supple and resilient. It also can prevent the minor disorders commonly associated with aging. Children can learn some principles of Whole Health Shiatsu and discover their body's needs. Shiatsu helps us share the process of discovering lasting good health.

Whole Health Shiatsu recognizes the interrelations of the body's complex systems. Full body treatment is the foundation of good health. When an area is treated in isolation the effects are more likely to be temporary.

One of the aims of shiatsu is to maintain balance for both giver and receiver. That is, the effect of both giving and receiving a treatment makes you feel more centered, more like yourself. It makes you feel whole and connected to the earth and to life.

Here are several suggestions for both the giver and the receiver of the treatment which will enhance both the enjoyment and effectiveness of the session. Not only should the receiver benefit from the session, the giver also must profit. For the giver, a successful treatment can be done only when sufficient energy is in reserve to be given away. This means that the giver must be in a state of good health. If the giver is fatigued or weak, the session will be unsatisfactory. The combination of proper eating, correct breathing, and adequate day to day movement will ensure the vitality necessary for good treatments. If the giver is eating too much meat, eggs, fish, and cheese, then his or her attitude can be tight and aggressive. It will be difficult to listen to the problems of others whom you are treating. The treatment itself can be given too roughly, making the receiver feel uncomfortable. If sugar, oil, chemicals, or other artificial foods are eaten the giver can easily become distracted, losing the ability to concentrate. The giver will not be able to focus on the treatment and can easily become depressed and negative.

Advice to the Giver

Cleanliness
Before using your hands and feet as tools of treatment, be sure that they are washed and clean. The fingernails should be cut short so as not to hurt the receiver.

Concentration

To center yourself, which will allow a greater focusing power, some time of meditation or controlled breathing exercise should be performed before you begin the treatment. This can be done at the beginning of each day.

Attention to Breath

Your breath should be rhythmic, deep, and slow. Breathing should come from the diaphragm. This will minimize fatigue as well as maintain mental clarity. Your attention should be on the breathing pattern of the receiver; watch his or her breath. A coordinated breath, where both the giver and receiver are breathing together, greatly increases the treatment's effectiveness. This type of breathing promotes relaxation especially for the receiver. If the receiver's breathing rate becomes too fast, you can adjust the treatment to slow it down to a relaxed rate. Tell the receiver to breathe in deeply and then give the command to breathe out. You can set the pace.

Clothing

For greatest flexibility of movement and for comfort, the giver should wear loose, cotton clothing. Natural fibers breathe and allow better air circulation next to your body. Jewelry should be removed.

Posture

Your body position is important both for the success of the treatment and for your good as well. The back should be straight and the hips and knees relaxed. Do not twist your body. If you become unbalanced, it is better to readjust yourself rather than stay in an uncomfortable position. When you lean over, as when you press the back, bend from the hips and not from the small of the back. Any hunched position puts stress on the vertebrae and nervous system. Most importantly, when you do a complete shiatsu, follow a specific routine. This conserves your energy.

Rhythm

The body of the receiver is a fine instrument. As with a piano, the giver, if attentive, can learn to play and harmonize with the instrument. If the giver and receiver are breathing well together a natural rhythm can be established. When shiatsu is given with a sense of harmony, the receiver feels very good. If the rhythm is off or the giver is insensitive to the receiver, then the receiver will not feel so good when the session is finished.

Support

When treating any part of the body always be attentive to how it feels to the receiver. Make sure that the receiver feels comfortable and secure. For example when rotating the head do not allow the shoulders to roll about. Stabilize the area that you are working on. You will then be able to maintain your focus on the treatment.

Stillness

The purpose of shiatsu is to use touch to create peace. Our direction in the session is to accomplish this goal. Do not argue during a treatment. Even further, it is best not to talk too much especially nonessential talk such as gossip.

Confidence

During shiatsu, and perhaps throughout our lives, if we have confidence in our action then we can be successful. If your condition is not good, or you are uncertain of your capability to treat someone's problem, then you better not try to do it. To be on the safe side, if you lack confidence do not treat the receiver.

Environment

Give shiatsu in a place that is quiet and as free from distraction as possible. The session can be done on clean, comfortable cushions or a blanket placed on the floor. A small natural fiber pillow can be used under the head.

After the Treatment

With the contact of shiatsu, there is an exchange of energy between the giver and receiver. Several simple methods can be used to clean the receiver's vibrations from you after the treatment. Vigorously shaking the hands or clapping them together several times will disperse the receiver's vibrations and clear the connection between you. Washing the hands is also effective.

Advice to the Receiver

Trust

When receiving a treatment, the body can relax very deeply where there is trust between the receiver and giver. If you cannot trust the family member or friend who is about to give you shiatsu, perhaps it is best not to receive the treatment. Without your trust it is difficult for them to touch you.

Clothing

When preparing for shiatsu you should remove any jewelry and socks or stockings. Thin cotton clothing is best to wear during the session. Women should remove any restrictive article of clothing such as a brassiere or girdle.

Cleanliness

In the home situation, perhaps a bath or shower can be taken before receiving shiatsu. This will relax the muscles. The warm water promotes better circulation as well.

General Information

It is better to wait two hours after meals before receiving shiatsu. Before the session, tell the giver any information about your present condition that seems useful. If you have had any past back or knee injuries, briefly explain the details. Any current problems should be voiced also. This information allows the treatment properly to be adjusted to suit you.

Female Concerns

Shiatsu can be given during menstruation or pregnancy if there are no complicating factors. If a woman usually has excessive menstrual flow, it may be best to skip shiatsu during this time. If the expectant mother has had a history of miscarriage, it would be best to avoid vigorous shiatsu. A light touch or laying on of hands would be appropriate.

Breathing
During the treatment, concentrate your breathing on the exhalation, especially when pressure is being given. Always coordinate your breathing with the giver so that you are inhaling and exhaling simultaneously.

Rest
If possible, after the treatment, continue to lie down and rest for ten to fifteen minutes. This will bring better results from the shiatsu.

Confidence
Whether the shiatsu treatment is given by a friend, family member, or professional, have confidence that the session will help you. Learning to relax allows your natural healing ability to surface.

A Word of Caution
Shiatsu is a safe, health-enhancing activity. As with all physical manipulative therapies, a few common-sense guidelines should be followed:

1. Before you treat, reflect on the age and, physical and emotional condition of the receiver.
2. Do not press too strongly or make the session last more than one hour.
3. Do not place the receiver in an uncomfortable position during treatment.

Avoid giving shiatsu when:

1. The receiver is too tired or exhausted.
2. The receiver is extremely hungry.
3. When the receiver has recently eaten.
4. When you do not have confidence to handle the receiver's problem.

That Special Touch

Shiatsu is easy to learn. You do not need much technical knowledge to complete an effective treatment. No tools or special equipment are necessary to help friends. Your hands, feet, and body are your tools. Using your hands during shiatsu treatments not only increases our own sense of well-being and health but also increases manual dexterity and sensitivity. The human hand is a marvelous tool.

The hand has many sense receptors located in the fingers, especially the fingertips, and the palms. These sensors can feel the difference between light touch, deep pressure, temperature changes such as hot and cold, and abnormal sensations like pain. With continued practice your hands become more and more sensitive to slight variations in texture, temperature, and skin elasticity. Understanding these variations help you to adjust your style to be appropriate to the needs of the receiver. This sensory information helps you to decide which touch method to use, how long to press, and where to press.

Whole Health Shiatsu uses the simplest techniques that we can develop. It is always easiest to allow natural force to do the work for us. The better our technique, the less effort we have to use. Our technical form is more important than the force of physical power. The degree of pressure applied depends on the condition of the area to be treated. Obviously, to overtreat or to undertreat lacks value. Giving abrupt, strong pressure to stiff muscles will cause needless pain and be counter-effective. Strong pressure is best preceded by quickly applied light pressure for a short time. With practice you will learn to observe changes in muscle condition and adjust the degree and type of pressure accordingly.

There are three types of pressure:

1. *Light pressure:* The body is barely touched. Used for diagnosis and light treatment.
2. *Medium pressure:* Penetrates more deeply into the muscles, producing a sensation of pleasurable discomfort.
3. *Strong pressure:* Deeper penetration that affects stiff muscles and may produce some pain. This releases long-term stagnation. The pain level is kept in the tolerable range for the receiver. When completed the pain is gone and the receiver feels better than before.

Shiatsu practitioners have developed and use many types of touching techniques. Each has its own effect. The styles I use are: palm healing, holding, vibrating, rubbing, patting, tapping, pounding, shaking, stroking, kneading, pulling, "leaning into it," pressing, adjusting, bending, and stretching. The energy that we use to accomplish our tasks comes from our body's center—the area located just below the navel. Called *Hara* in Japanese, this area is thought to be a principal storage place of energy as well as the physical center of the body. It is here that we have our balancing point. Before you even touch the giver, concentrate your energy in the lower abdomen and allow it to flow from there to your hands. Never just use the pressure from the fingers, hands, or feet. By leaning into the touch with an exhalation, the weight of your body brings about a beneficial effect.

Palm Healing, Holding, and Vibrating Methods

Use this method when we want to transfer or stimulate the movement of energy in someone. In palm healing, the hand is placed either on the receiver's body or away from it. The giver relaxes, breathes deep, rhythmic breaths, and concentrates on sending healing energy. This can be done with or without touching. This technique is used in cases of cancer, AIDS, or skin disorders such as burns, cuts, or rashes. Remember to send and extend your energy to the receiver.

Fig. 179 Palm Healing

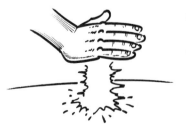

Holding can be used with anyone, especially with older people and children. Holding sustains the pressure and concentrates it in one area. One use is with children who have nausea or stomachache.

When doing the vibrating technique, keep your spine straight. You can either sit or stand. Lightly put your hand on the receiver's skin. Your arms should be extended. Inhale and exhale with a calm, long breath.

If you repeated this practice with concentration, a natural vibration occurs in your hand. This vibration comes from your center. The energy transmitted from the center through the hand moves like electricity into the receiver's body. Strong concentration and practice, coordinated with breathing, is necessary to be effective. This technique is different from shaking.

Rubbing Method

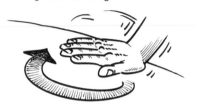

Fig. 180 Rubbing

Perhaps the most familiar form of touch is rubbing. When we are cold we rub the palms of our hands together. As it stimulates blood flow, rubbing is used to relieve fatigue and to improve the tone of the skin and muscles. When rubbing, place the hands flat on the body and maintain a steady pressure from the beginning to the end of the motion.

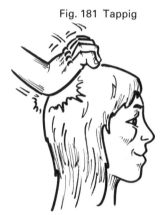

Fig. 181 Tappig

Patting, Tapping, and Pounding Methods

When we pat someone on the back or shake hands during an introduction, we are using touch methods. A repetitive hitting motion with the open palm is patting. This increases circulation.

Tapping can be done with the fingers, with the palm, with the side or back of the hand, or with the fist. This light pounding should be done rhythmically. Light tapping restores vitality to tired muscles and nerves.

Pounding can be done with fists or open palms together striking with the back side of the hands. This stronger style is applied on hard or stagnant surfaces such as the area between the shoulder blades. Excessively heavy striking will tire the muscles and nerves and cause pain.

Shaking Method

Fig. 182 Shaking with Foot

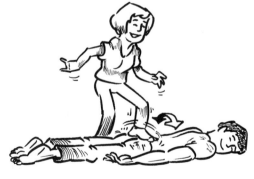

The shaking motion is used when there is a lack of vital energy within the body. This is the easiest way to loosen up any part of the body. It loosens and relaxes. The hands or feet can be used to do this simple technique. Placing the giver's foot on the sacrum of the reclining receiver and shaking the whole body brings relaxation. The giver can hold different parts such as the receiver's heel or wrist and shake. An exercise for whole body stimulation is to have the receiver lie on the floor on their back and raise both arms and legs into the air and vigorously shake. This warms the body and increases blood and lymph circulation to the extremities. It warms the hands and feet.

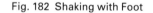

Stroking Method

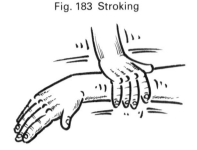

Fig. 183 Stroking

The stroking method is similar to rubbing but with more strength and squeeze power. The thumb and four fingers grip an area such as the arm and apply strong pressure while moving up and down. This technique is used on arms, legs, and back. This removes stagnation and is good for poor circulation.

Kneading Method

Fig. 184 Kneading

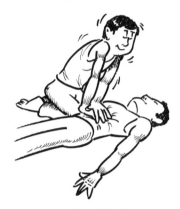

Using the thumb and index finger together or the whole hand, knead areas such as the tendons near joints, for example the knee or elbow. Kneading also can be used along the back or side of the neck and along the tops of the shoulders. This squeeze motion loosens stiffness and increases circulation in the area. In every shiatsu treatment I always knead the abdomen with the palms of my hands.

Pulling Method

Pulling various body parts releases joint stagnation. Common areas of application are the fingers and toes, arms and legs, pulling the arms over the head, and bringing the elbows back together while the receiver is in a seated position. One simple technique is for each finger and toe to be pulled during the Total Body Treatment. This stimulates circulation in all the meridians in the body.

Fig. 186 Leaning into It

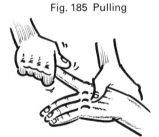

Fig. 185 Pulling

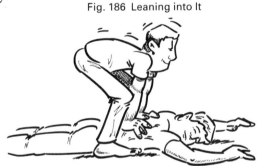

"Leaning into It" and Pressing Methods

This pressing technique is the one most frequently used in my treatment. With the palm of the hand, the sole of the foot, or the thumbs and fingers, the whole body leans into each movement. Each press is done with coordinated exhalations of both the giver and receiver. This makes the receiver's muscles relax and the giver can get in more deeply with greater effect. Pressure comes from the center of the body not just the fingertips or feet. These techniques are applied mainly on the back.

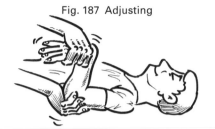

Fig. 187 Adjusting

Adjusting Method

Quickly adjusting stiff parts of the body stimulates a vigorous flow of energy throughout the body. It has a special effect on the body's joints. We can adjust the arms, wrists, fingers, legs, ankles, toes, and neck.

Bending and Stretching Method

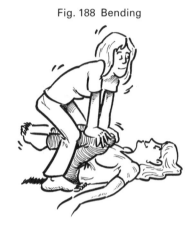

Fig. 188 Bending

These techniques are used to increase movement and flexibility and to relax the muscles and tendons of the joints. Upon awakening in the morning we all stretch; it is a natural process. This promotes circulation to all parts of the body. It also stimulates the body's energy channels and the acu-points simultaneously. Bending the knees to the chest with the receiver on the back stretches the low back area of the receiver.

Simple Total Treatment

This treatment is invigorating. It stimulates the entire system yet it balances internal organ function. I designed the treatment so that even the busiest of people can take advantage of it. It should take less than 30 minutes, therefore families and friends will be able to practice on each other regularly. Try it! You will discover the benefits are tremendous.

Receiver lies face down with arms extended out at the sides, palms down.

1. Relaxing the Body

Lightly hold the receiver's torso with your outstretched palms and gently shake the body as you move down from shoulder to waist (Figs. 189 and 190). Check the receiver's condition with this movement for less than 1 to 2 minutes.

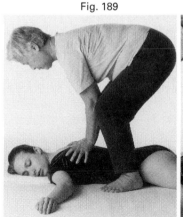

Fig. 189

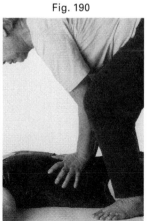

Fig. 190

2. Pressing the Back—with Open Palm

Stand over the receiver, with one foot on each side of the body, and place the heels of your hands together at your wrist on the spine near the top of the back. Your fingers are outstretched and perpendicular to the spine. Press from shoulder level down to the buttocks (Fig. 191–193). Lean your body weight onto the receiver as you exhale. Press with both hands, palm open. Breathe deeply with each exhalation. Take about 5 to 6 presses to do the entire back.

Fig. 191

Fig. 192

Fig. 193

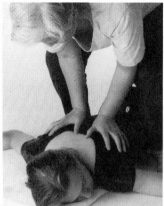
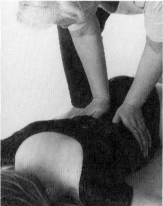
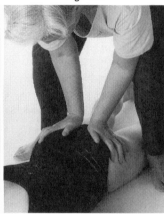

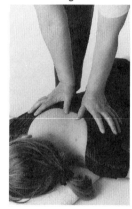

Fig. 194

3. Pressing the Back—with Thumbs

Use the thumbs to press the acu-points (*tsubo*) and meridians (*keiraku*) on the back. Beginning near the large bone (C7) at the shoulder level in the center of the back, place each thumb 1 1/2 inches apart from the spine. Breathe in with the receiver and on exhalation press straight down, leaning your body weight into the back. Hold each point for 3 to 5 seconds. Continue down each vertebra to the tailbone (Figs. 194 and 195). Carefully observe your body posture.

The Yu points located along the Bladder meridian flow down the back from the head. Each point relates to an internal organ. Usually, abnormal reactions, such as tenderness or sensitivity, will occur at these points if unusual activity is occurring in the respective organs. Consequently these points may be used in treating organ disorders. For example, treatment can be applied to Stomach Yu (BL 21) for stomach upset and gastric distress, and at Lung Yu (BL 13) for breathing difficulties.

Fig. 195

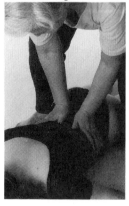

These back Yu points also can be used with diseases of the sense organs. Each of the five senses relates to an internal organ. When the sense organ is distressed its controlling organ is likewise affected. When the eye has trouble, treat Liver Yu (BL 18) and when the hearing is impaired, treat Kidney Yu (BL 23).

The Back Yu Points

Organ	Acu-point (*Tsubo*)	Location
Lungs	BL 13	T_3
Heart Governor	BL 14	T_4
Heart	BL 15	T_5
Liver	BL 18	T_9
Gallbladder	BL 19	T_{10}
Spleen	BL 20	T_{11}
Stomach	BL 21	T_{12}
Triple Heater	BL 22	L_1
Kidneys	BL 23	L_2
Large Intestine	BL 25	L_4
Small Intestine	BL 27	S_1
Bladder	BL 28	S_2

Relationship of Sense Organs and Internal Organs

Sense Organ	Internal Organ	Acu-point	Location
Eye	Liver	BL 18	T_9
Mouth	Spleen	BL 20	T_{11}
Ear	Kidneys	BL 23	L_2
Nose	Lungs	BL 13	T_3
Tongue	Heart	BL 15	T_5

Fig. 196

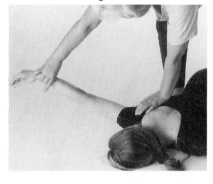

4. Arm Shoulder Stretch

Place your left hand at the receiver's right shoulder. Your thumb is near the armpit with the other fingers firmly lying on the shoulder blade (Figs. 196 and 197). Exhale and press the shoulder blade down as you lift the right arm from the floor stretching the two against each other (Fig. 198). Hold wrist from top.

Next, after stretching the arm, rotate in both clockwise and counterclockwise directions (Fig. 199).

Fig. 197   Fig. 198   Fig. 199

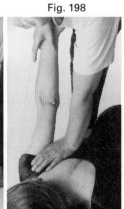
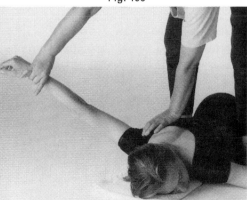

Fig. 200

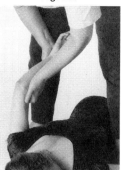

5. Shoulder Blade Press

Bend the arm at the elbow and place the hand as far up on the back as is comfortable (Figs. 200 and 201). Hold the receiver's right hand with your left hand (Fig. 202). Place your open right hand directly on the shoulder blade. Brace your elbow against your knee (Fig. 203). Exhale and press the shoulder blade toward the heart (Fig. 204). Be sure to push toward the heart and not up toward the shoulder. Pushing up toward the shoulder could create pain and be dangerous. Repeat 2 to 3 times. Do other side.

Fig. 201	Fig. 202	Fig. 203	Fig. 204

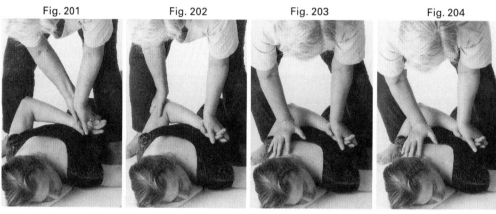

Fig. 205	Fig. 206

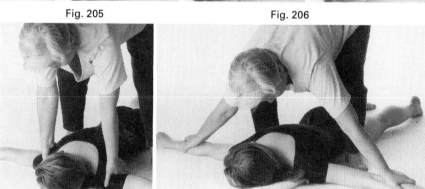

6. Extended Arm Press

Lean forward and with open palms press along the receiver's arms from the shoulder to the hands (Figs. 205 and 206). Your thumb should be on the top side of the shoulder. Repeat several times.

7. Upper Body Lift

Pick up the receiver's arms at the wrists. Ask receiver to lift and support own head. Exhale as you lift the upper torso from the floor (Figs. 207 and 208). Hold for several seconds.

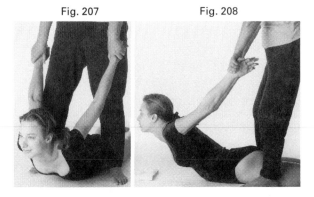

Fig. 207   Fig. 208

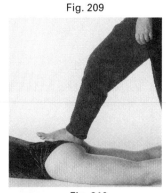

Fig. 209

8. Foot Press on Coccyx and Inner Thigh

Stand between the receiver's legs, facing the head. Place the center of your foot on the tailbone (coccyx) and gently press this area (Figs. 209 and 210). Push up toward the head and shake the spine (Fig. 211). Lift your foot off the tailbone and press on and off as you treat the inner thighs (Fig. 212). Do both sides 2 to 3 times.

Fig. 210

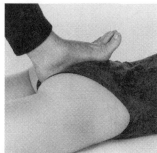

Fig. 211   Fig. 212

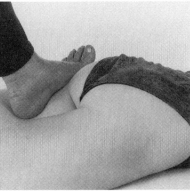

Fig. 213

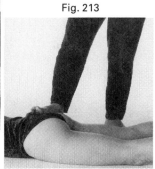

Fig. 214

9. Foot Press on Hip and Outer Thigh

Stand to the right side of the receiver. Place your right foot firmly on the large muscles of the lower buttock. Press on and off and gently rock the hip area (Fig. 213). Press from the buttock down the leg (Fig. 214). Move your right foot down the outer thigh pressing every 6 to 10 inches. Repeat 3 to 5 times until receiver is relaxed. Do other side. Do not press the back of the knee.

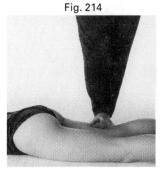

Fig. 215

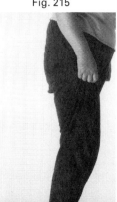

10. Walking on the Feet

Stand between the receiver's legs, facing outward, and walk on the bottoms of both feet simultaneously, walking from arch to heel several times (Figs. 215 and 216). Do not walk on the toes. Shift your weight from one side to the other. Your toes are on the floor; your heels do the pressing.

Fig. 216

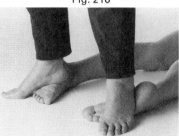

Fig. 217

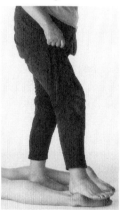

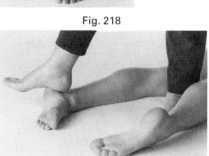

Fig. 218

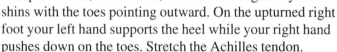

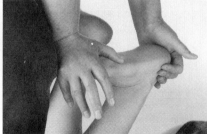

11. Heel Stretch

Press out the heel with your foot. Catch the receiver's left ankle with your right foot and press down and outward lightly, diagonally stretching out the ankle (Figs. 217 and 218). Repeat on other side.

12. Bending Knees

At the foot of the receiver pick up both feet, bend knees, and rest them against your shins with the toes pointing outward. On the upturned right foot your left hand supports the heel while your right hand pushes down on the toes. Stretch the Achilles tendon.

Fig. 219

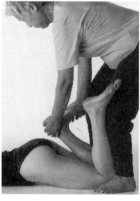

Fig. 220

Exhale and bend the knee moving the foot toward the buttocks as you continue to exert pressure on the toes (Figs. 219 and 220). Hold then release. Repeat 2 to 3 times.

Fig. 221

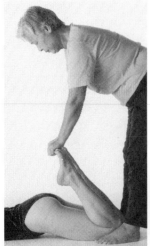

Next grab toes with your fingers gripping the toes firmly (Fig. 221). Exhale and lean your body weight on the receiver's legs pushing the legs to the buttocks (Figs. 222 and 223).

Fig. 222

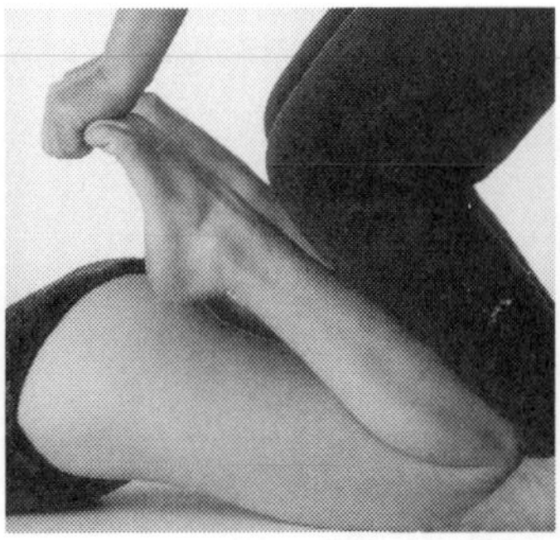

Fig. 223

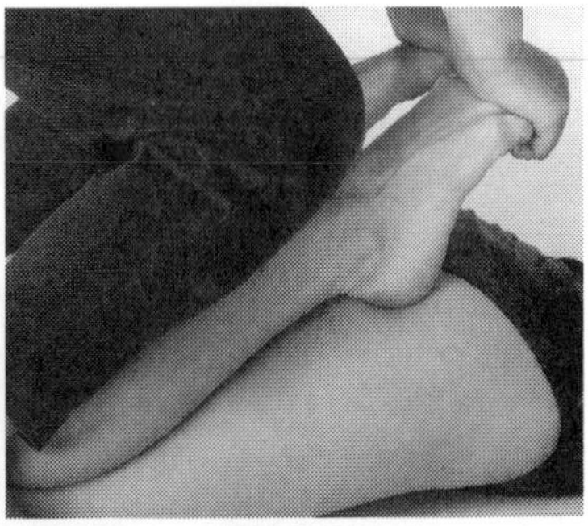

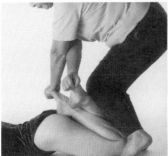

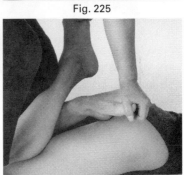

Fig. 224

Fig. 225

Then, release, cross the ankles while holding the toes, and push the legs down, with right foot on top, toward the buttocks again (Figs. 224 and 225). Release, cross the ankles with left foot on top, and press toward buttocks like before.

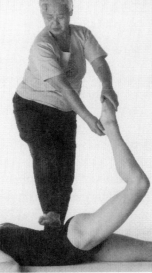

Fig. 226

Fig. 227

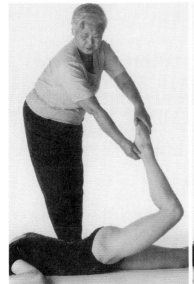

13. Foot on Back Diagonal Leg/Hip Stretch

If you feel the receiver will benefit from this stretch and you have confidence that you can do it accurately, then proceed. If not, skip this routine.

Pick up the left ankle, lift leg, and walk to the right side of the receiver (Fig. 226). Place your right foot lightly on the hips (sacrum). You should be standing at the receiver's side near the waist (Fig. 227).

Fig. 228   Fig. 229   Fig. 230

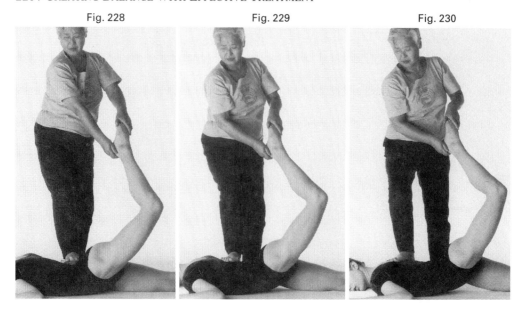

Exhale, lean back, and lift the leg toward yourself at a diagonal (Fig. 228). Release, move your support foot on the back, and lightly place it 2 to 3 vertebrae up from first position (Fig. 229). Exhale, stretch, and release. You can continue up the back until between the shoulder blades (Fig. 230). Pick up other leg and repeat. Do this routine only once.

Fig. 231   Fig. 232

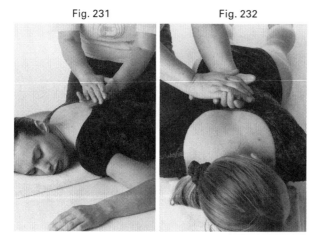

14. Pounding the Back

Kneel at the receiver's right side. Place your left hand with palm up and the right hand with palm down, loosely touching each other. With a pounding motion, let your hands bounce off the back (Figs. 231 and 232). Move from hip to upper back and back again.

15. Rotating and Adjusting Hip

Have the receiver turn over onto the back. Stand at the feet. Place your hands on the knees (Fig. 233). You must hold ankles together with your knees (Fig. 234). Exhale and rotate legs in a clockwise direction 3 to 5 times (Figs. 235–237). Release, exhale, and rotate in a counterclockwise direction 3 to 5 times. Be sure that you correctly support receiver's ankles and knees. Exhale, bend, and at the end of the breath, push toward receiver's chest by placing your body weight on the receiver's shins.

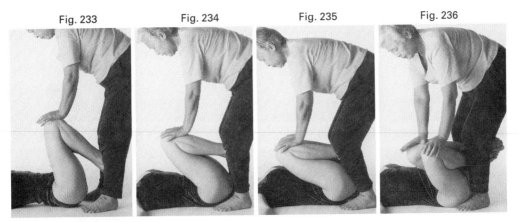

Fig. 233   Fig. 234   Fig. 235   Fig. 236

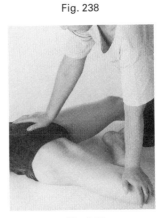

Fig. 237

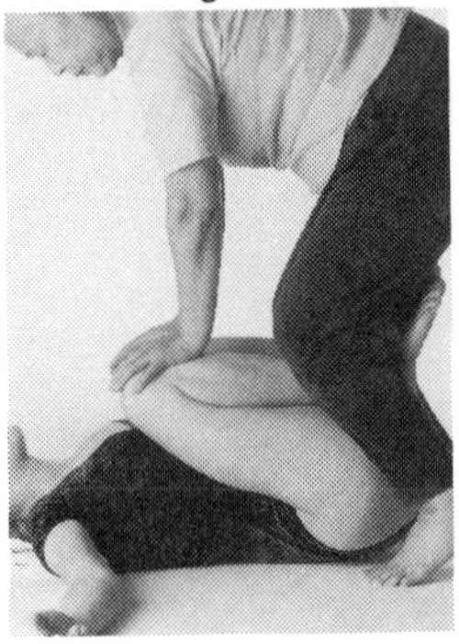

Fig. 238

16. Inner Thigh Stretch

Bend the right knee placing the foot near the groin area (Fig. 238). Place your right hand on the receiver's left hipbone and support it while your left open palm is on the right knee. With your body weight centered, stretch the two hands apart.

Move your left palm up the inner thigh pressing with each exhalation (Figs. 239 and 240). Repeat 3 to 5 times. Go on to next routine, then return and repeat on other leg.

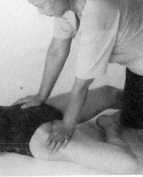

Fig. 239   Fig. 240

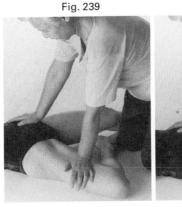

Fig. 241

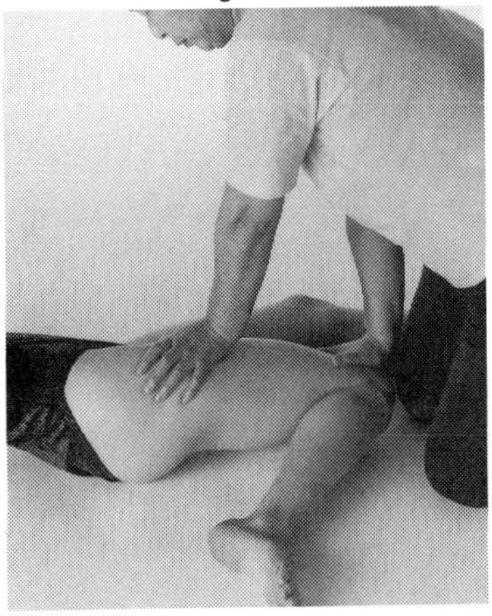

17. Outer Thigh Stretch

Bend the right leg and let the knee move inward. Your left hand supports the receiver's right hip while your right open palm is on the right knee (Fig. 241). Center your body weight and stretch your hands apart. Release, exhale, lean onto the leg, and move your left hand down the outside of the thigh,

Fig. 242

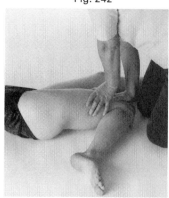

pressing with each exhalation (Fig. 242). Repeat 3 to 5 times. Do previous routine on other leg, return, then do this routine on left leg.

18. Knee Adjustment

Bend right knee with foot flat on the floor. Grab ankle from the outside with your left hand. Support receiver's right knee with your right hand (Fig. 243). Exhale and pull ankle out parallel with floor straightening the leg (Fig. 244). Gently drop outstretched leg on floor. Do other side.

Fig. 243

Fig. 244

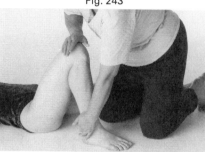

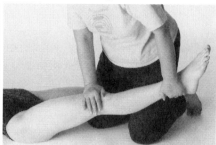

19. Elbow Adjustment

Move to the left side of the receiver. Sit between outstretched arm and torso. Pick up hand with palm down at wrist with your right hand. Your left hand should support the elbow from underneath. Bend the elbow by bringing the hand closer to the body (Fig. 245). Gently pull hand outward with a one, two, three pumping action. On three straighten arm (Fig. 246). Continue to next routine. Repeat on other side after Rubbing/Kneading *Hara* (Routine Number 21).

Fig. 245

Fig. 246

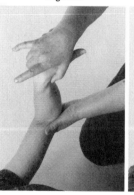

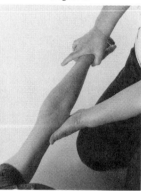

20. Hand Pressing Arm

With your hand touching the lower abdominal area, press the arm with your right open palm from the shoulder down to the wrist (Fig. 247–249). Repeat this routine several times. Continue to next routine. Repeat on other side after Rubbing/ Kneading *Hara* (Routine Number 21).

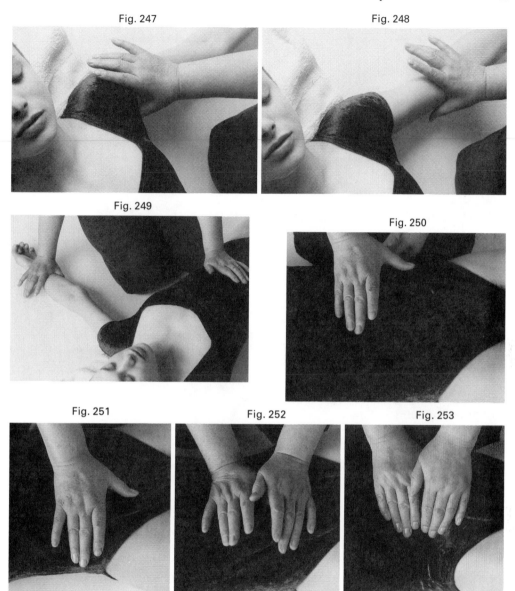

Fig. 247   Fig. 248

Fig. 249   Fig. 250

Fig. 251   Fig. 252   Fig. 253

21. Rubbing/Kneading *Hara*

With the heel of your right hand placed directly on the abdomen, massage in a clockwise direction. Work in the area between hips and ribs. You can make large spirals and small spirals (Figs. 250 and 251). Continue for 30 seconds to 2 minutes.

Next, with both hands together knead the intestines as you lean your weight into the receiver's navel area. Push with the heels and pull with the fingertips (Figs. 252 and 253). Warm and loosen the abdomen for 30 seconds to 2 minutes.

22.—Go to right side and repeat Elbow Adjustment, Hand Pressing Arm, and Rubbing/Kneading *Hara* (Routine Number 19 to 21).

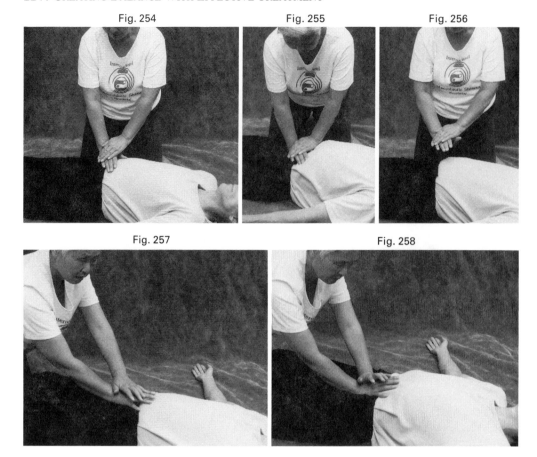

Fig. 254   Fig. 255   Fig. 256

Fig. 257   Fig. 258

23. *Hara* Breathing

The lower abdominal area, named *Hara*, in Japanese, is very important in diagnosis and treatment. Traditional Oriental medicine teaches that the energy of all internal organs affects and is reflected in this area. That is why the following *Hara* breathing treatment has such a powerful effect. It is especially good for recovery in children and seriously ill people. When you guide the receiver to breathe deeply several positive responses occur. They will increase the oxygen content of the blood. Automatically, the nervous system relaxes and the internal organs function better. General body circulation improves. This technique calms the emotions and can be useful in reducing pain. As the practitioner, during this segment of the treatment you can figure out if the treatment will be successful or not. By observing the receiver's response you should be able to sense if positive changes are occurring. This is such an important part of the treatment, do not fail to do it well!

Kneeling on the receiver's right side place both open palms on abdomen (Fig. 254). Coordinate your breathing with the receiver's breathing. On exhaling, press down gently until you feel resistance (Fig. 255). Hold for 1 to 2 seconds. Release and lift the palms off (Fig. 256). Repeat up to 10 times. This is powerful for both giver and receiver. Optionally *Hara* can be treated from the foot position (Figs. 257 and 258).

24. Back of Neck Stretch

Move to behind the receiver's head. Lace fingers together and place under the neck (Fig. 259). Exhale and pull the neck toward yourself then rotate left and right (Fig. 260). Repeat 2 to 3 times.

Next, pick up the head with both hands and stretch the neck by moving the head toward the chest (Fig. 261). Try to touch the chin to the chest. Repeat 1 to 2 times. You can stretch the head at both right and left diagonals. This stimulate upper spine to cervical region.

Fig. 259

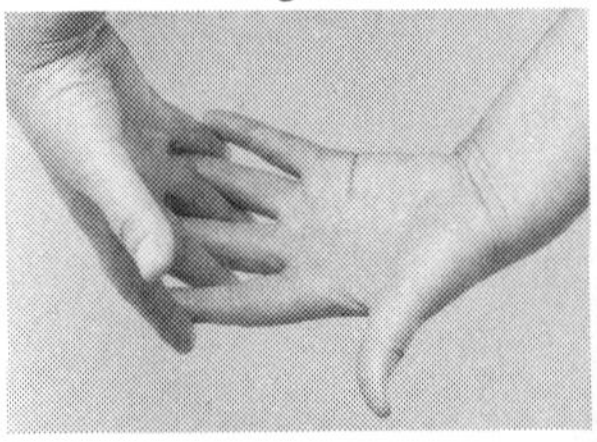

Fig. 260

Fig. 261

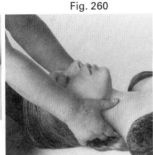

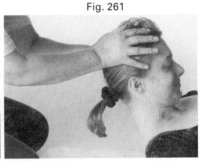

Fig. 262

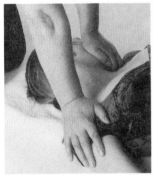

25. Side of Neck Stretch

Have the receiver look to the left. Place open palm of your right hand on the receiver's right shoulder and your left palm on the chin with fingers pointing to the floor. Exhale and gently stretch your hands apart (Fig. 262). Do not force stretch. Repeat 1 to 2 times. Turn head and stretch other side.

26. Thumb Pressure on Neck

On right side of the receiver's neck use your right thumb to press from below the ear down the tendons of the neck to the shoulder (Figs. 263 and 264). Hold each point for 1 to 3 seconds. Repeat thumb pressure

Fig. 263

Fig. 264

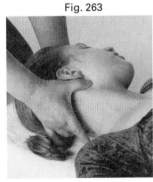

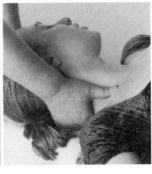

Fig. 265

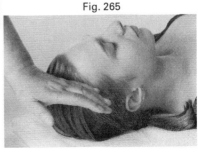

along this line 3 to 5 times. Turn the head so receiver is looking to the right and repeat on left side using left hand and thumb.

27. Tapping Head

Open your left palm, reach across to the right

Fig. 266

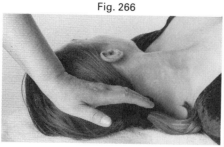

Fig. 267

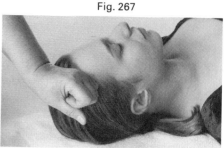

side of the receiver's head, and lightly tap rhythmically (Fig. 265). Tap along the entire side of the head. Continue for 30 seconds to 2 minutes. Turn the head to side and continue (Fig. 266). Turn the head to the other side and repeat.

Fig. 268

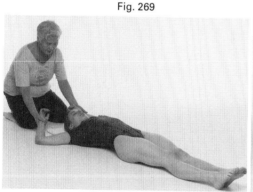

As a variation you can tap with a loosely held fist in a similar way (Figs. 267 and 268).

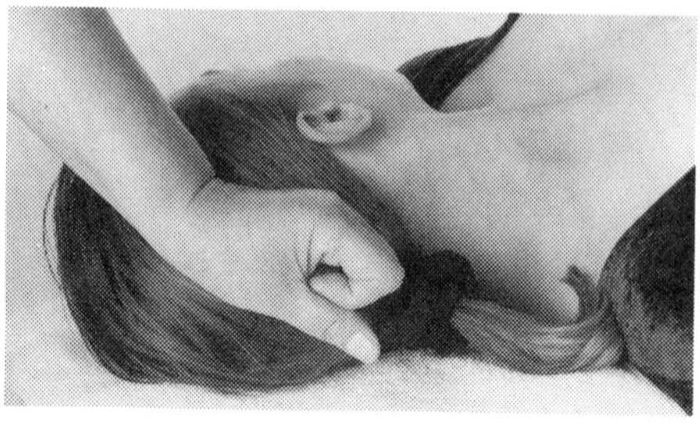

28. Overhead Body Stretch

Holding the arms at the wrist, have the receiver breathe in (Fig. 269). On an exhalation, pull the arms overhead, while the receiver pushes the heels away. The toes are pointed back toward the body (Fig. 270). Hold for a few seconds. Repeat 2 to 3 times. Release arms and gently drop them to the sides at the receiver's waist.

Fig. 269

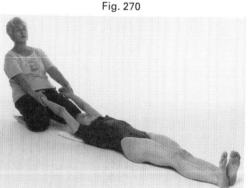

Fig. 270

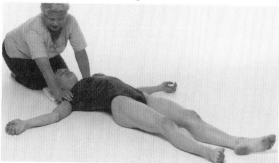

Fig. 271

29. Pushing Shoulders

Place your open palms on the receiver's shoulders and alternate pushing away right shoulder then left shoulder (Fig. 271). Shake up the whole body. Continue for 10 to 20 seconds.

Simple Seated Treatment

Shiatsu treatment can be performed in many positions. Circumstances such as pregnancy, automobile or other injuries, tumors, or recovery from operations limit the posture that the receiver may be able to assume. Lack of mobility or pain may restrict the traditional face-down position. When any such situations arise do not hesitate to do a shiatsu session in the seated position.

Generally for the first 4 to 5 months of pregnancy the expectant mother can receive shiatsu in a lying down position. But after that time the abdomen enlarges to such a degree that lying down is uncomfortable. In this case shiatsu is best administered from both seated and side positions. For this seated shiatsu the receiver can be either on the floor in a relaxed crossed legs position, or in *seiza* posture (legs folded under), or on a chair. If you use a chair position the receiver so that the back of the chair does not interfere with the treatment. The following series of techniques will loosen and stimulate the receiver to sufficiently bring about noticeable positive changes. Done at a leisurely pace these 9 techniques take approximately 10 to 20 minutes.

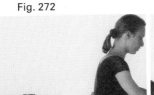

Fig. 272   Fig. 273 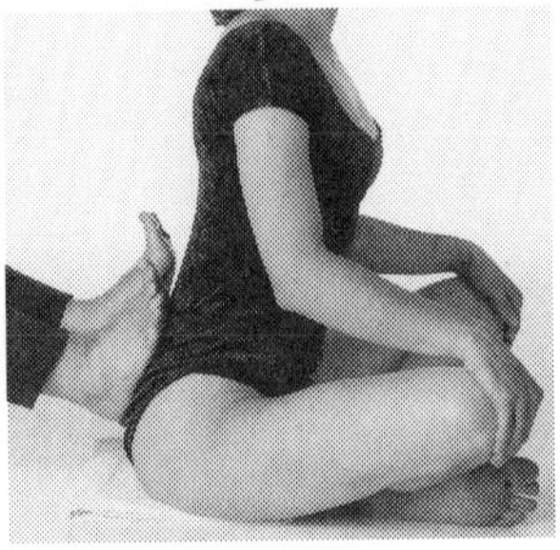   Fig. 274

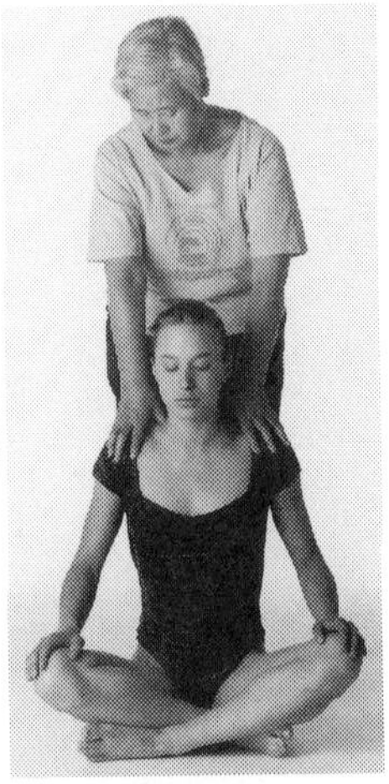

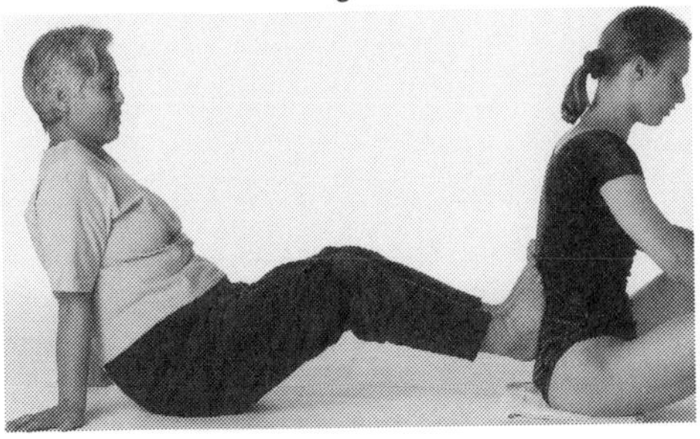

Fig. 275

1. Loosening the Back with Feet

Sit behind the receiver and place both feet firmly on the back near the hipbones (Fig. 272). Press the side of the spine with your heels and/or balls of your feet. Start at the hip and work your way up the back (Fig. 273). The hip and lower areas receive most of the treatment. This relaxes the entire body and stimulates the central and autonomic nervous systems. Continue up and down for 1 to 3 minutes.

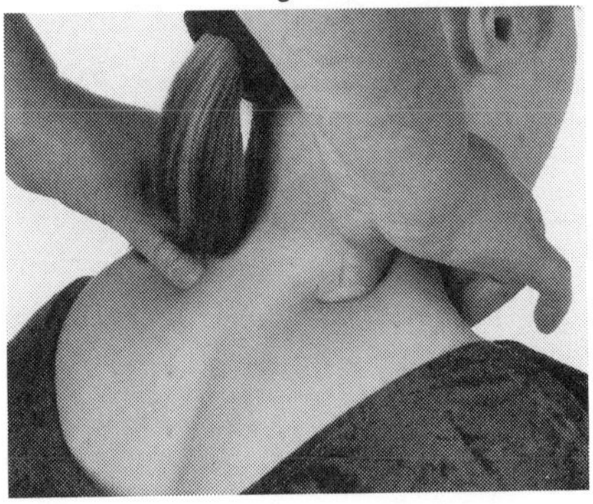

2. Pressing Shoulders

Stand in back of receiver and place palm on edge of shoulders. Alternate pressing down right side then left side (Fig. 274). Starting near the center knead the large muscles (Fig. 275). With thumbs press shoulder muscles, holding each point for several seconds (Fig. 276). Press from the neck toward the

Fig. 276

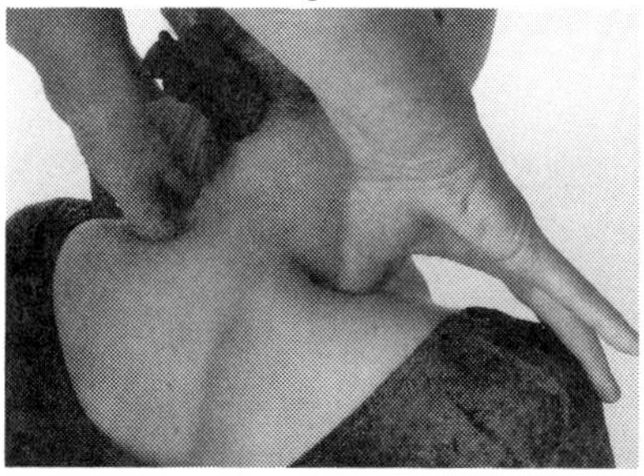

Fig. 277

Fig. 278

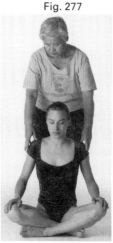

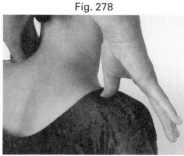

Fig. 279

shoulder tips (Figs. 277–279). If you find particularly knotted muscles hold knotted point and breathe slowly and deeply for up to 2 minutes. Maintain pressure the entire time. Move to next point. If necessary, return to difficult areas and repeat.

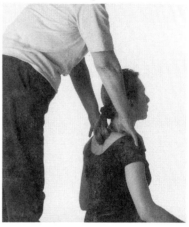

Fig. 280

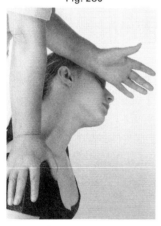

3. Stretching the Neck

Place your outside hand, with palm open and fingers outstretched, on the receiver's shoulder tip. Place your other hand with the back of the palm directly on the side of the head above the ear (Fig. 280). As the receiver exhales stretch down and away, opening the neck.

Fig. 281

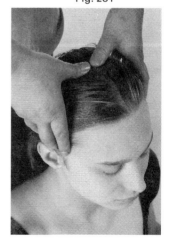

4. 100 Meeting Point

With both thumbs press 100 Meeting Point (GV 20). This is found on the midpoint of the line that connects the tips of the ears and the center of the head (Fig. 281). This point has tonic qualities and has been traditionally used for mental disorders, aftereffects of stroke, headache, dizziness, ringing in the ears, blurred vision, nasal congestion, hemorrhoids, and prolapse of the rectum.

5. Neck Press and Rotation

Sit slightly to the side of the receiver, place your left hand on the forehead, and hold. Place your right hand at the base of the neck. Press the large muscle with your thumb

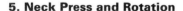

Fig. 282

Fig. 283

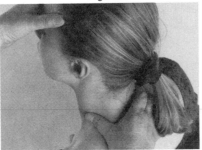

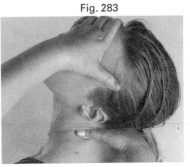

Fig. 284

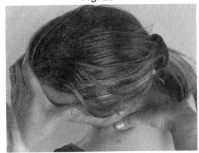

from below the ear to the bottom of the neck at the shoulder (Fig. 282). With slow deep exhalation, rotate the head in a clockwise direction (Fig. 283 and 284). Move to other side and repeat rotation in counterclockwise direction.

Fig. 285

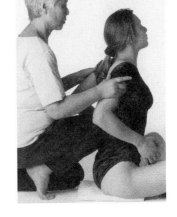

6. Rotating Shoulders

Firmly hold upper arms. Lift and rotate the shoulders in both directions (Fig. 285). First forward 3 to 4 times, then backward 3 to 4 times.

7. Releasing Tension between the Shoulder Blades

Hold elbows with receiver's palms up. Breathe in together (Fig. 286). As you both exhale pull the elbows back while the receiver's head brings her own head back (Figs. 287 and 288). Hold arms parallel with the floor until the exhalation is 80 percent complete, then let go quickly. The arms and shoulders will bounce. This technique creates a strong focus to the area between the shoulders. This is a very common site of stored chronic tension. Repeated use of this technique

Fig. 286

Fig. 287

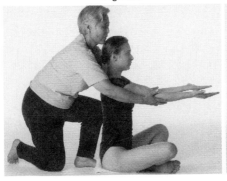

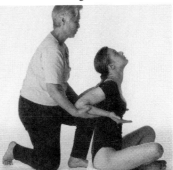

Fig. 288

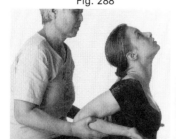

will increase circulation here and relax overly tense muscles that restrict blood and energy flow to the neck and head.

Fig. 289   Fig. 290

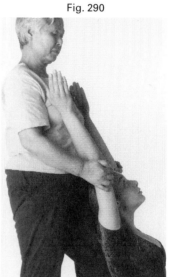

8. Overhead Stretch
Breathe in and hold the receiver's arms at elbow. Your knee is in the center of receiver's back. Lift arms over head (Fig. 289). As you both exhale, push chest open by pulling elbows toward you guiding the receiver to arch their back against your supporting knee (Fig. 290). Hold for 3 to 5 seconds. Repeat 2 to 3 times. This stretches the upper and mid-back and underarm area.

9. Spinal Twist
Have receiver open legs. The treatment giver is at the side. Put one leg between the receiver's legs. One arm goes under far shoulder. The other arm's elbow is braced against your own body for support with your closest hand placed on the receiver's shoulder blade (Fig. 291). Inhale and on the exhalation twist the body away from you (Fig. 292).

Fig. 291   Fig. 292

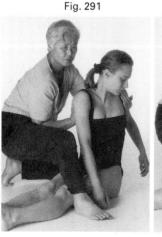
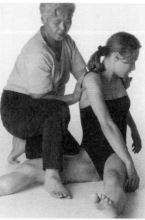

Simple Side Treatment

Treatment from the side can be used in a general session or when there are special circumstances such as pregnancy and back or neck problems. Often times the side treatment is combined with Seated Shiatsu as many similar conditions require the use of both. The following series of techniques will loosen and stimulate both the upper and lower portions of the body. Done at a leisurely pace 13 techniques take approximately 10 to 20 minutes.

Have the receiver lie on their side. Tell them to use their own hand under their head for pillow-like support. Bend the upper leg at knee with lower leg straighten but still slightly bent.

Fig. 293

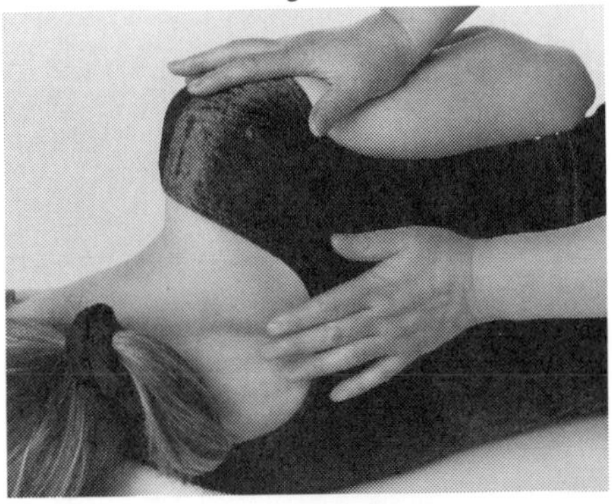

1. Loosening the Back with Hand

Sit to the receiver. Press the side of the spine with your left hand (Fig. 293). Start below the neck and work your way down the back (Fig. 294). This relaxes the entire body and stimulates the central and autonomic nervous systems. Continue up and down 1 to 3 times.

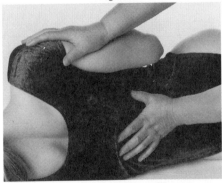

2. Pressing the Head

Hold temple point with thumb for several seconds. Release and press several times more (Fig. 295). This point calms and relaxes the body. It is also good for headache and eye problems.

Fig. 294

3. Pressing the Neck

Press below the ear to the base of neck along large muscle with thumb (Fig. 296 and 297). Hold each point along the line for 2 to 5 seconds.

Fig. 295

Fig. 296

Fig. 297

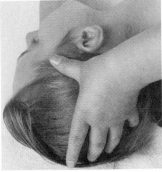
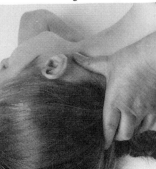
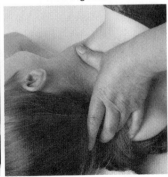

Fig. 298

Fig. 299

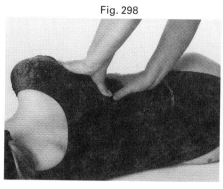

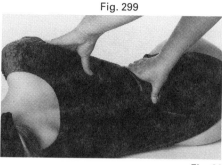

Fig. 300

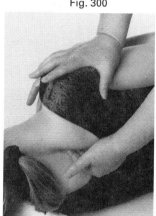

4. Two Hand Rib Press

Place upper hand near shoulder blade with the other hand next to it, thumbs almost touching (Fig. 298). Press along side near spine with lower thumb moving down toward waist (Fig. 299). Hold each point for 2 to 5 seconds.

5. Cleaning under Shoulder Blade

Place fingertips along contour of shoulder blade and press (Fig. 300). Try to dig under shoulder blade.

6. Upper Arm Press and Rotation

Firmly hold upper arm and elbow. Press and rotate the shoulder (Figs. 301 and 302). This releases tension in neck, shoulder joint, and shoulder blade.

Fig. 301

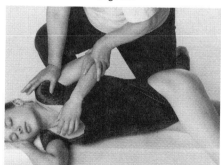

7. Shoulder/Arm Stretch

Firmly hold upper arm and elbow. Press your upper hand up and lower hand down, stretching the arm and shoulder (Fig. 303).

8. Kneading Arm

Press and squeeze along upper arm with whole

Fig. 303

Fig. 302

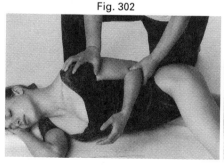

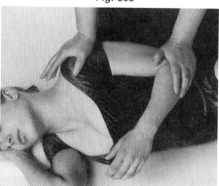

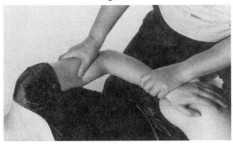

Fig. 304

hand and thumb (Fig. 304). Hold each point along line for 2 to 5 seconds. You can also briskly rub up and down along area.

9. Holding Elbow Point

Locate point at midway of bend in elbow. When the elbow is flexed, the point is in the depression at the end of the crease. Hold point with one hand as you move other hand, using the elbow joint (Fig. 305). This

action increases stimulation. Hold for 5 to 10 seconds. Large Intestine 11 literally means curved pond (known as *Kyoku-Chi* in Japanese and *Quchi* in Chinese). Clinical uses include: headache, hypertension, diarrhea, rashes, hemorrhoids, sore throat, vomiting, abdominal pain, pain and paralysis of upper extremities, and tennis elbow. Its major use has been to discharge excess heat from the body.

Fig. 305

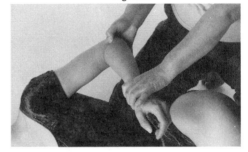

Fig. 306

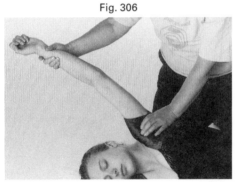

10. Inner Arm Press and Stretch

Lift arm over head. With your inner hand press underarm and armpit (Fig. 306).

11. Hip and Thigh Press

Squeeze and press with open palm from hip to knee, stimulating the large thigh muscle (Figs. 307 and 308).

Fig. 307

Fig. 308

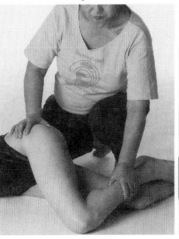
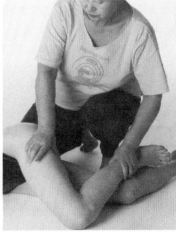

12. Arm Pull

Stand behind the receiver and hold hand and wrist. Breathe in and on exhalation pull the arm toward you (Fig. 309). Release quickly. This bounces the body and relaxes it.

Fig. 309

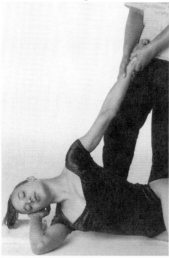

13. Spinal Twist

This is an optional technique. Only attempt this technique if you have experience and confidence in your abilities.

Fig. 310

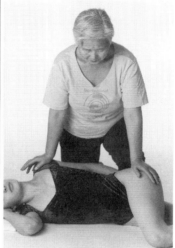

Place one hand on the receiver's shoulder with other hand on hip. Brace one knee on back of hip. Inhale and as you exhale press the shoulder back while you press hip with knee and hand forward (Fig. 310). Release immediately. This action twists the body and releases spinal tension. Sometimes there is a cracking sound.

Treating the Head

Fig. 311

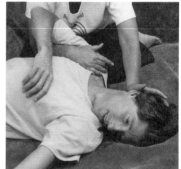

1. Side Neck Stretch

Receiver is lying face up. Practitioner on side uses supporting arm to brace body by reaching underarm and hold shoulder. Practitioner places open palm on base of receiver's neck. On an exhalation practitioner pushes with active hand and pulls shoulder with other hand, stretching and opening neck (Fig. 311). Move to other side and repeat.

2. Lifting Head

Move to behind the receiver. Pick up head. Exhale and lift head so that chin touches chest (Fig. 312).

Fig. 312

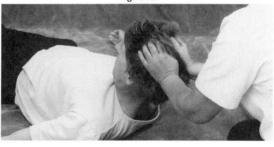

Fig. 313

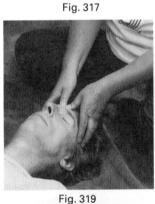

3. Rotating Head

Hold head and rotate in circular movement (Fig. 313). Rotate in both directions.

Fig. 314   Fig. 315

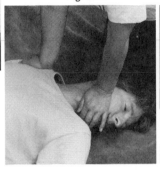   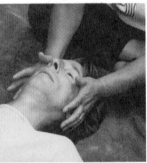

4. Simple Neck Stretch

Practitioner kneels and places one hand on shoulder with fingers pointing away from body. Opposite hand rests on jaw. Exhale and press down, stretching neck (Fig. 314).

5. Holding Temple

Concentrate on thumbs and press temple (Fig. 315). Send your energy through your hands.

Fig. 316

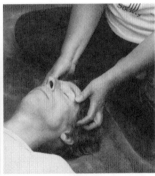

Fig. 317   Fig. 318

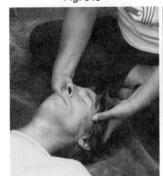

6. Pressing Neck with Thumb

Press neck area below ear to shoulder on large muscle (Fig. 316). Repeat 3 to 5 times.

7. Stimulating Eyes

With thumbs press bony rim above eyes (Fig. 317). Continue pressing until outer rim (Fig. 318). Press temple area with thumbs (Fig. 319). Place tip of index finger on solid rim near inner corner of eyes and press (Fig. 320). Hold for 2 to 5 seconds. Repeat 3 to 5 times.

Fig. 319   Fig. 320

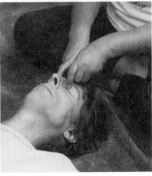

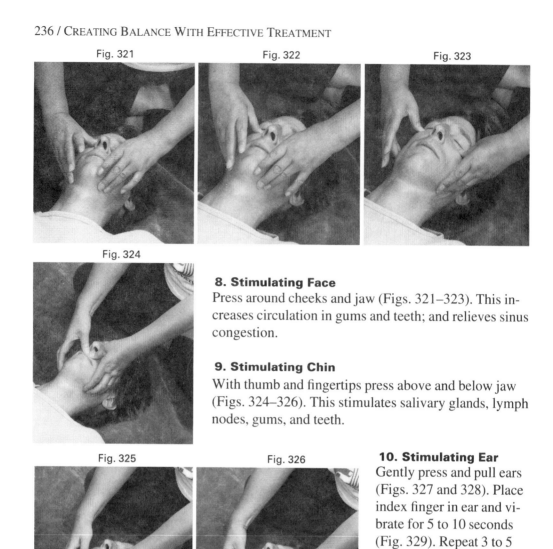

Fig. 321   Fig. 322   Fig. 323

Fig. 324

8. Stimulating Face
Press around cheeks and jaw (Figs. 321–323). This increases circulation in gums and teeth; and relieves sinus congestion.

9. Stimulating Chin
With thumb and fingertips press above and below jaw (Figs. 324–326). This stimulates salivary glands, lymph nodes, gums, and teeth.

Fig. 325   Fig. 326

10. Stimulating Ear
Gently press and pull ears (Figs. 327 and 328). Place index finger in ear and vibrate for 5 to 10 seconds (Fig. 329). Repeat 3 to 5 times.

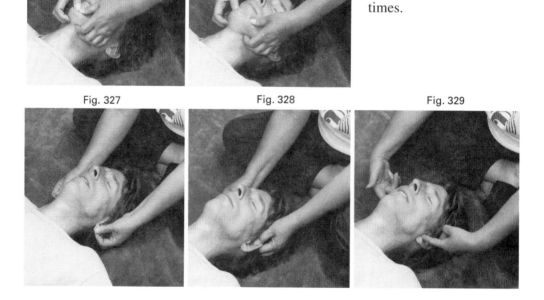

Fig. 327   Fig. 328   Fig. 329

Fig. 330

Fig. 331

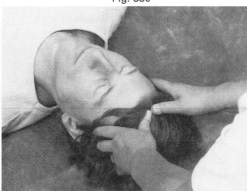

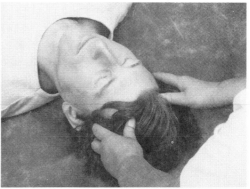

Fig. 332

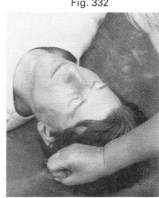

11. Pressing Top of Head
Press all over top of head with thumbs (Figs. 330 and 331). Hold each point for 1 to 3 seconds. Repeat as many times as you feel it is necessary. This relaxes whole body and balances nervous system.

12. Tapping Head
Turn the receiver's head to side. Make a fist and gently

Fig. 333

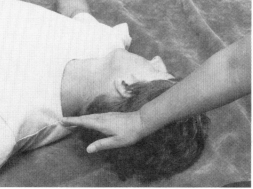

Fig. 334

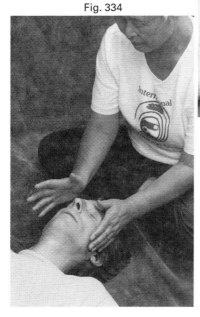

tap same side and top of head (Fig. 332). Reach across with opposite hand to tap. Turn head to other side, switch hands, and continue tapping. Tap with side of open hand (Fig. 333). Do both sides.

13. Waking up Face
Gently slap face with open palms (Fig. 334). This increases blood circulation and makes more youthful skin.

Treating the Foundation—The Hips and Spine

The physical position of the hipbones makes them extremely important in the mainte-nance of overall well-being. The bones that make up the hips support the rest of the body's bony structure. This in turn supports and protects the internal organs, muscles, nerves, and blood and lymph vessels. Internal function as well as physical movement is dependent on the positioning of the hips.

The spine extends from the hips and is supported by the hip. If the hip is off-centered, the spine will adjust to compensate and also be off-centered. The spine is like a central pole that in turn supports the same organs and functions mentioned earlier. The efficient functioning of the entire body, to one degree or another, is dependent on the position and support of the hips and spine combined. At the top of the spine rests the skull and brain. Can you imagine the influence the hips and spine have on the brain, thinking, and consciousness?

The relative balance of the body's seven main energy distribution centers—*chakra*—relies on the stability of the physical structure, namely the hips and spine. Any out of balance position influences the *chakra* system. The effects of gravity and long-term physical condition can be seen by viewing the hips and spine. If one bone is in a wrong position, the whole system suffers. The spine and hips are very important. If you loosen up the spine you can achieve a tremendous positive effect on the nervous system and on a person's mechanical and structural balance. The following exercise treatments are designed to positively effect the hips and spine. They are divided into four different positions: standing, seated, and lying down both face up and down. Each affects the hips and spine in a different way. In your recommenda-tions to patients, you can choose the ones you feel appropriate. For many people the entire series is beneficial.

Standing

1. Crossed Leg Walk
Cross one leg over the other as the arms and elbows move in opposite directions (Fig. 335). Quickly walk forward, alternating from side to side (Fig. 336).
Focus: Loosens spine, espe-cially middle part.

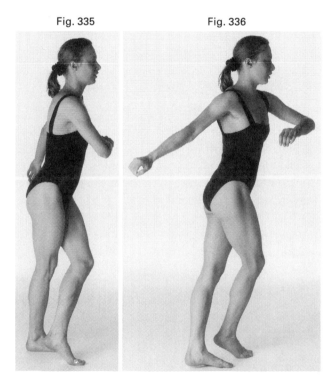

Fig. 335   Fig. 336

2. Over the Shoulder Twist

With one arm and elbow up at shoulder height and the other low at waist height, twist from side to side (Figs. 337 and 338).
Focus: Loosens spine, especially middle to upper portions.

Fig. 337

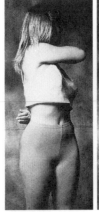

Fig. 338

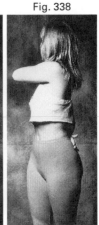

3. Upper Torso Twist

Hold a pole across the top of the shoulders (Fig. 339). Lean to one side as you exhale (Fig. 340). Inhale and lean to opposite side as you exhale (Fig. 341). Repeat 5 to 10 times. Return to beginning posture and turn

Fig. 339

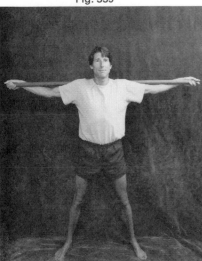

Fig. 340

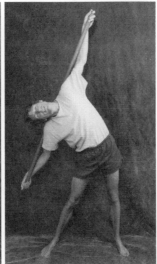

to one side as you exhale, fully stretching the spine (Fig. 342). Do the same movement on opposite side. Repeat 5 to 10 times.
Focus: Loosens spine and hips, relaxes and stretches side muscles.

Fig. 341

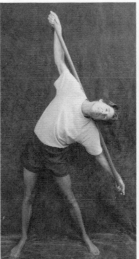

Fig. 342

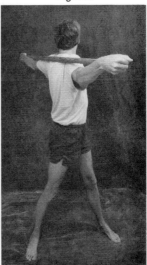

Fig. 343

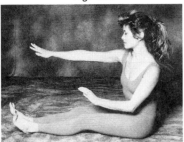

Fig. 344

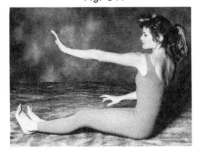

Seated

4. Scooting Forward and Backward

With arms and legs outstretched in front, scoot one hip forward. At the same time the arm and leg on the same side moves forward. Continue scooting forward alternating both sides (Figs. 343 and 344). After 10 to 15 scoots, scoot backward and return to beginning position. For variation, move to the side.

Focus: Loosens hips and lower spine.

Fig. 345

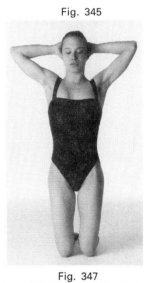

5. Hip Up and Down

Interlock hands behind head and kneel with your hips raised up (Fig. 345). Sit to one side (Fig. 346). Return to starting position and sit to other side (Fig. 347). Inhale as you return to beginning position and exhale as you sit down. Continue going from side to side for 5 to 10 times. If you have a curvature of the spine (scoliosis) repeat the difficult side many times daily. For variation, arriving at seated position twist the upper torso inward.

Focus: Whole spine and hips.

Fig. 346   Fig. 347

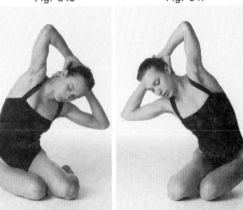

Lying Down—Face Up

6. Shaking Spine

Lie on back resting arms at your sides with palms up. Use your hips to shake spine and body (Fig. 348)

Focus: Loosens whole spine.

Fig. 348

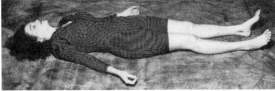

7. Hip Up and Down

Place interlocked fingers behind your head. Bend your knees (Fig. 349). Inhale, hold your breath, and

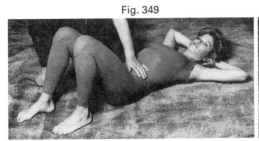

Fig. 349

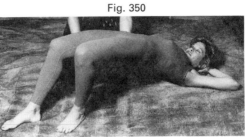

Fig. 350

lift hips up as you exhale (Fig. 350). Hold for 3 to 5 seconds. Repeat 5 to 10 times. For variation, doing same technique, at the end of hip up let the hips drop to the floor. This pounding stimulates the base of the spine and loosens hip joints.
Focus: Lower spine.

8. Spine Bend
Stretch heel out, hands behind head, exhale, and bend to one side (Fig. 351).
Focus: Upper spine.

Fig. 351

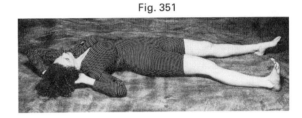

Fig. 352

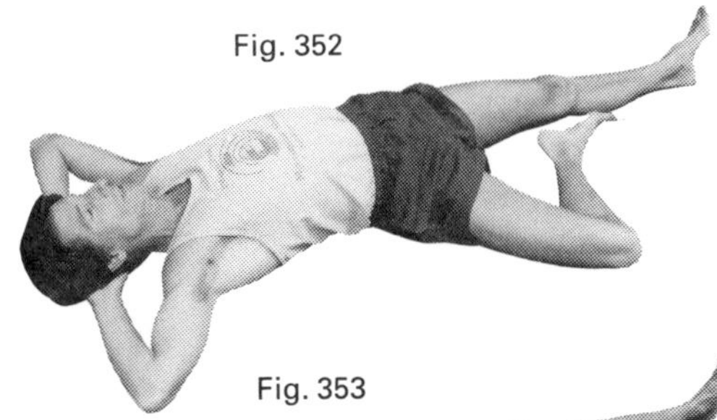

Fig. 353

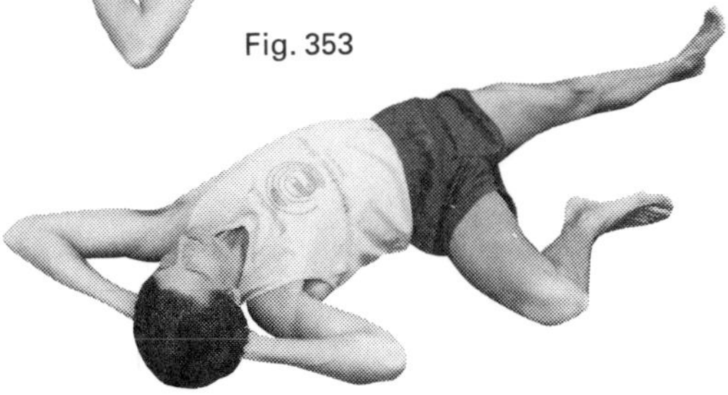

9. Side Stretch
Lie on your back with hands clasped together behind your head. Extend your left leg and stretch out your heel by pulling your toes back. Bend your right knee and place your right foot near your groin area (Fig. 352). Exhale as you stretch your right knee up toward the head and you bend your head toward the knee trying to make the two meet (Fig. 353). Relax and repeat this side 3 to 5 times. Reverse body position and do other side.
Focus: Neck and upper and lower spine.

Fig. 354

Fig. 355

10. Rocking
Grab knees, push heels away (Fig. 354), and try to sit up (Fig. 355).
Focus: Whole spine.

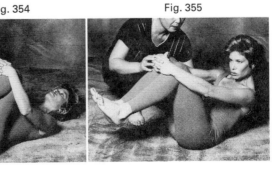

Fig. 356

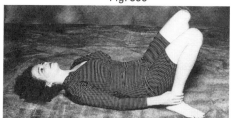

11. Hip Joint Stretch

Lying on your back grasp your ankles (Fig. 356). Bend your right knee inward as you exhale (Fig. 357). Alternate with left knee (Fig. 358). Repeat 3 to 5 times.
Focus: Lower spine.

Fig. 357

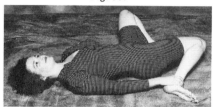

Fig. 358

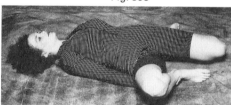

12. Leg Lift

Lift legs up 1 inch (Fig. 359). Hold long enough to feel tension in your lower abdomen. Repeat 5 to 10 times. Rest when tired. Gradually open legs with following lifts (Fig. 360). For variation, bicycle or shake side to side.
Focus: Legs together—center of spine; legs open—low spine.

Fig. 359

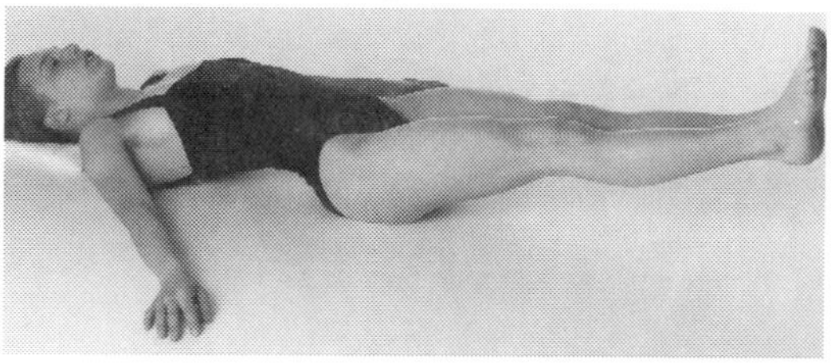

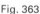

Fig. 360

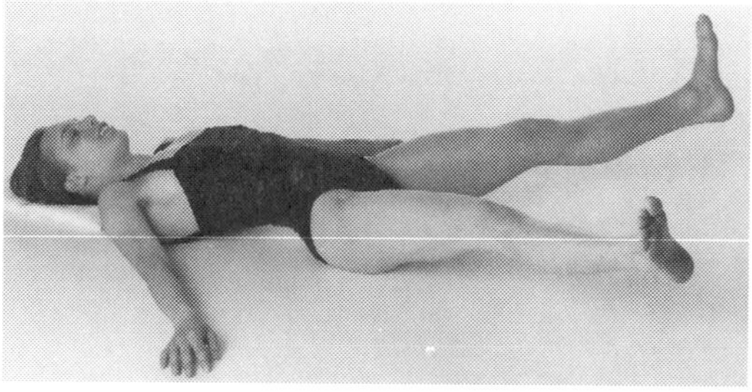

13. Hip Side to Side I

Keep heels and feet together, bend

Fig. 361

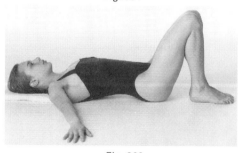

knees, and hold floor with palms down (Fig. 361). Allow knees to move to one side (Fig. 362). Bring up and move to opposite side (Fig. 363). Repeat 5 to 10 times.
Focus: Middle of the spine.

Fig. 362

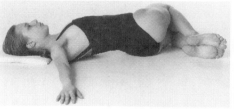

Fig. 363

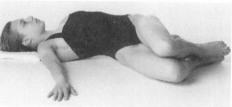

Fig. 364

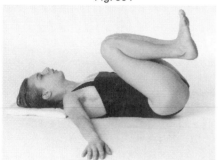

14. Hip Side to Side II

Keep heels and feet together, bend knees deeply, and hold floor with palms down (Fig. 364). Allow knees to move to one side (Fig. 365). Bring up and move to opposite side (Fig. 366). Repeat 5 to 10 times.
Focus: Middle and upper spine.

Fig. 365

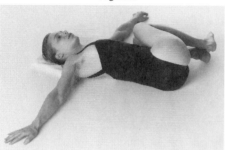

Fig. 366

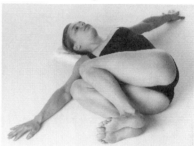

Fig. 367

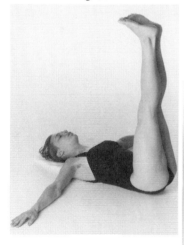

Fig. 368

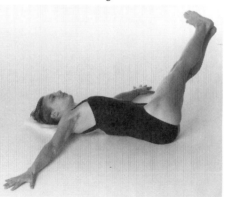

Fig. 369

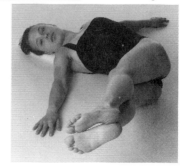

15. Abdominal Power

Keep heels and feet together, extend legs up, and hold floor with palms down (Fig. 367). Allow legs to move to one side almost touching floor (Fig. 368). Return to beginning position and let legs drop to opposite side (Fig. 369). Repeat 3 to 10 times.
Focus: Whole spine and abdominal muscles.

Lying Down—Face Down

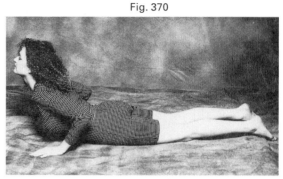

Fig. 370

16. Spinal Cobra

Push up into the cobra posture (Fig. 370). Inhale and as you exhale twist to one side by looking over your shoulder (Fig. 371). Twist and look to other side. Repeat 3 to 10 times.

Focus: Hip and upper spine.

Fig. 371

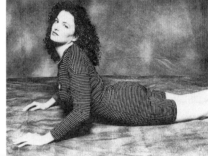

17. Spinal Cat

Start with all fours on floor. Bend toes in, go forward with hands, and stretch out arms and chest. You can bounce your chest trying to touch the floor (Fig. 372). Hold for 15 to 60 seconds. Repeat 2 to 3 times.

Focus: Progressively the lower, middle, and upper spine.

Fig. 372

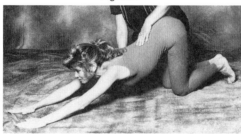

18. Baby Crawling

Lie on floor. Bend your elbows, hand under chin. Use your elbow to crawl forward. Move your hips side to side (Figs. 373 and 374).

Focus: Whole spine, especially middle and upper portions.

Fig. 373

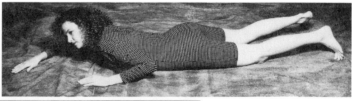

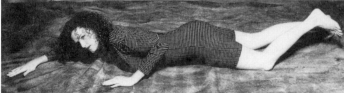

Fig. 374

19. Infant Crawling

Get on all fours. Crawl forward using hands and knees (Fig. 375)
Focus: Whole spine.

Fig. 375

Fig. 376

Fig. 377

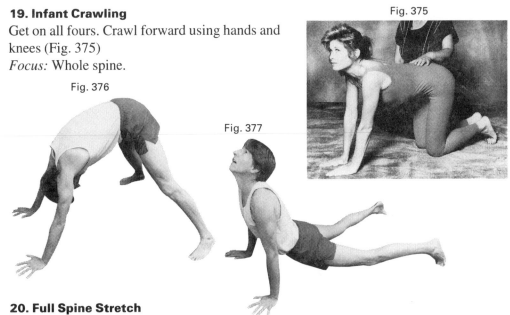

20. Full Spine Stretch

Stand with legs spread one and a half times waist width, feet parallel to each other. Slowly bend forward, keeping the knees straight. Place your hands on the floor with fingers spread apart, pointing forward. The arms should be straight and stretched out as far as possible in front of the shoulders (Fig. 376). Inhale and as you exhale lower the hips near to the floor arching the head and upper torso up and back (Fig. 377). Keep the arms straight. Repeat this procedure 3 times.

Treating the Hands and Feet

The yin and yang relationship of Oriental medicine is fascinating. The energetic and diagnostic systems of old that continue to the present day exhibit many examples of what at first glance appear to be unrelated connections. The effect of treating the hands and feet is one of the best examples of these not-so-obvious connections. The inner-outer relationship explains why treatment on these areas can be so powerful. This principle states that what exists on the inside shows itself on the outside; the more deep inside the source, the more peripheral outside will be the effect. What this means is that treating the hands and feet stimulates the deep aspects of the internal organs in a direct way.

Fig. 378

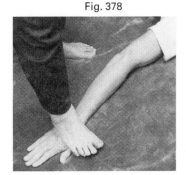

Treatment for Hands and Arms

1. Walking on Hand

Receiver lies face down. Press the back of the hand with your foot (Fig. 378).

Fig. 379   Fig. 380   Fig. 381

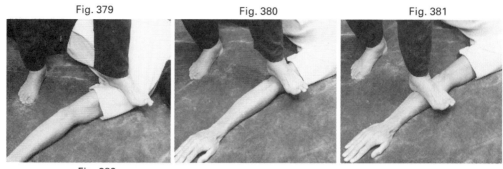

Fig. 382

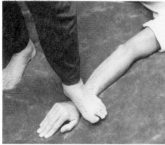

2. Upper Arm Press

Press the upper part of the arm with your inside foot beginning at the shoulder joint (Fig. 379). Continue pressing the length of the arm (Figs. 380–382).

Fig. 383

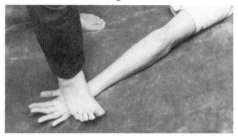

3. Palm Press with Foot

Turn hand palm up and press with foot (Fig. 383).

Fig. 384   Fig. 385   Fig. 386

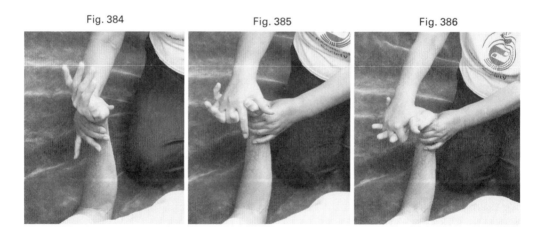

4. Loosening Hand

Receiver turns over and is face up. Hold wrist with your hand and shake back and forth (Fig. 384).

5. Stretching Fingers

Interlace your fingers between receiver's fingers and stretch backward (Figs. 385 and 386).

6. Squeezing Hand

Firmly hold receiver's hand with both of your hands and squeeze (Fig. 387).

7. Pressing Top of Hand

With your thumbs press the top of receiver's hand vigorously (Fig. 388)

Fig. 387

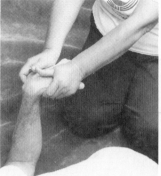

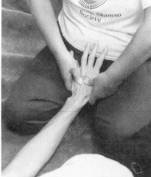
Fig. 388

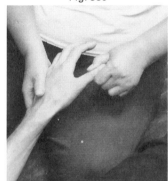
Fig. 389

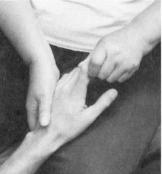
Fig. 390

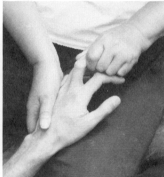
Fig. 391

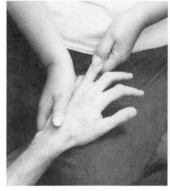
Fig. 392

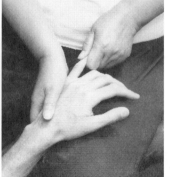
Fig. 393

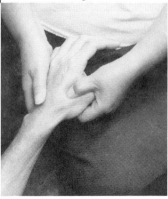
Fig. 394

8. Manipulating Fingers

Press each of the receiver's fingers firmly. Stimulate top and bottom, and side to side. Move from base of finger to end several times (Figs. 389–393).

9. Large Intestine Point

With your thumb press Large Intestine 4 point (Fig. 394). Hold for 3 to 5 seconds and release. Repeat 5 to 10 times.

10. Palm Press

With receiver's palm up, insert your little finger between the last fingers at both ends of receiver's hand (Fig. 395). With thumbs press the center and periphery of open palm (Fig. 396).

Fig. 395

Fig. 396

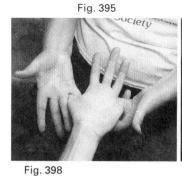

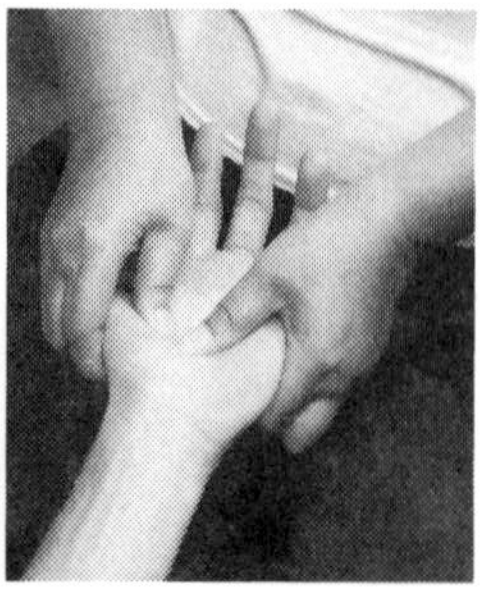

Fig. 397

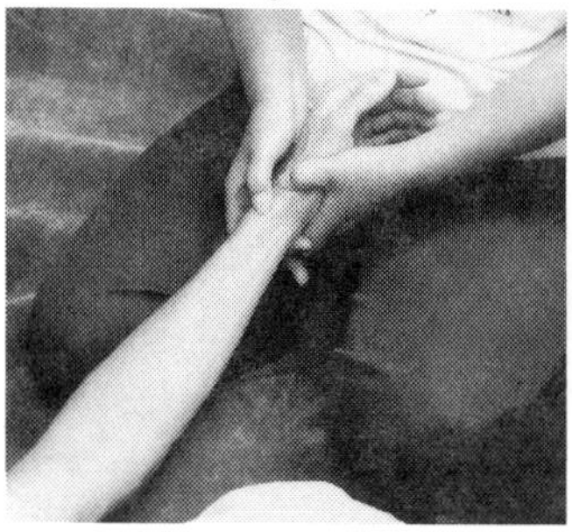

Fig. 398

Fig. 399

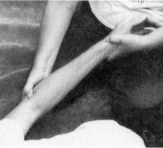

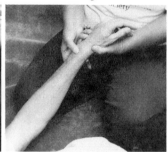

Fig. 400

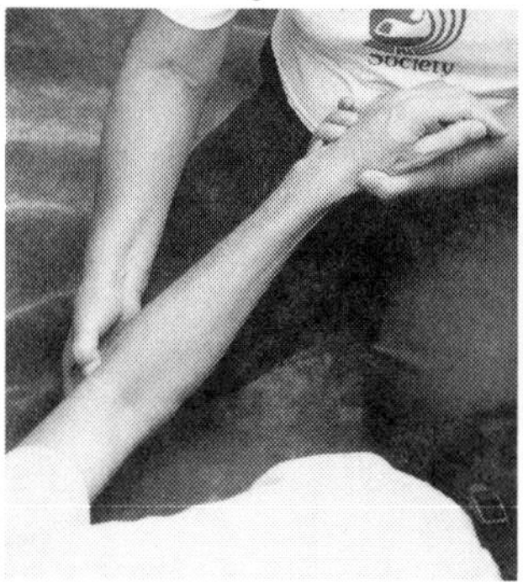

Fig. 401

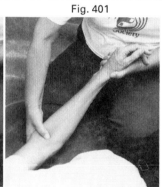

11. Lower Arm Press

Hold receiver's wrist like a handshake with your left hand. Press from wrist to elbow with the thumb of your right hand on top of bone (Figs. 397 and 398). Turn palm down and press the outside of forearm from wrist to elbow (Figs. 399 and 400). Finally press the inside of forearm from wrist to elbow (Fig. 401).

12. Upper Arm Press

Reach and grab shoulder muscle. Press down with thumb outside of the upper arm to elbow (Figs. 402 and 403).

Reach inside and press in armpit. Press down the inside of the upper arm to elbow (Figs. 404 and 405). Reach to top of shoulder and press on top ridge to inside elbow (Figs. 406 and 407). Repeat each of the three lines several times.

Fig. 403

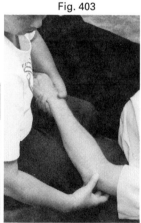

Fig.402

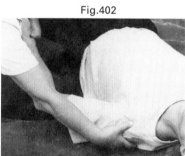

Fig. 404

Fig. 405

Fig. 406

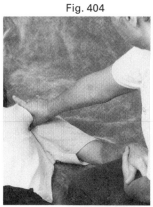

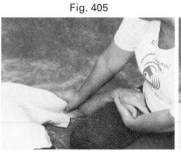

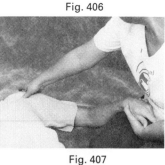

Fig. 407

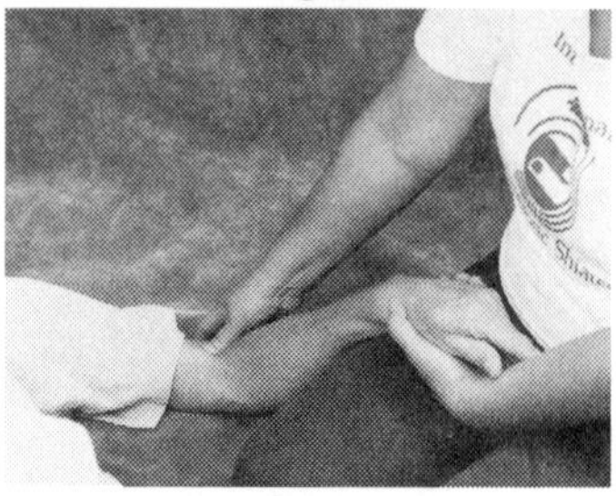

Fig. 408

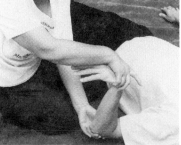

Fig. 409

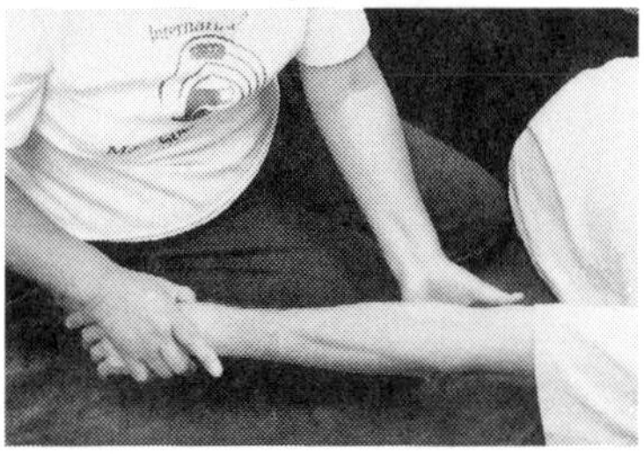

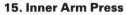

13. Arm Adjustment

Sit between outstretched arm and torso. Pick up receiver's hand at wrist with palm down with your right hand. Your left hand should support the elbow from underneath. Bend the elbow by bringing the hand closer to the body (Fig. 408). Gently pull hand outward with a one, two, three pumping action. On three straighten arm (Fig. 409).

Fig. 410

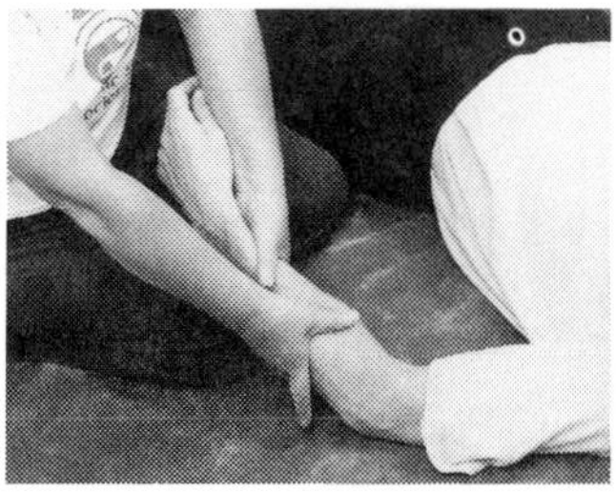

Fig. 411

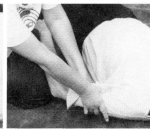

14. Squeezing Arm

Reach up with both hands and squeeze receiver's upper arm. Continue squeezing as you come down to the wrist (Figs. 410 and 411).

Fig. 412

15. Inner Arm Press

With your open palm press the receiver's arm from the shoulder down to the wrist (Fig. 412). Repeat this routine several times.

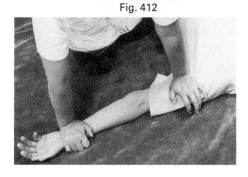

Repeat above all techniques on other side.

Treatment for Feet and Legs

Fig. 413

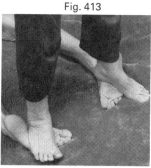

16. Walking on Feet

Receiver is face down. With your toes on the floor use middle and heel part of your foot to press the bottoms of the receiver's feet (Fig. 413). Alternate your weight from side to side.

17. Ankle Stretch

With closest foot catch receiver's heel and stretch out (Fig. 414). Do not hold more than 1 second.

Fig. 414

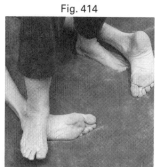

Fig. 415

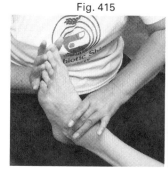

Fig. 416

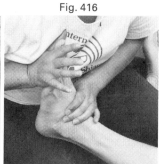

Fig. 417

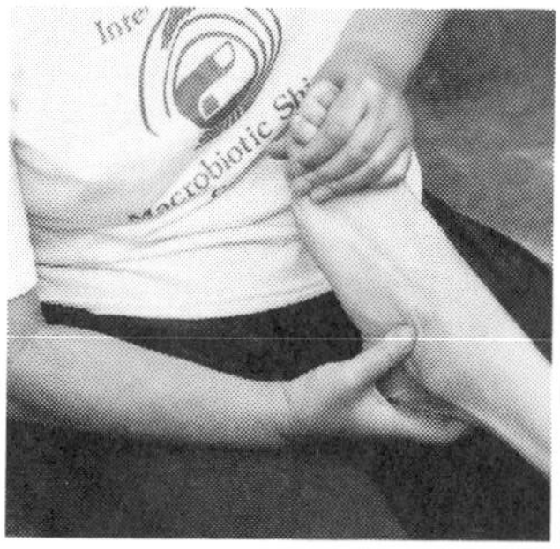

Fig. 418

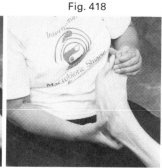

Fig. 419

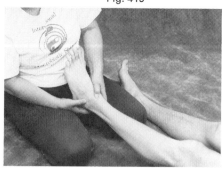

18. Stretching Ankle with Hand

Support ankle with one hand while you grab toes with other (Fig. 415). Stretch toes toward body, stretching ankle (Fig. 416).

19. Outside Ankle Press

Press around ankle with thumb (Fig. 417 and 418).

20. Lower Leg Press

Press up center of leg and end up at Stomach 36 (Figs. 419–421). Press outside of leg from ankle to knee (Figs. 422–424). Finally press inside of leg from ankle to knee (Figs. 425–427).

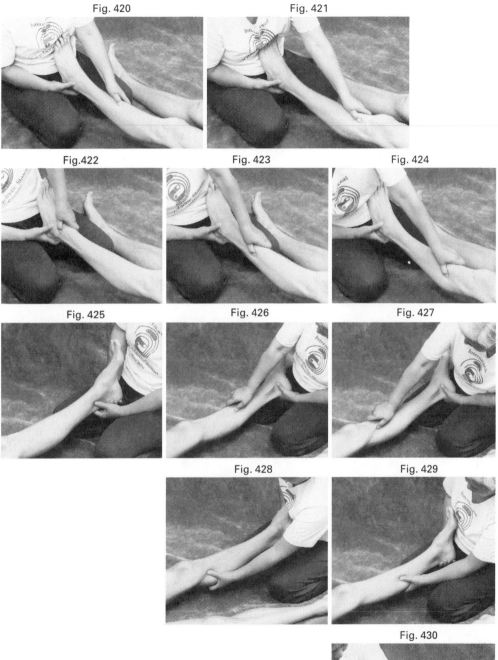

Fig. 420   Fig. 421

Fig.422   Fig. 423   Fig. 424

Fig. 425   Fig. 426   Fig. 427

Fig. 428   Fig. 429

Fig. 430

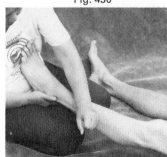

21. Squeezing Calf

Grab calf muscle and squeeze (Fig. 428). Move hand
down leg and squeeze along the way (Fig. 429).

22. Pounding Outside of Leg

Make a fist and lightly pound on the outside of the leg
(Fig. 430). Move from knee down to ankle. Repeat 3 to
5 times.

23. Bending Toes
Place one hand directly on receiver's toes supporting at heel with other. Bend forward and backward (Figs. 431 and 432). Do this 3 to 5 times.

Fig. 431

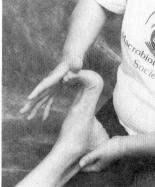

Fig.432

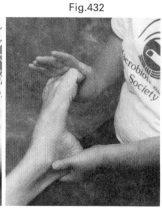

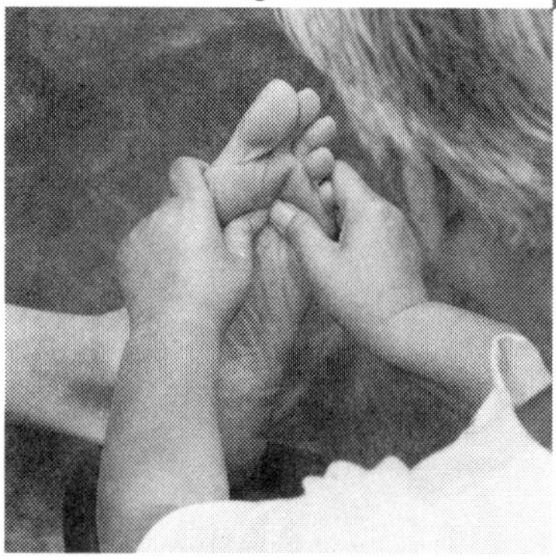

Fig. 433

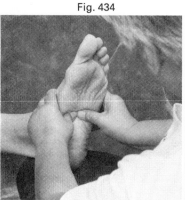

24. Pressing Bottom of Foot
Press the bottom of foot with your thumbs. Follow 3 lines from toes to heel (Figs. 433 and 434).

25. Pounding Bottom of Foot
With a fist pound the bottom of foot (Fig. 435). Continue for 5 to 15 seconds.

Fig. 434

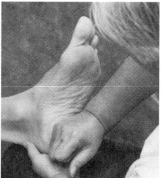

Fig. 435

Fig. 436

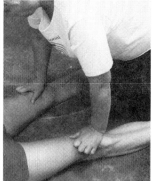

Fig. 437

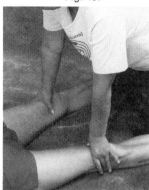

26. Rotating Kneecaps
Place your hands firmly on kneecaps and rotate in a circular direction (Fig. 436).

27. Pressing and Squeezing Thigh
Open hands and place directly above kneecaps. Squeeze thumb and fingers together and lift (Fig. 437). Move hands up thighs repeating this process. Press upper thighs with open palm (Figs. 438 and 439).

Fig. 438

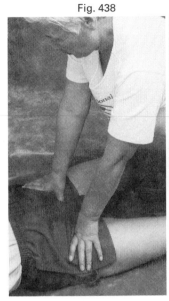

Fig. 439

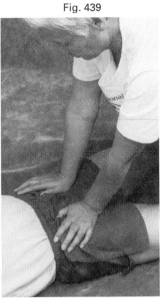

Fig. 440

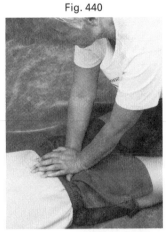

Fig. 441

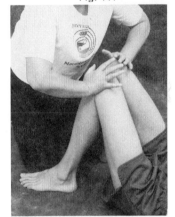

28. Low Abdominal Breathing
Place one hand on the other hand with palms down on lower abdomen. Ask receiver to breathe in. Receiver's belly should rise. On an exhalation gently press down and slightly up toward umbilicus (Fig. 440). Repeat 3 to 5 times.

29. Outward Leg Resistance
Bend receiver's legs so that knees are up. Place your hands on the outside of knees. Ask receiver to breathe in. On an exhalation receiver tries to separate knees while you hold them together creating resistance (Fig. 441). Resistance is maintained only for the length of one exhalation. Repeat up to 10 times.

Fig.442

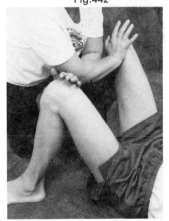

30. Inward Leg Resistance
Place your hands on the inside of receiver's knees. Ask receiver to breathe in. On an exhalation receiver tries to bring knees together while you hold them apart creating resistance (Fig. 442). Resistance is maintained only for the length of one exhalation. Repeat up to 10 times.

Special Arm and Leg Points

Source Points
Each of the twelve regular meridians has a Source point in the extremities where the original Ki is retained. In the yang meridians of traditional Oriental medicine, the

Source points coincide with the Stream points. The Source points are of great significance in diagnosis and treatment of diseases of the meridians and the internal organs.

Connecting Points

Each of the twelve regular meridians has a collateral in the extremities connecting a definite pair of yin and yang meridians which are externally and internally related. For example there is a pathway that connects the Lung meridian with the Large Intestine meridian. A Connecting point is used to treat diseases that involve either of the two related meridians and also diseases in the area supplied by the two meridians.

Accumulating Points

The Accumulating point is the site where the Ki of the meridian is deeply converged. Each of the twelve regular meridians has an Accumulating point. The Accumulating points are used in treating acute disorders and pain in the areas supplied by their respective pathways and those in their respective organs.

Energy Flow

Along each of the twelve regular meridians, below the elbow or knee, lie five specific points. They are Well, Spring, Stream, River, and Sea points. They are arranged in the above order from the distal ends of the limbs to the elbow or knee. These names have traditionally brought to mind the image of flowing energy along the meridian, much like the movement of water.

- The Well point is the location where the energy (Ki) of the meridians starts to bubble.
- The Spring point is the location where the Ki of the meridian starts to flourish.
- The Stream point is the location where the Ki of the meridian flourishes.
- The River point is the location where the Ki of the meridian increases in abundance.
- The Sea point represents the confluence of rivers in the sea, where the Ki of the meridian is the most flourishing.

Relationship of Points and Meridians

The treatment of hands, arms, feet, and legs stimulates all the points located in these areas. In general, each meridian has an effect on a particular part of the body, while the combination of meridians, such as the three located on the inner arm, have another effect. The following explains these relationships.

The three yin meridians of the hand:
- The Lung meridian treats disorders of the lungs and throat.
- The Heart meridian treats disorders of the heart.
- The Heart Governor meridian treats disorders of the heart and stomach.
- The three combined treat disorders of the chest and mental illness.

The three yang meridians of the hand:
- The Large Intestine meridian treats disorders of the face, nose, mouth, and teeth.
- The Small Intestine meridian treats disorders of the neck, ear, and shoulder blade region.
- The Triple Heater meridian treats disorders of the ear, temple, and abdomen.
- The three combined treat disorders of the head, eyes, and throat, and febrile and mental diseases.

The three yin meridians of the foot:
- The Spleen meridian treats disorders of the spleen, stomach, and intestines.
- The Kidney meridian treats disorders of the kidneys, intestines, lungs, and throat.
- The Liver meridian treats disorders of the liver and external sexual organs.
- The three combined treat disorders of the abdomen and urogenital organs.

The three yang meridians of the foot:
- The Stomach meridian treats disorders of the face, mouth, teeth, throat, stomach, and intestines.
- The Bladder meridian treats disorders of the neck, eyes, and low back region.
- The Gallbladder meridian treats disorders of the eyes, ear, temple, and abdomen.
- The three combined treat disorders of the head, and febrile and mental illnesses.

Special Neck Treatment

The neck is the bridge between the body and the central computer—the brain. Treatment to loosen stiff muscles and joints is useful. If the receiver is experiencing stiffness, a limitation in motion or tenderness in the upper back or neck these techniques can be used. They relax muscles, increase blood supply to the area, and often adjust spinal corrections. However, if the receiver complains of extreme pain (before or during treatment) or has an extreme traumatic injury, see a professional. Do not attempt stretches.

1. Rubbing Neck
With inside of index fingers gently rub side of neck (Fig. 443). Continue for 10 to 20 seconds.

2. Shoulder Press
Place forearms on shoulder near neck and lean your body weight into it (Fig. 444). Hold for 5 to 10 seconds. Repeat 3 to 5 times.

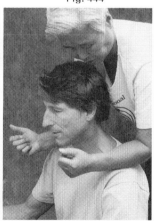

Fig. 443   Fig. 444

Fig. 445

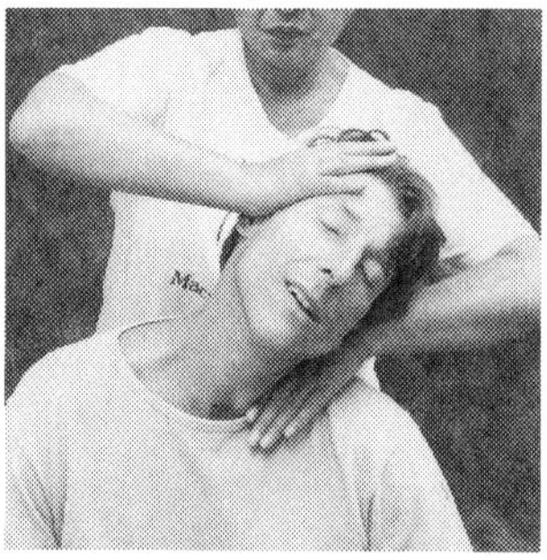

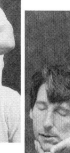

3. Side Neck Stretch

Place left hand at base of receiver's neck, with thumb on back side and other fingers in front. Place right hand on opposite side of head above the ear. Inhale and as you exhale push the hands toward each other (Fig. 445). Your left hand is moving from left to right while your right hand is moving from right to left. Gently take the head until you feel resistance then quickly take it a bit further and release immediately. Do only once. Repeat on other side (Fig. 446).

Fig. 446

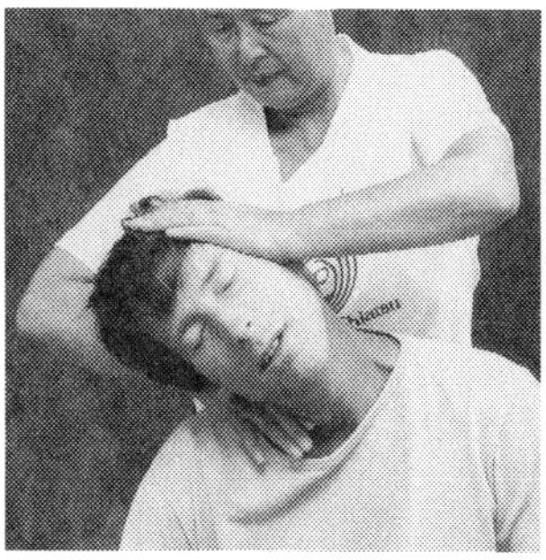

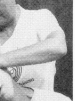

Fig. 447

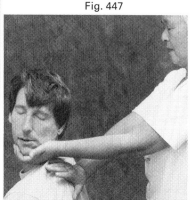

Fig. 448

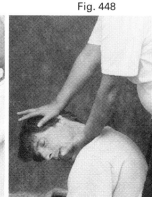

Fig. 449

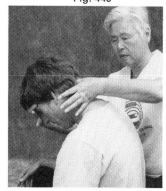

4. Over the Shoulder Stretch

Have receiver look over left shoulder. Place left hand on chin and right hand at top and back of receiver's left shoulder. Inhale and as you exhale pull with left hand (on chin) while you push with right hand (on back near shoulder) (Fig. 447). Gently bring the neck back until you feel resistance then quickly take the neck back a bit further and release immediately. Do only once. Repeat on other side.

5. Dropped Head Stretch

Have receiver drop head and look to left. Place left hand on chin and right hand on side of head above ear. Inhale and as you exhale gently take the head as far as it will go until you feel resistance then quickly pull! the chin toward you and release immediately (Fig. 448). Do only once. Repeat on other side.

Fig. 450

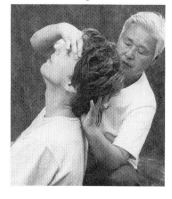

6. Medulla Press

Kneeling off center in back of receiver, find the medulla oblongata indentation at the base of skull or top of neck.

Place your thumb and index finger on the temples. Place your other thumb in the hollow (Fig. 449). Gently rock the head back onto the thumb and hold for 3 seconds (Fig. 450). Brace your elbow on your knee. Repeat 2 to 3 times.

7. Squeezing and Pressing Neck
From same position with Medulla Press, squeeze neck muscles (Fig. 451). Press large muscle on side of neck with thumb (Fig. 452). Move and repeat on other side.

8. Over the Shoulder Stretch—Standing Position
Stand over the receiver as he lies face down. Place left hand on chin and right hand at top and back of receiver's shoulder. Inhale and as you

Fig. 451

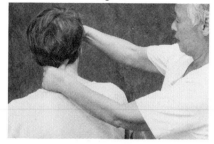

Fig. 452

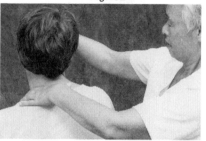

Fig. 453

Fig. 454

Fig. 455

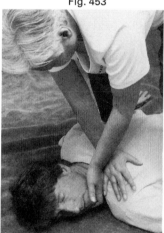
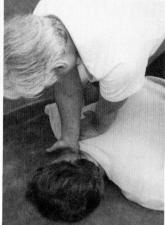
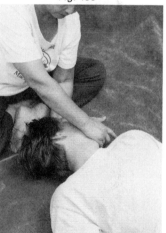

exhale pull with left hand (on chin) while you push right hand (on back near shoulder) (Fig. 453). Gently bring the neck back until you feel resistance then quickly take the neck back a bit further and release immediately. Do only once. Repeat on other side (Fig. 454).

9. Over the Shoulder Stretch—Lying Position
Have receiver lie on back and look to left. Place your left hand covering receiver's left ear, supporting head. Your hand is resting on the floor with the receiver's head resting on your hand. Place your right hand on chin. Inhale and as you exhale gently stretch the neck until you feel resistance then quickly take the neck a bit further and release immediately (Fig. 455). Do only once. Repeat on other side.

The Power of Food

Is it possible to alter the function of the body through diet? Does food have a power to change that goes beyond ordinary energy supplied by calories? In the past many people could not accept the idea that there are naturally occurring substances in foods that affect the body's processes in measurable ways, both beneficially and adversely. The idea of a power or energetic influence in food is foreign to a modern scientific society. However, on the harmful side, toxic residues from foods are known to involve the nervous system, immune system, cardiovascular system, skin, urinary tract, and many other systems, organs, and tissues. Not only acute poisonings, such as mushroom poisoning, but chronic long-term disease may be produced by food ingredients. Some elements that are found in foods can even cause behavioral and attitude changes. Several everyday foods contain chemical compounds that adversely affect us such as potatoes that contain solanin. Solanin may cause acute toxicity at times and arthritis on a chronic basis in some individuals. Coffee containing caffeine is another example. Contaminants such as aflatoxins, a fungus found regularly in peanuts, can cause cancer. Common sugar has been linked not only to changes in tooth structure (caries) but also to behavior. Most teen offenders in juvenile detention centers are found to have large blood sugar swings from sugar and "junk food" consumption. It is estimated that at the time of their crimes they were experiencing hypoglycemia, a blood sugar disorder. For these youths temporary symptoms included feelings of paranoia, anger, and hostility, the same emotional states of criminals that allow them to be antisocial.

Genetic abnormalities can cause the inability to tolerate specific foods that makes these foods toxic to the eater, thus leading to chronic illness. An inability of the body to manufacture specific enzymes for milk products or shellfish is an example. Another factor relevant to food toxicity is the interaction between foods when several foods are eaten simultaneously. An example is the reaction of nitrites and nitrates, found in prepared meats such as bacon and sausage, that join with amines to form nitrosamines; very potent cancer producers.

Foods, indeed, have power. In the above cases they have the power to cause damage. We should not forget that it is estimated that 70 percent of all cancers are linked to diet and nearly 100 percent of heart and vessel disease is preventable with food.

Looking at the Power of Food—East and West

In the West diet and foods are considered for their protein, calorie, carbohydrate, vitamin, and other nutrient content, but in the East, diet and foods are considered for their flavors, energies, and actions. Diet is considered an important influence on health and illness in traditional Chinese medicine. As the stomach receives food and the spleen transforms it into Ki and blood, these two organs are most affected by diet.

Hundreds of years ago Chinese medical experts recorded that foods create many effects on the body. Excessive eating and eating late before bedtime causes stagnation in the digestive system. This leads to symptoms of abdominal distention, sour stomach, belching, or diarrhea. Having too much raw and cold foods has been known to generate internal cold and dampness throughout the digestive system. This is seen as chilliness systemwide, diarrhea, inability to digest grains, a complaining attitude, and sluggishness. Too much fatty and greasy foods, alcohol, or sweets can produce dampness and heat. This may be seen as itch, rash, or hemorrhoids. Chinese dietary therapy describes the medical qualities of foods in a similar way that Chinese medicine describes the qualities of herbs. There is a fine line between herbs and foods.

Solid Foods

Material substance is needed to build the body, make good the deterioration of life's wear and tear, and to act as fuel for the production of heat and energy. The body depends on solid, liquid, particle, and vibration forms of food. Solid sources of food contain large quantities of calories, protein, carbohydrates, and fats. These macronutrients are the primary sources of energy. At one time or another humans have eaten everything on the planet. This consists of whole grains, land vegetables, sea vegetables, foods from animals such as flesh and milk, beans, seeds, nuts, and fruit. Even unusual items such as grasshoppers, larva, and bird's nests have been on the human dinner table. In times of famine or shortage, humanity created dishes that may repulse most of us. Yet because of this ability to be inventive and the strength of the human digestive system, mankind survives today.

Liquid Foods

Water forms two-thirds of the weight of the body. It is essential to well-being, and deprivation of water is more immediately serious than any other article of diet. It forms a large part of the tissues. It dissolves many substances and so helps the chemical changes in the digestive system. It maintains the normal salt concentration of the tissues, thus regulating many processes of the body and rendering the process of osmosis possible. Water is taken as food, soups, teas, beverages, and water. A large proportion of solid food is composed of water, particularly fruits and vegetables, which contain from 75 percent water, as in potato. Many fruits contain over 85 percent water, and melon 95 percent or more.

Many believe you must drink seven or eight large glasses of water per day. Is this true? Urologists dealing with patients eating animal protein foods daily discovered the extra water dilutes toxic waste product levels in the blood that if unchanged can cause damage to the kidneys in the form of stones and disease. However, people who do not eat standard amounts of beef, eggs, chicken, milk, cheese, and other animal proteins and who do not consume excess protein from bean sources, need not consume such large liquid volumes. In fact, excessive liquid consumption dilutes the blood (a yin condition) and stimulates urine production and elimination. Not only do you lose valuable disease neutralizing and blood stabilizing minerals, you feel cooler than normal. It is best to follow your body's protective mechanism and meet your individual liquid requirements. If you are active and sweat your requirements will be greater than if you are inactive. When satisfying body needs it is important that you always use the best quality organic foods and pure water. I like to recommend spring and well water. But, depending on where you live this may be bad advice. With the widespread use of chemicals and seepage into the ground water, most water sources are unsafe. City tap water is bacteria-free because of the addition of chlorine—a known cancer causing agent, therefore I cannot recommend it. The popular alternative is bottled water. The bottled water company has purified the water by running it through a carbon filtration system. You can do the same at home, at a fraction of the cost, with a solid carbon purification system such as MultiPure. Distilled water is without minerals and is not recommended. One rule of thumb is "Eat When Hungry, Drink When Thirsty."

Particle Foods

Minerals

There are many particle substances that give food its power. For our purposes, particles are small items such as the minerals, vitamins, and enzymes. Minerals make up 4 percent of the body. When calories, proteins, and vitamins are provided in sufficient quantity by the various food groups, the mineral requirements are usually met automatically. It is not helpful to any of the body systems to have a mineral surplus on hand. In fact, body functions are hampered or even destroyed by an excess.

Minerals serve very important functions in the metabolism. They maintain an acid-base balance in the body by shifting easily into plasma or out of plasma into bone or muscle. Minerals slide around readily to provide the narrow tolerance we have for a change in acids or bases in blood or tissues. Minerals buffer (attach to and neutralize) harmful acids or bases allowing them to leave the body via the urine. This important function helps to maintain life.

Minerals provide a medium for nerve transmission and muscle contraction. The shifting of sodium, potassium, chloride, calcium, and various hormones and enzymes make it possible for muscles to carry electrical currents and move. The most common mineral requirements are for: calcium, sodium chloride, iron, iodine, potassium, and phosphorus.

Calcium is required by all tissues, is carried by the blood serum and its use is regulated by parathyroid gland secretion. It is particularly necessary for the strengthening of bones, the formation of teeth, and the clotting of blood. Sources include: cabbage, carrots, sea vegetables, sesame seeds, and the bones of small fish (*chirimen*).

Sodium chloride regulates osmotic pressure between and within cells. When you eat too much salt and retain fluid in your fingers, face, or feet it is because fluids move easily to accompany minerals. Fluid is trapped in the tissue. While it is present in most foods it is also supplied as table salt. Because of excess consumption of salt, generally in the forms of animal foods, processed and junk foods, salt has a bad reputation. It is said that it leads to kidney, vessel, and heart disease. Many official sources concerned with health advise to greatly reduce or eliminate salt. For the average person who eats those foods along with refined salt, this is good advice. But if you have eaten a dairy-free vegetarian diet for over two years you must reevaluate this advice. Once the body has eliminated stored excess salts it becomes important to supply daily requirements. Bacteria, yeast, and virus thrive in a salt-free environment. Salt purifies the blood. Sea vegetables also are another good source. Unrefined sea salt supplies a good balance of sodium chloride and other trace minerals.

Iron is needed for the composition of hemoglobin, and in combination with it oxygen is distributed to the body. A deficiency leads to iron-deficiency anemia. Foods high in iron include green leafy vegetables, beans, whole grains, and some dried fruit such as raisins.

Iodine balances the metabolic processes stimulated by the secretion of the thyroid gland. Certain geographical areas, usually far from the sea, may be deficient in iodine. Deficiency causes goiter. This enlargement of the thyroid has disappeared since iodized salt was introduced. Natural sources include: unrefined sea salt and sea vegetables.

Potassium is the most abundant salt in intracellular tissue fluid. It is found in all vegetables.

Phosphorus is present in every cell in the body. It is essential for the production of muscular and nervous energy and for the correct composition of hard tissues such as bone and teeth. It is found in green vegetables.

Vitamins

Discovered about the turn of the century, vitamins are compounds that are essential to life, health, and growth. They are concerned with the well-being of body metabolism. These compounds, classified according to their solubility as fat-soluble and water-soluble vitamins, are normally absorbed in the small intestine.

Vitamins promote the rate and ease with which essential chemical reactions take place in the body. They regulate metabolism. They help in converting fat and carbohydrates into energy. They assist in forming bones and tissue. They also prevent deficiency diseases. Less than one hundred years ago the causes of diseases such as rickets, beriberi, scurvy, and night blindness were unknown.

Fat-soluble Vitamins: Fat-soluble vitamins include vitamin A, D, E, and K.

Vitamin A is needed for maintaining normal mucous membranes, proper night vision, normal growth, and tissue repair. It increases the defense mechanism against infection. Increased protein intake increases the need for vitamin A. Large doses of vitamin C and E reduce the availability of vitamin A in the body. Sources are: green leafy vegetables, carrots, sweet potato, cantaloupe, green peas, and lesser amounts in other vegetables and fruits. Vitamin A is highly toxic at doses not much higher than the recommended daily allowance. Symptoms include: skin lesions, itching, hair loss, blurred vision, and headache.

Vitamin D is essential for the growth of bone and teeth as it promotes calcium absorption. It prevents rickets. It is synthesized in the skin on exposure to sunlight. Children are more susceptible to serious injury from vitamin D deficiency, as their bones can be permanently deformed if the deficiency occurs while the bones are being formed. Vitamin D is readily stored in the body, and children should obtain a long exposure to sunlight on every sunny day in winter, even fully clothed. In summer, children should store plenty of vitamin D if they live in areas that are cold, and cloudy in winter. As a backup for children in northern countries fish fat and oils have substantial vitamin D.

Vitamin E reacts with harmful compounds that damage body tissue. It slows deterioration of the body and influences blood coagulation. It is found in many natural foods such as green vegetables, whole grains, nuts, beans, some seeds, and fruits. Large losses of vitamin E occur in milling of grains and in freezing foods.

Water-soluble Vitamins: Water-soluble vitamins include the B-complex, vitamin C and P. The B-complex group of vitamins includes B_1 (thiamine), B_2 (riboflavin), niacin, biotin, B_6 (pyridoxine), choline, pantothenic acid, folic acid, B_{12}, and para-aminobenzoic acid.

Vitamin B_1 regulates normal appetite and digestion and is essential in carbohydrate metabolism. Mental concentration, learning, cheerfulness, and being organized are dependent on thiamine. Deficiency leads to beriberi with stiffness, weakness, tissue swelling, abnormally slow heart rate, congestive heart failure, loss of appetite, nausea, and inflamed or irritated nerves. Chlorinated water destroys thiamine.

Vitamin B_2 deficiency causes dermatitis, cracks, and fissures about the lips and nose. Sources include whole grains and beans.

Niacin is the anti-pellagra vitamin. Pellagra is characterized by dermatitis, diarrhea, and dementia. Since the amino acid tryptophan can be used to make niacin in the body, any food containing significant amounts of tryptophan will prevent pellagra. Niacin can be synthesized by certain bacteria in the intestine. A vegetarian diet promotes this process more easily than a meat centered diet. Sources include green leafy vegetables and all grains. Corn is low in tryptophan.

Biotin is essential for the health of the skin and mucous membrane. Deficiency causes dermatitis and conjunctivitis. Sources include greens, beans, whole grains, fruits, and vegetables.

Vitamin B_6 is active in the production of blood, in central nervous system metabolism, and in amino acid metabolism. Deficiencies may cause anemia and convulsions. Oral contraceptives cause vitamin B_6 deficiency in about 25 percent of users.

Vitamin B_{12} is important for blood formation, central nervous system and gastrointestinal functions. Deficiency leads to pernicious anemia. It is a rare disease with the overwhelming number of cases occurring in non-vegetarians. Malabsorption, increased need, or increased elimination have been accepted as the most likely causes of cellular deficiency of B_{12}. Known causes of malabsorption are a lack of intrinsic factor and hydrochloric acid in the stomach, the removal of the second part of the ileum, and competition for B_{12} by microorganisms or intestinal parasites. Sources include all animal products. Vegetarian sources include bacteria found in fermented foods and on the outside of some root and stem vegetables. One study reports B_{12} found in bacterial growth in the mouth. Up to 0.5 micrograms daily can be obtained from this source. Daily needs are about 0.1 micrograms. Vegetarians' low protein intake reduces the need for B_{12}. Excess amounts of B_{12} feed the growth and spread of cancer cells and rheumatoid arthritis. B_{12} levels have been found to be higher than average in patients with ulcerative colitis and leukemia. Some people require larger than average amounts of B_{12}: meat eaters, drug users; those who take multi-vitamins; those with pernicious anemia, atherosclerosis, or diabetes that causes malnutrition; those with excessive blood levels of protein, calcium, and vitamin C; women who take contraceptives; those with liver disease, cancer, or chronic infection; those with intestinal parasites; and those with low thyroid function.

Vitamin C is essential for the healthy development of all connective tissues. It raises immunity to infection and assists in the healing of wounds and fractures. Deficiency causes scurvy. Vitamin C also helps to maintain blood vessel integrity and assists in the absorption of iron and the formation of hemoglobin. As with all nutrients there is an optimal level of intake; you can take too little as well as too much. Excess vitamin C irritates the gastrointestinal tract, interferes with B_{12} absorption, can increase blood sugar levels, and possibly form kidney stones. Sources include all fruits and vegetables.

Vitamin P (hesperidin) aids in maintaining normal capillary resistance. Deficiency may result in subcutaneous bleedings. It is found in greens, rose hips, and fruits.

Vibration Foods

Sunshine, weather, cosmic radiation, and even the rotation of the earth are powerful vibrations. These exert an effect on all life on earth. Although generally considered non-material things, they consist of minute particles of subatomic matter. These forces, including air that contains oxygen, must be considered as a source of food.

Thoughts, reading, investigation and study, and conversations with ourselves or others are further examples of food. Nature provides the means to feed both body and mind. When you are sensitive you can feel the vibrations of people and places. These sensations also feed us.

Using the Power of Food

The use of food in healing dates back several thousand years before Christ. Traditional Oriental medicine classifies foods by their effect on the body, their taste, and the direction in which energy moves inside the body. The following are many food remedies that I use.

Internal Use

Grains

Brown Rice Cream

In a cast-iron skillet dry roast 1 cup of brown rice until it is golden color. Do not use oil. Put rice in a pot, add 7 to 10 cups of purified water (not chlorinated tap water) and bring to a boil. Cover, lower the flame, and simmer for 3 to 4 hours. It is quicker to use a pressure cooker. Reduce water to 5 cups and pressure cook for 2 hours. Set aside. Squeeze cooled contents through a cotton cheesecloth and save. Add sea salt to your portion as you use it. It can be eaten as is or topped with sesame salt or nori.

Uses: For recovering from sickness, fatigue, and lack of appetite.

Brown Rice Soup

Add 1/4 to 1/2 cup of cooked rice to miso soup. Have only soup for the meal.

Uses: Good when sick or weak and in the inability to digest heavy meals.

Pearl Barley (*Semen Coix*)

Make a soup using 1 cup of cooked pearl barley, carrots, onions, wakame, and enough water to make soup consistency. Season to taste. Eat 1 bowl per day. Another method of using pearl barley is to add 10 percent pearl barley to brown rice. Eat regularly.

Uses: For hemorrhoids, warts, moles, some cancers, and the side effects of chemotherapy and radiation. Pearl barley, known as Job's tears and *hato mugi* in Japanese has been used to reduce tumors, swelling, inflammation, and heat in the body. It has been used extensively in the Orient.

Brown Rice and Malted Barley Sweeteners

Add 1/2 to 1 teaspoon to morning porridge or as sweetener in desserts.

Uses: To supply calories and control appetite, better quality substitute sweetener for sugar and honey.

Brown Rice *Mochi*

Pound cooked sweet brown rice for a long time, until the grains are broken and begin to stick together or you can get it prepared in natural food stores.

Uses: Good for weak people, children, and people doing physical labor. Mochi increases breast milk. Mugwort mochi is a good source of iron—good for anemia.

Soup

Miso Soup

> 4 cups water
> 6-inch piece wakame
> 1/4 cup each of onion, carrot, green vegetables or wild greens
> 1/2-inch slice tofu, cubed
> 1/4 cup barley (or brown rice or *Hatcho*) miso

Place wakame and water in soup pot and bring to a boil. Simmer while cutting the vegetables to similar size and shape. Remove wakame, cool briefly, and cut. Return chopped wakame to pot. Add all ingredients to soup pot except miso and slow boil until done, up to 1/2 hour, depending on how vegetables are cut. Soup vegetables are well cooked so they melt in our mouth. A side dish of vegetables may be more lightly cooked. Dilute miso in a little of the hot soup liquid and add during the last 3 minutes of gentle simmering. It is important not to cook the miso at a rolling boil that would kill the beneficial bacteria. Use organic ingredients and 1 to 3 year old, unpasteurized miso.

Uses: For strength and stamina, and to support metabolism, prevent allergies, increase circulation, and purify blood.

Shredded Kombu Soup

Add 1 to 2 tablespoons of shredded kombu to miso soup. Or add to hot water, stir, season with tamari soy sauce, and eat.

Uses: For fatigue and to clean the blood.

Egg Drop Soup

Add one organic, fertilized egg to miso soup.

Uses: For weakness, anemia, vitamin B_{12} deficiency, and heart failure. Use only occasionally.

Carp Soup (*Koi-koku*)

> 1 pound fresh carp
> 1–1 1/2 pound burdock root

1 tablespoon oil
1/4 cup used *bancha* leaves
3/4 cup barley miso
1/4 teaspoon fresh grated ginger

Cut fish into l-inch pieces. Cut burdock into thinly shaved pieces, like sharpening a pencil with a knife. Sauté the burdock for 10 to 20 minutes in oil. Add the fish and cover with enough water to cover over fish with 2 inches. Tie some bancha or *kukicha* leftovers together in a cheesecloth. Add this sack to soup pot. The tea leaves or twigs will help soften the fish bones. Bring to a boil and cook for at least 2 hours (up to 4 to 8 hours) on a low flame. If you use a pressure cooker cook for 1 to 2 hours. Remove the tea bag and add miso and ginger. Season to taste. Simmer for 10 minutes. Garnish with chopped scallions. Eat 1 to 2 bowls per day. For variety, instead of carp with burdock, you can use snapper or trout with carrots.

Uses: To strengthen the whole system and for decreased energy, decreased sexual vitality, lack of mother's milk, and anemia.

Round Vegetable Soup

Chop several round or sweet vegetables such as winter squash, daikon, carrot, onion, turnip, cabbage, and wakame in similar pieces. Make soup as you normally would. Season with sea salt, miso, or tamari soy sauce.

Uses: To regulate desire for sweets and maintain constant blood sugar level. Therefore round vegetable soup is good for diabetes and hypoglycemia.

Vegetables

Upper Body Influence—Receives upward moving energy
General principle: Leafy green vegetables positively affect this upper area of the body. Everyone should have fresh cooked green vegetables 1 to 2 times per day. They are good sources of mineral and fiber. Examples are: kale, mustard greens, cabbage, dandelion, and so on.

Use wild plants occasionally such as nettle, wild onion, miner's lettuce, dandelion, watercress, and malva. Get a wild plant handbook or take classes to learn to identify nature's harvest. Mix together with salad or vegetables in small amounts.

Middle Body Influence—Receives balanced energy
General principle: Round vegetables positively affect the center segment of the body. It receives a blend of upward and downward moving energies.

All round vegetables contain this influence. Examples are squash and cabbage.

Azuki Beans with Squash and Kombu

1 cup azuki beans
2 cups squash, sliced into bite-sized chunks
2 6-inch pieces kombu
pinch of sea salt

Wash azuki beans. Cut soaked kombu into l-inch pieces. Place kombu pieces in the bottom of a pot and place azuki beans on top. Cover with water. Bring to a boil and simmer for 40 minutes. Add squash. Sprinkle with sea salt. Cover and cook for 30 minutes more. Be sure enough water is in pot. Season to taste with sea salt or tamari soy sauce.

Uses: Helpful in regulating the blood sugar level such as hypoglycemia and diabetes, useful in taming the sweet craving, and good for lack of vitality and any kidney problem. Some people enjoy it as a dessert.

Lower Body Influence—Receives downward moving energy
General principle: Root vegetables positively affect this lower portion of the body.

Examples are lotus root that also influences the lung area (coughs and breathing difficulties); burdock root that is a blood purifier (infections), good for constipation, and has strengthening action in the body (chronic fatigue syndrome and allergies); and daikon that serves as a diuretic and softening agent (inflammatory swelling like arthritis and edema).

Carrot Spread

> 2 cups (about 1/2 pound) carrots, cut in 1/2-inch chunks
> 1/4 cup water
> 2 tablespoons almond butter
> 1/2–1 tablespoon tamari soy sauce
> 1/4 teaspoon sea salt

Pressure cook carrots in water for 5 minutes (or boil until tender in water to cover). Drain, reserving broth. Purée carrots with remaining ingredients. Gradually add broth only if needed for creamy texture.

Uses: Carrot spread is a good energy source for weak people and those who have cold. It is easy to digest.

Carrot-Daikon Mixture

> 1/4 cup grated daikon
> 1/4 cup grated carrot
> 1/4 teaspoon fresh grated ginger
> 1/2 umeboshi or 1/2 teaspoon umeboshi paste
> 1 cup twig tea
> 1 teaspoon green nori flakes

Mix daikon, carrot, ginger, and umeboshi or umeboshi paste well. Pour twig tea over mixed ingredients and add green nori flakes. Take on empty stomach before breakfast. Wait 30 to 60 minutes before eating.

Uses: To break up accumulated fat, good for fat people to skip breakfast, this way they will lose weight quickly.

Sea Vegetables

Kombu Soaking Water

Place 1 piece of kombu in 2 quarts of water to soak overnight. Use water for everything from soups and teas, to steaming broth and water for your plants.

Uses: All sea vegetables are effective in dealing with environmental pollutants including radiation. They are also good sources of iodine and positively affect the thyroid gland.

Sautéed Hijiki and Vegetables

    1/2 cup hijiki
    2 cups water
    1 teaspoon–1 tablespoon sesame oil (optional)
    1 cup onion, thinly sliced
    1 cup carrot, thinly sliced in matchsticks
    2 tablespoons natural tamari soy sauce
    2 tablespoons parsley or green onion tops

Soak hijiki in water for about 20 minutes until reconstituted. In a large skillet, heat oil and sauté onion and carrot briefly. Push vegetables to side of pan and transfer hijiki to pan. Put vegetables on top of hijiki. Pour hijiki soaking water over vegetables and hijiki to a depth of 1/2 inch. Take care to avoid using the last bit of water where sand or other particles may have settled. Cover and bring to a boil. Turn the heat to medium-low and simmer for about 15 minutes until done. Broth should be evaporated. Add tamari soy sauce and parsley or green onion tops and cook a couple of minutes more, uncovered. You can substitute arame for hijiki.

Uses: Good for osteoporosis and other bone illnesses because of high calcium content, anemia, high blood pressure, allergies, arthritis, rheumatism, and nervous disorders.

Nori Condiment

Tear up 3 to 4 sheets of nori into a frying pan. Add a little water and tamari soy sauce to moisten. Bring to a boil and simmer for approximately 15 minutes until smooth so that very little liquid remains. Eat 1 teaspoon of this paste per day on rice.

Uses: Good for lack of strength, fatigue, and lack of appetite. Nori condiment cleans the blood by supplying minerals.

Shio Kombu

Start with leftover kombu from soaking. Chop into 1-inch squares. Cover with a half-and-half mixture of water and tamari soy sauce. Bring to a boil and cook until soft. Be sure enough liquid is present to prevent burning. When it is ready all liquid should be allowed to evaporate. Use 1 to 2 pieces of shio kombu per meal.

Uses: For fatigue, mental weakness or dullness, and lack of concentration. Shio kombu strengthens the immune system.

Roasted Sea Vegetable Powder

Preheat the oven to 350°F. Place whole package of sea vegetable on cookie sheet and bake at 350° F for 3 to 5 minutes for most sea vegetables, or up to 10 to 15 minutes for wakame. Overcooking makes it taste bitter. Pulverize into powder with your hands or a mortar and pestle (or *suribachi*). Two cups of dry sea vegetables, baked and pulverized, yields just 1/2 cup flakes or 2 tablespoons powder. Store in tightly covered container. Use in soups or on grains and vegetables.

Uses: Good for fatigue, helpful in chronic fatigue syndrome, and excellent source of minerals the body can assimilate. Roasted sea vegetable powder helps to stop bleeding.

Roasted Sea Vegetable Powder with Seeds

> 2 cups dry dulse, wild nori, or wakame, or 1/4 cup packaged nori or dulse flakes
> 1 cup seeds (sunflower, pumpkin, or sesame)
> 1/2–1 tablespoon natural tamari soy sauce

Preheat the oven to 350° F. Place sea vegetable on cookie sheet. Bake at 350° F for 3 to 5 minutes for most sea vegetables, or up to 10 to 15 minutes for wakame. Overcooking makes it taste bitter. Pulverize into powder with your hands or a mortar and pestle (suribachi). Then bake seeds in the same oven for 10 to 15 minutes, checking seeds after 8 minutes. Sprinkle or spray seeds with tamari soy sauce, stir, and return seeds to oven to toast for about 2 minutes more until dry. Instead of baking, a dry skillet may be used on stove-top, but this method demands constant attention. Crush seeds with a rolling pin and mix with crumbled sea vegetables. Store in tightly covered container. Use in soups or on grains and vegetables.

Uses: Good for fatigue, helpful in chronic fatigue syndrome, excellent source of minerals the body can assimilate.

Special Foods

Umeboshi

- Cook umeboshi with brown rice instead of using sea salt.
- Add umeboshi pieces to center of brown rice balls to be used as a snack or travel food.
- Eat as is.
- Add umeboshi pieces to hot water or tea.

Uses: Umeboshi is a powerful and useful food, and good for food poisoning, upset stomach, water contamination, diarrhea, constipation, motion sickness, headache, and to decrease fatigue.

Baked Umeboshi or Umebosh Pits

Roast the umeboshi plum or saved pits in the oven at a very high temperature. Crush them into a black powder. Store in sealed container. Use 1/2 to 1 teaspoon charred powder mixed with 1 cup water or tea. If you crush the pits you will find a seed inside.

Eat this seed. It contains vitamin B₁₇ (laetrile)—an anticancer agent. Baking umeboshi is a very yang preparation.

Uses: To get rid of unfriendly intestinal bacteria, painful gas buildup, intestinal cancer, peptic ulcer, colds, and diarrhea; good for strengthening the immune system.

Shiitake Mushrooms

Cook with other vegetables or add to soup. Dried shiitake mushrooms, reconstituted with water and cooked, can be used 2 to 3 times per week.

Uses: Shiitake mushrooms are good source of protein, contain anticancer agents, break up fat, eliminate cholesterol, and relax an over-tense or stressed body. It is not a good idea to eat any variety of mushrooms raw.

Black Soybeans

Soak black soybeans overnight and cook 10 percent black soybeans in with brown rice. Eat 2 to 3 times per week. Black soybeans can be used in a soup.

Uses: Good for constipation, female troubles such as menstrual irregularities, and hardening or swelling of the breast.

Sesame-*Kuzu* Pudding (*Goma-dofu*)

Dilute 1/4 tablespoon of sesame butter with 2 1/2 tablespoons of pure water until thin. Add 1 heaping tablespoon of kuzu root powder and stir. Cook for 5 to 10 minutes until it becomes creamy. Place in mold to set up. Mix 1 part tamari soy sauce to 1 part water and use as dip sauce.

Uses: Sesame-kuzu pudding is easy to digest for those with weak intestines and general weakness.

Gomashio

Roast 1 to 3 teaspoons of unrefined sea salt in a skillet for about 1 to 2 minutes until dry. Place roasted salt in mortar or suribachi. Add 1 cup of whole (unhulled) sesame seeds in the skillet and stir over medium heat for 5 to 10 minutes until they taste good, are dry, or crush easily between the pressure of 2 fingers. If seeds pop a lot, heat is too high. Grind salt, then add sesame seeds and grind together for about 5 to 10 minutes until half the seeds are pulverized. Store in a sealed container. Use 1/4 to 1/2 teaspoon on grains and vegetables.

Uses: To stimulate the appetite, relieve tiredness, and strengthen the nervous system. Gomashio tastes good and is good for overacidity.

Tekka

Tekka is a mixture of burdock root, carrots, lotus root, grated ginger, miso, and sesame oil, roasted together for a long time in a cast-iron skillet. You can buy prepared tekka seasoning at natural food stores. Use 1/4 to 1/2 teaspoon of tekka on grains and vegetables.

Uses: Tekka is used for fatigue and anemia. It is good as a tonic, influences asthma and diarrhea, and strengthens the heart.

Shiso

Shiso is the purple red leaf that comes in umeboshi and that gives the plum its distinctive color and flavor. The leaf is high in calcium, iron, and vitamin A, B₂, C. Use as sprinkling on grains and vegetables.

Uses: For anemia, cough, lack of urine production, irritability, and common colds.

Small Dried Fish (*Chirimen*)

Sprinkle small portion of ground up *chirimen* (obtained from Oriental markets) on grains. You also can soak in water for 15 to 30 minutes until soft, and add to moist wakame. Season with brown rice vinegar and tamari soy sauce for salad.

Uses: Good for poor digestion, osteoporosis, and lack of calcium, mineral, and protein source.

Beverages

Brown Rice Tea

In a cast-iron skillet, dry roast 1/2 cup of washed brown rice. Roast until it becomes golden yellow in color. Place it in a saucepan and add 1 quart of water. Bring to a boil and simmer for 20 to 30 minutes. Add a pinch of sea salt during the cooking process. Strain and use 1 cup per serving.

Uses: Brown rice tea serves as a nutrient source for those with inability to digest well and is good for heating the body during winter.

Barley Tea

In a cast-iron skillet, dry roast 1/2 cup of washed barley. Roast it until golden brown. Place it in a saucepan and add 1 quart of water. Bring to a boil and simmer for 20 to 30 minutes. Add a pinch of sea salt during the cooking process. Strain and use 1 cup per serving.

Uses: Barley tea serves as a nutrient source for those with inability to digest well and is good for cooling the body during summer.

Barley-Azuki Drink

> 1/4 cup pearl barley (hato mugi)
> 1/4 cup azuki beans
> 1 6-inch piece kombu
> 1 quart water

Mix all ingredients together in a saucepan. Bring to a boil and simmer for 30 to 40 minutes. Strain and use broth.

Uses: To increase circulation to the skin and cleanse the kidneys. Barley-azuki drink is easy to absorb nutrient source for weak and underweight people. It positively affects spleen and lymphatic system.

Kombu Tea

Boil a 6-inch strip of kombu in 1 quart of water for 15 minutes.

Uses: To clean and strengthen the blood, and strengthen and calm the nervous system. Kombu tea positively affects the immune system.

Sweet Vegetable Drink

Dice and mix 4 kinds of round and sweet vegetables to make 1 cup. Use winter squash, cabbage, carrot, onion, and kombu. Add assorted 1 cup of vegetables to 1 quart of water. Simmer for 10 to 15 minutes. Strain and use liquid. Take 1/2 to 1 cup broth 1 to 2 times per day.

Uses: To maintain constant blood sugar level; helpful for diabetes and hypoglycemia. Sweet vegetable drink reduces craving for sweets and affects positively the pancreas and spleen.

Fresh Squeezed Carrot Juice

Juice organic carrots to make 1 cup fresh carrot juice or buy fresh carrot juice from a good source.

Uses: To supply easy to absorb vitamins, minerals, and calories and satisfy craving for sweet taste.

Lotus Tea

Grate a 2-inch piece of fresh lotus root. Squeeze out its juice through a cheesecloth. Add 2 to 3 drops of ginger juice and a few grains of sea salt or drops of tamari soy sauce. Add equal volume of water and simmer for a few minutes. Or you can prepare from dried lotus root or lotus root powder. If you use dried lotus root, boil 6 to 10 slices in 1 cup of water for 15 to 20 minutes. Add ginger juice and sea salt, and serve. For lotus root powder, use 1 to 2 teaspoons and 1 cup of water, simmer for 5 minutes, add ginger juice and sea salt, and serve.

Uses: Lotus tea positively affects respiratory system, calms irritated mucous membranes of the lungs, and is good for bronchitis, asthma, cough, and sinus congestion and infections.

Fresh Lotus Juice

Crush fresh lotus root and squeeze out the juice. Drink 1/2 cup.

Uses: To stop nosebleeds, vaginal bleeding, discharge of blood from anus, and vomiting of blood.

Kombu-Shiitake Broth

Soak 2 to 4 shiitake mushrooms and a 6-inch piece of kombu for 30 minutes. Bring to a boil and simmer for 20 to 30 minutes.

Uses: To clean blood, soften hard condition such as stress, and add mineral to the body. Kombu-shiitake broth can be used as a broth for soups or stews and adds nutrition and flavor.

Shiitake Tea

Soak 1 to 2 dried shiitake mushrooms for 1 hour or until it is soft. Cut it in quarters, add 2 cups of water, and bring to a boil adding a pinch of sea salt. Simmer for about 15 to 20 minutes until 1 cup of tea is left. Drink half a cup at a time.

Uses: To eliminate the residue of excess protein and salt from the body, relax a tense condition, reduce high blood pressure, and increase urine.

Ume Concentrate

Mix 1/4 teaspoon of ume concentrate (product found in natural food stores) in 1 cup of boiled water or twig tea. Stir and drink.

Uses: To strengthen and alkalize the blood; good for diarrhea, constipation, upset stomach, lack of appetite, headache, and minor food poisoning.

Barley Green Beverage

Mix 1 to 2 teaspoons of barley green powder (product found in natural food stores also known as *green magma*) in 1 cup of water. Stir and drink.

Uses: To reduce heat and inflammations from the body such as inflammatory arthritis, hemorrhoids, and rash; to reduce stress and calm the body; to supply easy to digest nutrient base of vitamins, minerals, and chlorophyll; and to reduce toxicity and side effects of radiation and chemotherapy.

Reishi Tea

Boil 4 to 8 grams of reishi mushrooms (*Ganoderma lucidum*) with a small amount of licorice root in 1 quart of water. Bring to a boil, cover, and simmer for 1 hour. Drink 1/2 to 2 cups per day.

Uses: Useful as general tonic; good for allergies; to enhance immune system; to reduce blood pressure and increase circulation to the lungs; and good for asthma. Reishi tea positively affects chronic fatigue syndrome, AIDS (acquired immune deficiency syndrome), and ARC (AIDS related complex), and has anticancer effect.

Ume-Sho-Bancha Drink

Pour 1 cup of bancha twig tea over the meat of 1/2 to 1 umeboshi plum and 1 teaspoon of tamari soy sauce. Stir and drink hot.

Uses: To strengthen the blood, regulate the digestion, and stimulate circulation.

Umeboshi Kuzu Drink

Dissolve a heaping teaspoon of kuzu root powder into 1 cup of cold water. Add 1/2 of an umeboshi plum and a dash of tamari soy sauce. Bring the mixture to a boil, reduce the heat, and simmer stirring constantly until the liquid becomes a transparent gelatin. A little bit of fresh grated ginger can also be added.

Uses: To strengthen digestion, increase vitality, and relieve general fatigue.

External Use

Brown Rice- or Barley-Green Plaster

Mix 70 percent cooked grain with 30 percent raw green leaves in a mortar and pestle or suribachi. Add 1/2 teaspoon of fresh grated ginger. Crush this mixture together. Spread on cotton towel approximately 1/2 inch thick and place on body area to be treated. The grain-green mixture touches the skin directly. Secure in place for 4 hours or overnight. Continue until you feel better.

Uses: To reduce swelling and inflammation, pain, and itch; good on boils, sore spots, insect bites, lymph nodes, breast, and bruises.

Buckwheat Plaster

Mix buckwheat flour with enough warm water and knead it to obtain a stiff dough that is not too wet. Spread 3/4 inch layer directly on the skin and hold it in place with a piece of cotton cloth. Remove after 1 to 2 hours, or when the dough has become soft and watery. Replace the plaster with a fresh one. This plaster must be applied often to get results.

Uses: To draw out swelling and remove excess water. Buckwheat plaster can be used on the abdomen, pleural cavity, or on joints and can be applied on the bladder area to increase possibility of urinating.

Green Plaster

Mash up 2 to 3 leaves of cabbage or other available green leafy vegetable. Place directly on affected area. When leaves become warm, replace with fresh compress.

Uses: To draw heat out of the body, in inflammatory conditions such as mumps.

Green Cap

Place leaf of cabbage or other broad-sized greens directly on the head, wearing it like a cap. While it may look silly it is helpful at drawing out excess head heat.

Uses: Good for fevers and some types of headaches.

Lotus Plaster

Grate fresh lotus root with a cheese grater. Mix with 1 teaspoon of fresh grated ginger-root and enough white flour to make it all stick together. Spread on towel approximately 1/2 inch thick. Place towel on forehead with moist material directly touching the skin. Secure in place and leave overnight.

Uses: To dissolve mucus deposits in the throat and bronchi. Lotus plaster is also good for nasal congestion and sinus irritation or inflammation.

Lotus Root Plug

Place small piece of lotus root up into nostril. Do not force it. Allow it naturally to settle into a comfortable position. Keep in place while you sleep.

Uses: To clear up sinus congestion.

Scallion Plug

Place l-inch piece of the white part of a scallion into nostril. Allow it to remain in place as you sleep. This onion family of vegetables calms the nerves.

Uses: Good for sinus congestion and excessive mucus buildups; helpful with insomnia.

Ginger Compress

Bring 3 to 4 quarts of water to a boil. Place about a golf size of fresh grated gingerroot in a cotton, cheesecloth, or a handkerchief. Fold the corners to make a little bag and close it with the string. Put this bag into the boiled water that is now just below the boiling point. Do not let the liquid boil again as this lessens its effectiveness. The mixture is now ready to use. Dip a towel into the hot ginger water trying to keep the ends dry, as the liquid is very hot. Hold by the ends of the towel and dip in the center portion. Wring it out and place directly on the area to be treated. Place a second dry towel on top to reduce heat loss. Apply a fresh hot towel every minute or so and continue for about 15 to 20 minutes until the skin becomes red.

Uses: For muscle tension and to promote circulation of body fluids such as blood and lymph fluid. Ginger compress has a stimulating effect and reduces stagnation, used for 3 to 5 minutes before a following taro plaster is applied to the warm area.

Taro Plaster

Wash 3 to 4 taro potato roots and peel off the skins. Grate the internal white part of potatoes and add enough white flour to bind the mash. You do not want the mixture to be too dry. If it is too dry it will lose its drawing power. Add 1 teaspoon of fresh grated gingerroot. Spread mixture on a damp cotton towel or cheesecloth about 1/2 inch thick. Place plaster on affected area so that the taro mixture is directly on the skin. Secure and keep on for 2 to 4 hours.

Uses: Taro plaster is a cooling agent to reduce heat or inflammation, reduces trauma induced swelling and pain, and is helpful in reducing hardness and size of tumors.

Potato Plaster

Peel and grate regular white potatoes. This makes a moist paste. Mix with enough white flour to make it stick together. Add 1 teaspoon of fresh grated gingerroot. Spread mixture on a damp cotton towel or cheesecloth about 1/2 inch thick. Place plaster on affected area so that the potato mixture is directly on the skin. Secure and keep on for 2 to 4 hours.

Uses: Potato plaster is a cooling agent to reduce heat or inflammation, reduces trauma induced swelling and pain, and is helpful in reducing hardness and size of some tumors. This plaster is less strong than taro plaster.

Miso Plaster

In a saucepan, heat up miso mixed with water, and simmer to reach a consistency like cottage cheese. Pour liquid onto towel and place on area you want to treat such as the abdomen. Cover with a dry towel to retain heat longer. Warm again when cool.

Uses: For any cold conditions and swollen abdomen.

Miso Used Externally

Spread miso paste directly on the skin.

Uses: For bleeding, itchy skin diseases, any kind of swelling, and for burns. Put on minor burns after soaking burn part in salted cold water. Immediately apply miso to shut air out.

Sea Vegetable Bath

Add 1 package of kombu to 1 gallon of water. Bring to a boil and simmer for 15 to 30 minutes. Strain and put liquid into already filled hot bathtub. Soak for 10 to 20 minutes.

Uses: Good for rough, irritated, or dry skin. Sea vegetable bath softens skin and is a mineral source.

Kombu Plaster
Soak large piece of kombu. When it is fully reconstituted place directly on affected area.
  Uses: To calm down heat, burns, and cuts.

Ginger Oil
Mix 1 part sesame oil and 1 part fresh squeezed ginger juice together. Store grated ginger remaining on a cheese grater in refrigerator. Using small amount, rub on the skin and/or spine.
  Uses: To increase skin circulation, warm body, and stimulate spine and nervous system.

Sesame Oil
Sesame oil is my favorite. Toasted sesame oil is tasty. For variety use regular, toasted, and dark toasted sesame oil.
  Uses: Good for burns, after soaking minor burn area in cool salted water, dry skin, and cracked nipples. In the eye, first boil the sesame oil, then strain it through sterile gauze. With an eye dropper, put 2 to 3 drops in eye before sleep. It stings then pushes excess water out of the eye.

Salt Bath
Add 3 cups of sea salt to hot water in normal sized bath. Keeping very warm, sit in bathtub and relax for 10 to 20 minutes.
  Uses: To relax an over-tense body, increase circulation especially in lower portions, and draw toxins out of the body.

Salt Pack
Roast 1 to 1 1/2 cups of sea salt in a frying pan until hot and then wrap in a thick cotton linen or towel. Apply to the troubled area. Change when the pack begins to cool.
  Uses: For abdominal cramps, menstrual cramps, diarrhea, and ear pain such as after swimming. Salt pack can be used to warm cool area.

Salt Water Compress
Mix sea salt with pure water to the taste of the ocean. Dip towel into solution. Slightly wring out and place on affected area. Change before it becomes warm.
  Uses: To sanitize area; helpful with burns.

Salt Water Wash
Dissolve small amount of sea salt in pure water. Taste should be salty like the ocean.
  Uses: For inflamed or sore throat, gargle with mixture; for nasal congestion and tendency toward excess mucus production and nasal trouble, rinse the sinuses by sniffing salt water up the nostrils; and for eye redness, burning, and allergy reaction, wash eyes

with solution by placing water in an eye cup, placing over one opened eye for 3 to 5 seconds, and repeat with other eye.

Cold Water Shower

After taking a hot bath or shower and your body becomes comfortably hot, finish with a brief cold shower. Turn hot water completely off so that only cold water remains, take a deep breath, and step in the stream of water. Start with water on the top of the head first then let it splash the rest of your body as you turn around slowly several times. Remain in shower from 30 seconds to 5 minutes. It is an easy process to do after the first few times. Surprisingly, you are always warm after the shower.

Uses: Good for poor circulation and for people who have cold frequently. Cold water shower increases blood flow, stimulates the nervous system, and strengthens the body's ability to adapt.

Macrobiotic Shiatsu Consultation

The combination of Whole Health Shiatsu techniques and dietary and lifestyle information creates the essence of the Macrobiotic Shiatsu consultation. This section is designed for those interested in learning how to give professional counselling sessions. Also it can be useful for nonprofessionals and "family shiatsu experts" to understand the depth of macrobiotic shiatsu. This section lays the foundation for the step-by-step procedure resulting in a complete macrobiotic shiatsu consulting session.

Learning about the Problem

Getting to know someone is always an interesting yet oftentimes unnerving process. For the professional shiatsu therapist it is necessary to obtain information that is critical to your treatment procedures. How you will treat someone's problem and what suggestions you will recommend to them is based on this first encounter. Before you can play the role of treater you must first be something of a host. You must be successful at making the receiver feel as relaxed and comfortable as possible in this unfamiliar situation. Undoubtedly it is your reputation and skills that have brought the person to you. Yet everyone is a little uncomfortable, I hope just once, in a new encounter. If you can imagine how you felt the first time you visited your dentist, doctor, or massage therapist, you will ease the tensions that many people have.

In this meeting with the new patient it is essential that you allow him or her to explain the details of their problem. Why has he or she come to see you? What are their major symptoms? When did they first notice the symptoms? Have them explain briefly and clearly about the nature of the problem or problems, including types of pain, duration, when it occurs, and so forth. Some people are shy to talk about themselves so you must be encouraging to discover the nature of the problem. Others are all to eager to talk about themselves, therefore you must limit this segment of the consultation to ten minutes. Be courteous but firm with the individual in trying to keep to your time schedule.

Keeping Records

It is a good idea to keep records of each person that you treat. Generally people will come to you more than once. The easiest and most accurate ways to note progress are to keep records. No one's memory is perfect therefore you cannot expect to remember the details of each person that you work with. Over the years, if you continue in this field, there will be thousands of cases. Some individuals that you will work with will have memorable characteristics. Their problem or personality may be unique in one way or another. In these cases it is easy to remember them. This is not so for most people that you will see. There are many routine problems that will be seen repeatedly. Without help you probably will forget the details. But, because each individual is in fact unique, it is much easier for you to rely on records taken earlier to refresh your memory. This simple technique also displays a sense of professionalism.

As we are not medical doctors and this is not a medical consultation in the generally accepted sense you need not keep extensive records of the receiver's medical history. However, the information that you keep should be relevant to you and should allow you to remember the specifics of the individual's condition well into the future, say for example one or two years from now. It also will allow you to be able to explain in simple terms what the person's problem is, as you see it, and what the direction as well as the specifics of treatment that you would like them to do. To do this you must experiment with your form of record keeping that over the years should be simplified to minimize the time required to keep things up to date. You may find the following suggestion useful as a model.

On a lined card record: name, address, telephone number, age, and date of birth. Leave a space for comments. You may want to number each card as this will give you at a glance a running total of the number of individuals that you have seen at any given time. This record keeping system also may be useful for future reference if you decide to computerize your files. It will serve as the foundation of a data base. You also should include on the cards the reason for the visit, an explanation of treatments the patient has already received and when they were received, and any results. You should include a space for the receiver's comment about the source of the problem, your comments concerning diagnosis, and treatments suggested. There should be a dated entry each time you see the individual with an update, especially of results and treatments given.

Say for example that Roberta Jones comes to see you Friday, September 20, 1994. After introductions you discover and record:

Name: Roberta Jones
Today's date: 9/20/94
Age: 48
Date of birth: 3/26/46
Address: 1856 Highland Road, Buffalo, NY 14222
Telephone: 716-485-6272 (home), 716-485-2290 (work)
Reason for visit: menstrual pain and cramping, on and off since 1988
Prior treatment: none
Comments: she seems likable, mother of two boys, speaks slowly with hesitation, and looks a bit pale.

During this information gathering segment is an excellent time to observe the patient's facial features, coloration, speech pattern, energy level, and the intangible diagnostic clues that you sense about someone. The following segments will help you figure out if your impressions based on inner feelings can be collaborated with the five senses.

Touch Examination

The examination portion of the macrobiotic shiatsu session is extremely important. Receiving physical feedback via your touch is the single most important source of diagnostic information. Your ability to interpret these tactile findings accurately is crucial. Your understanding of the receiver's condition is the foundation upon which you should base your dietary suggestions. Have the receiver lay on their back on a mat or blanket.

Arm

Pick up and hold the receiver's right hand. With your fingertips lightly brush up the arm from the wrist to the elbow, sensing the texture of the skin. Note if the skin is dry, rough or has any resistance against your hand movement. This is a highly subjective experience. Only after eating a sensible diet for a long time and touching many thousands of people will you be able to discern the energetic quality that this subtle form of diagnosis reveals. Though you may not feel or sense much continue to practice with each person that you treat. This is the only way to learn.

Fig. 456

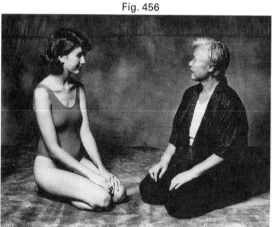

Fig. 457

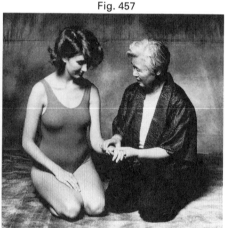

Skin to Skin Test

Lightly pinch the receiver's skin on the top of the forearm midway between wrist and elbow. Beneath the skin is fat. The size of skin that is picked up reveals the fat content below the skin. This indicates general body fat content. If what you picked up is small you can assume body fat content is low. If on the other hand the pinch is thick (more than 1/3 inch) you can assume body fat content is greater than normal. Fat content on the arm may be an indication of fat content in or around the internal organs. This may reveal why the internal organs functions as they do.

The skin to skin pinch test also reveals the elasticity of the skin. When you release the skin it should return to a normal position quickly. It is abnormal if the skin appears loose or stretched. This suggests the system is too expanded—too yin.

Look at the fingers and palm of the hand. Color, temperature, and dryness should be appropriate for the individual. If anything catches your interest note it on your records.

Abdominal Palpation

Check the internal organs such as liver, gallbladder, stomach, pancreas, small intestine, large intestine, bladder, lungs, and heart by touching the skin of the abdomen and pressing in the appropriate locations. A good understanding of anatomical locations is essential. Even with study individual differences make abdominal palpation difficult. You must take your time and try to visualize below the skin and imagine the internal organ's condition. Like any art this is not easy. Practice on everyone that you treat. With experience you will perceive subtle differences that differentiate between health and illness, stagnation and flaccidity (being too soft). For women, assess the condition of the ovaries by pressing on the lower abdomen below the umbilicus to the right and the left. The uterus can be found just up from the pubic bone. For men, the prostate gland's influence is found just up from the pubic bone.

Tongue

Check the flesh and coating of the tongue to discover the body's general condition. Note any distinguishing characteristics in your records.

Eyes

Look into the eyes observing the pupil, iris, and sclera (eye white). Pull down the lower eyelid and check blood vessels of the conjunctiva for correct color. Lighter than normal may suggest anemia.

Pulse

Take the pulse and note beats per minute. If you have a blood pressure device you may want to check the blood pressure. When you take the pulses check for energy movement in the three main sections of the body. Note any remarks in your records.

Record remarks:

After examining Mrs. Jones it is apparent that her appearance of normal body weight is deceiving. She has plenty of fat beneath the skin, her body fat content is excessive. Her coloring is pale with red highlights on her cheeks and forehead. Her energy level is low. She complains of chronic cold hands and feet, even when it is not cold. Her abdomen is soft, elastic, and spongy; signs of expanded intestines and cold in the interior. She is chronically constipated. There is a layer of fat sitting just inside both hipbones. The left side is thicker and harder.

Mrs. Jones' tongue is coated with a thick white coating, and the fleshy body of the tongue appears light pink, lighter than normal.

Her pulses are slow, without much force. The third finger on both wrists over the Kidney pulses barely feel the beat. The second finger on the right hand over the Pancreas pulse can suppress the beat entirely; a sign of digestive deficiency. Clearly she is tired, cold on the inside, without much energy or reserve.

Treating the Problem

Have the receiver turn over. Press along the spine. The right side of the back reflects the liver and gallbladder; while the left side reflects the pancreas, stomach, and spleen. Move near the low back and check the kidneys (at the last rib and below). Note any significant confirmations in your records.

Do parts of the simple total treatment shiatsu technique on the back, legs, arms, abdomen, and head.

Educating about the Problem

After compiling information from all sources such as the initial interview, patient's explanation of major complaint along with their history, touch diagnosis including abdominal palpation, acu-point diagnosis, touching the spine, and actual treatment, you should have a good idea what their condition is and what is going on. Many people arrive with a medical diagnosis when they come to see you, for example a diagnosis of osteoarthritis or diabetes, but you still must confirm for yourself to discover how arthritis or diabetes has affected this individual. Do not be satisfied with disease names. What are the patient's strengths and weaknesses, where lies the imbalance? Remember the cause of every trouble is an imbalance between yin and yang energies. Chapters 1 and 2 should supply you with abundant information on which to base the final part—education.

Sharing what you have discovered is the most meaningful portion of the consultation. You must be able to explain in simple terms the essence of what you discovered, what it may mean physically, emotionally, and even spiritually, in both the short and long terms, and you must make useful suggestions that the patient will be able to achieve. It does not do the patient much good if they leave the session without understanding their problem.

The current condition of the body represents the effect of eating, drinking, thinking, in short, lifestyle habits. The present lifestyle habits support the illness. In the body's wisdom it has allowed a problem to exist only because it is maintained by some attempt at balance. Symptoms of inflammation, pain, tumor growth, and so forth are examples of the body trying to maintain a relative balance. Instead of breaking down and expiring, the body adapts and produces an uncomfortable balance—that we call symptoms.

After explaining to the patient why and how the problem is allowed to continue to exist and where, in your opinion, the major imbalance is, diet is the most important aspect to discuss. By now you should be familiar with the necessity of a diet containing high carbohydrate, high fiber, low fat, and adequate protein foods. Discuss these points with the patient. Explain how these items relate to them personally. Once the basics are covered, discuss any special dishes, beverages, herbal formulas that may adjust the condition or help to speed up recovery.

Additionally, particular treatments used as homework are valuable to keep the effects of treatment and the new lifestyle direction ever present in the patient's focus. Breathing and exercise routines greatly increase change. They affect metabolism and consolidate new gained energies. Some people may benefit from a course of ginger compresses on the kidneys or abdomen, while others may find moxibustion applied to a number of tonifying acu-points useful. This is the time to share how you think the patient can best use their time and energies to help themselves.

Comments:
Although Mrs. Jones claimed to be eating a healthy diet, a fact when compared to most, she still was not in very good shape and her symptoms made life uncomfortable. Suggestions for her are: discontinue all fruit and fruit juices; discontinue the small amount of cheese and yogurt she eats from time to time; chicken and eggs should be eliminated as they affect the pancreas adversely and depletes energy (she does not eat beef or red meat).

On the positive side she should include warm foods daily (mostly cooked vegetables such as carrots, turnips, onions, kale, cabbage, and so on) with salad only if she craves it; whole grains such as millet and pressure-cooked brown rice should be included in sufficient volume but not so much as to feel tired after a meal; use fish a couple of times a week, but no shellfish; the occasional cup of coffee while not the best for her may be continued for the time being, maximum 1 cup per day as a special treat, until energy flow is stable and the artificial boost that coffee brings to a sluggish system is unnecessary; learning how to cook and chewing what she eats is essential to success.

Using Mu tea regularly and the special Chinese herbal formula of Women's Precious pills (also known as *8 Flavor Tea*) will help increase circulation in the lower regions of the body especially around the ovaries.

Taking more exercise to stimulate the metabolism and soaking in a hot salt bath in the evening rounds out the list of helpful suggestions for Roberta Jones.

In the first session there is less time to give shiatsu because of the time taken in examination and explanations. But, in subsequent sessions more time is spent on treatment with approximately 25 percent or 15 minutes taken to reacquaint yourself with the remaining problems and discussions. Modified or new suggestions should be given then.

At first it is unreasonable to expect the novice to perceive many subtleties of assessment. Touch is very subjective. The touch sensations of diagnosis are based on long-time experience. Certainty comes with the confirmation of a master. Being an apprentice to someone who already has achieved mastery is the only way to learn and achieve certainty quickly. Without direct training the serious student must persist in their studies, realizing that mastery will come with experience. Working alone always takes longer than with others who possess skill. Reading how to do anything is always more difficult compared to being shown how by a master who can teach.

The final portion of time spent together should always touch on the mental, emotional, and spiritual aspects of life. At times this means discussing beliefs and concepts that limit the patient's progress, but most of the time it is accomplished below the surface by encouraging the receiver to do their best and sharing your experience, optimism, and energy with them. Remind the patient that problems do not go away immediately. Their blood and body must change. This can take at least two to three years. Encourage them to have patience and to continue carrying on. Have them keep in contact with you, perhaps on a monthly basis. If you feel it is appropriate you may want to share the following Five Phases of Body/Mind Changes with the patient. This will give them a realistic timeline of what to expect. Being non-judgmental with the patient (which comes from tapping into your feelings of love for life and humanity) let's the patient leave the consultation with a renewed spirit of hope, and practical, useful techniques to help them achieve their desired goals.

The Five Phases of Body/Mind Changes

There is a transformation process that elevates individuals from confusion and lack of certainty to one of clarity; from illness to one of health. At one time or another all of us have been inspired to achieve a goal beyond our apparent capacity. One day we may step on a scale, cry when we see the registered weight, and make a firm commitment to lose it. We may experience some trouble and go to the doctor only to receive the news of the presence of cancer. At that moment we resolve to reverse our life's direction and save ourselves. We may have a brush with death in a near fatal auto accident and survive to become a new person who appreciates the little things in life. The transformation process comes in many sizes and packages, but the outcome is the same. You are a different person, a more whole person, after the process. In my research I have discovered five phases the process travels through. In a near death experience all five phases occur quickly. But for most people who adapt lifestyle changes the phases are distinct with periods or plateaus at each stage.

Phase I: There is a subjective sense of feeling better. You are more comfortable being you. Your body begins to feel good to you. You lose surface water and fat so the body begins to become slimmer and you lose weight.

Phase II: The body makes physical adjustments.
1. There are better bowel movements. Chronic constipation or diarrhea normalize as elimination becomes regular and easy.
2. Skin tone and texture become smoother with a silkier texture. The skin color becomes normal with blotches and color abnormalities diminishing.
3. Pains in the muscles and joints begin to decrease. Symptoms of arthritis, rheumatism, low back and other pains diminish in frequency and intensity.
4. The body becomes more flexible. You gradually want to do more and be active.

Phase III: After two to three years there is a turning point in your practice. There is a big adjustment and often a big discharge. There are a series of symptoms that may arise to test your faith in your new lifestyle. Not every symptom happens to everyone.
1. You begin to feel tired for no apparent reason.
2. You lose more weight.
3. You experience severe cold symptoms and sometimes spit up large volumes of mucus.
4. Skin eruptions appear such as pimples, boils, eczema, and psoriasis.
5. You may become emotionally unstable and have fits of anger and fear. At this stage without faith you will stop the diet or eat very widely and go backward in

your training. As much as you have promoted the diet and lifestyle to family and friends for the last couple of years you will question if this way of living is good for you after all.

6. You may pass kidney stones or gallstones.
7. For women, there may be a time of discharging excessive menstruation and clots from the uterus.

Phase IV: This is the stable period occurring between three to seven years. Mentally you are clearer. Your brain functions smoothly and easily. You are sharp. You remember dates, details, people's names, and so forth easily. Inside feels peaceful. Your breathing is deeper and easier. Your internal organs are cleaner and their function is smoother. (However, their cleansing is not complete at this time.)

Phase V: Your concern goes outward beyond yourself and your immediate world. This occurs between seven to fifteen years. Your body is very stable. You do not feel your body so much because there are few pains and troubles. Instead your attention is directed toward helping others. Emotionally you are very stable. You are not quick to react or anger. You feel at peace. You have a sense of truly becoming a free person. In daily activities you choose quality. You look for the best in products as well in people. You are not preoccupied about food or exercises, you know that you are caring for the physical body on a day-to-day basis and look more deeply in the emotional and spiritual aspects of your life. Your instinct is becoming stronger and your judgment better. Everything goes smoother in relationships and business. Naturally, others come to you, trust you, and put you in a position of leadership. You observe your personality as improving and feeling grateful, you want to help others even more. The phase continues and deepens for the rest of your life.

At any phase, all five phases can repeat themselves in varying degrees. In other words, within the first year of change there can be feelings of spiritual awakening and at the fifteenth year there can be sinus discharge. But at each time frame the depth of experience and understanding is different.

Caution: Do not expect the qualities described above to occur only with the passage of time and minimal attention to healthy living patterns. The timeline outlined is an average I have discovered from tens of thousands of people. Some people have severe amounts of hardened fat lining the small intestine. Even after fifteen years they may begin to discharge this physical accumulation. Others have experienced traumatic childhoods with poverty, alienation, or physical, emotional, or sexual abuse. While eating and living well supply the physical foundation for this transformation process, the individual must be attentive and willing to grasp life's opportunities as they arise. This means emotionally working and risking the loss of old habit patterns with the adventure of living in new ways. This means different things to different people. Each person must take a chance on themselves and work to allow the loving spirit within to surface. This takes courage. We can bolster our courage and our "stick-to-itive attitude" if we remember the natural state of humanity is to be happy. Every human has the capacity of living and experiencing happiness. The transformation process helps us regain our birthright.

Special Thoughts for Consideration

If you continue in your studies and develop a professional practice of macrobiotic shiatsu you will encounter new challenges. As your experience deepens you will be faced with an increasing number of seriously ill and even terminally ill patients. This is a difficult position to be in. When questions come up concerning the use of immune suppressing therapies such as chemotherapy, radiation, and surgery, how will you respond? Earlier I reported research that states some cancer patients who receive standard medical treatment do not fare as well as those who receive no treatment at all. Yet, most people believe that cancer therapies can cure them. What do you do when a patient wants to take radiation and asks your opinion?

The answer to this question lies in how you view your role. We are not physicians nor is the purpose of Whole Health Shiatsu to provide only medical care. Our purpose is to help people to become whole in body, mind, and spirit. Our principle concern is for the integration of the individual. We must respect the wishes of the patient and work closely with them to accomplish their goals. They have come to us for information and practical solutions. If you have established a bond of trust between you and the patient, you should honestly tell them what you think. They want to hear your opinion but do not practice medicine nor make medical decisions. You should ask yourself, "How can I support this person at this time?" If you bring clarity to them in this situation you are serving your purpose. It is important to promote cooperation and help the patient work with medical care providers whom they have faith in if they decide to do so.

In a similar way when someone comes to you with a terminal diagnosis how will you handle it? This is a question that cannot be easily answered. You must assess each individual's condition yourself and discover if they indeed appear to be terminal. If you have no experience in determining if someone is terminal this is an opportunity to discover what does "terminal" mean? If you are experienced and feel the person is terminal you must explain your observation to the family. The power of the mind is great as well as the power of healing. We never know with certainty who will survive and who will not. These areas are in the realm of divine providence. Therefore we should realistically explain the difficulties facing the patient. At the same time we should never give up hope. Encourage the family to give good food as long as there is an appetite. If the person is going to die, I feel eating well will minimize pain and make a smoother transition into the next realm. If the person is open and you feel they have given you permission, discuss with the individual what death means to them. Help the individual to clearly see their beliefs about life and death. If necessary you should help to dispel any doubts or fears. If you are not comfortable in this area you can suggest they seek guidance from others with more experience.

Appendix A: Case Histories

1. Elaine Nussbaum

In April 1980 I was diagnosed with uterine cancer. It was a mixed tumor, a carcinosarcoma, and it was embedded in the muscle of the lining of the connective tissue of my uterus. I was treated with external and internal radiation, oral and intravenous chemotherapy, and hormone therapy. In August 1980 I had a radical hysterectomy. I continued to take chemotherapy.

In May 1982, I started having pain in the lower back, which was diagnosed as a compression fracture. Despite medication, the pain got progressively worse. I could neither sit nor lie down. In August, after a few days of standing up all day and night, sleeping only on my husband's shoulder in a standing position, I consulted an orthopedist. The orthopedist confirmed the compression fracture and noted that I also had a partially collapsed vertebrae. In order to prevent a total collapse of my backbone, I was put into a brace which extended from below my chest to below my pelvis and wrapped around my back. I wore the brace all day and night.

The pain got worse and spread to my legs. When I could no longer stand, I was placed in a reclining chair where I stayed in a semi-reclining position taking strong pain-killers around the clock. Nothing stopped the pain.

In September, I was carried back to the hospital for more diagnostic procedures. These tests showed that, in addition to the collapsed backbone, I had cancer on my lumbar spine, cancer on my thoracic spine, and multiple metastatic deposits in both lungs.

I was given radiation again, then chemotherapy, then more radiation treatments, then more chemotherapy. The protocol was for ten rounds of chemotherapy, given at three to four week intervals. Each chemotherapy treatment required an overnight hospital stay. I was tired, weak, nauseous, and in pain. My husband rented a hospital bed where I lay motionless. I could not move nor turn because of the pain. When a bedpan was necessary, two people were needed to lift me. My parents moved in to help take care of me, the children, the cooking, and so on so that my husband could go to work. My mother stayed three months; she would not leave until I was able to get off the bed.

Toward the end of January 1983, after four cycles of chemotherapy, I cut my finger on an envelope. Because my blood levels were so depressed from the chemotherapy, I was unable to fight the infection that set in. The paper-cut resulted in a ten-day hospital stay, which included massive doses of intravenous antibiotics, four blood transfusions, and three days in isolation. The doctors decided that the chemotherapy I was getting was too strong for me; I would be put on something less toxic.

Diagnostic procedures performed during the hospital stay showed unchanged metastatic cancer in both lungs, and increased activity and progression of the the cancer in my spine.

It was then that I realized that conventional medicine was not helping me, and I began to consider an alternative. I chose macrobiotics, based mostly on my reading of other people who had healed themselves with this approach.

In February 1983 I began to practice macrobiotics. I completely eliminated from my diet all meat, poultry, eggs, dairy foods, and sugar. I reduced to zero the thirty-eight pills I was taking every day. I decided to stop all chemotherapy, hormone therapy, antibiotics, and vitamin supplements. I started to eat brown rice and cooked vegetables.

I began macrobiotics in a hospital bed, a wheelchair, and a brace, and in pain. The pain gradually subsided, and I never took another pain-killer. After a short time, I was able to take a few steps with the help of a walker, then with two canes, then with one cane. In April, a urinary problem that plagued me for three years (a result of the original radiation) disappeared. In mid-May I took off the brace. On May 22, I walked for the first time all by myself!

In June, I put away my wig; my hair, which had all fallen out from the chemotherapy, had grown back enough to be presentable. I returned the hospital bed. I started driving again. I resumed my studies toward my masters degree. Within six months I had changed from a sick, depressed, pill-popping invalid to a happy, optimistic, pain-free, and very very grateful person.

In November 1983, my macrobiotic advisors told me that the symptoms of cancer were gone.

It is now nine years that I have been living the macrobiotic way, and I continue to enjoy good health. I completed the Master's of Science degree in Nutrition, my thesis was titled "Macrobiotics: An Alternative Treatment for Cancer." I continue to study, practice, and teach macrobiotics. I have an active consulting practice, and I also offer macrobiotic cooking classes. My book *Recovery: From Cancer to Health through Macrobiotics* (Tokyo and New York: Japan Publications, Inc., 1986) has inspired thousands of people to improve their health with macrobiotics.

Some important factors in my recovery have included accurate practice of macrobiotic recommendations (no cheating), regular visits with a macrobiotic counselor, shiatsu massage, love and support from family and friends, a lot of prayer, and a positive optimistic attitude. My experiences, both personal and professional, have shown me some of the wonderful changes that can occur when living the macrobiotic way.

2. Rosemary Stark

I first met Shizuko in the Spring of 1986. I had been macrobiotic one year and had several consultations with Bill Spear, Lino Stanchich, and Michio Kushi. At that time I was fifty-five and had been under constant medical care since I was eighteen for allergies, depression, pneumonia, vaginal hemorrhages, staphylococcal infections, sinus infections, stomach and intestinal spasms, and corneal abrasions. In thirty years I had been hospitalized twenty-one times and had several D and C's, a Caldwel-Luc sinus surgery, a hemorroidectomy and an appendectomy. I had also been diagnosed with lupus, a terminal blood disorder and was recovering from alcohol and drug addiction. I was confused, depressed, and disoriented and my relationships were in turmoil. It was suggested to me that Shizuko could help my body to discharge all the excess toxins that were stored in the various cells and tissues. I know now that I also needed personal contact with a nurturing woman and the touch of a sympathetic and encouraging friend.

When Shizuko touched the various parts of my body she told me she felt many cysts and hard calcium deposits around the pancreas and much excess accumulation of hard fatty tissue although I was only eighty-seven pounds. She diagnosed stones in both kidneys and a very hard and nonfunctioning pancreas. She kneaded my body and pulled and pushed like someone kneading bread. She told me she had to "tenderize" me. I shrieked and screamed and cried a great deal. Shizuko talked to me and told me to hang on and to believe I could get well. Often she held me and rocked me as I got in touch with old and painful emotions. She kept assuring me I was going to get well, that I was very sick but that I could recover and that I should tell my story to the world. She asked me to keep a journal so I could help others with my story. It seemed endless and overwhelming but we continued every week and I did daily scrubs and exercises and ate as Shizuko directed.

A friend, Rochelle, came every week also and Shizuko had us helping each other. After eight months, Rochelle died and I almost gave up. Shizuko told me we were both like flowers, only Rochelle was bent over too far to lift up again and that I would have to recover for Rochelle. It was an inspiration to see how Shizuko cared for Rochelle, calling her and encouraging her every day. During my first year of shiatsu, I passed a kidney stone and had a major skin discharge. Michio Kushi also diagnosed pancreatic cancer and blood tests seemed to confirm this, although I refused more invasive diagnosis. I had much support from all the counselors, Dr. Martha Cottrell and Dr. Wally Burnstein. Many macrobiotic cooks came and cooked for me and I studied intensely at the New York Center. In the spring of my third year I had an intense lung discharge and broke several ribs from coughing and ran high fevers. In my fourth year I had a deep discharge from the uterus and two fibroid tumors disappeared. I was diagnosed with uterine cancer but after three months the tests were negative and so were my lupus tests.

I saw Shizuko steadily for three years and adhered strictly to her suggestions. My skin became softer and my body was more pliant. I was able to do Yoga with ease and felt more centered and clear. My energy levels and my weight increased and my emotions became more stable. The nicest part of all is that I now laugh and enjoy life and have wonderful relationships. Shizuko has been my teacher, my guide and a truly dear and compassionate friend. I am deeply grateful for my new life.

3. Sarah Deslauriers

In May 1977, I applied for an insurance and was refused. I was told to visit my Doctor, that my level of sugar was high. I made an appointment with a general practitioner.

After examining me and using a diastolic measurement, he told me that he was referring me to a diabetic specialist. As I entered the specialist's office he said, "My nurse will be with you shortly and she will start you on insulin." But I said, "Doctor you didn't examine me or run any test on me, you didn't ask me for my name, address or telephone number for your records. With all due respect, I refuse to be under your care under these conditions."

Six months later I went to see an acupuncturist because I had been coughing ever since I can remember with no help from doctors. I also mentioned to him my level of sugar. He recommended that I try a few sessions and see what happens, so I did. My cough did not disappear and my level of sugar was considerably high according to diastolic measures from the drugstore. The acupuncturist recommended that I visit a European specialist for diabetes. Then I started to take diabetes pills. According to my diastolic measurement I went up and down like an elevator. After awhile I decided not to renew my prescription.

In spring 1982, I woke up one morning, my middle toe of my right foot felt as if someone tied a tight string around it and felt awfully uneasy. I went to see a naturopath, who concluded that my circulation was a big problem and to use hot and cold treatments, he also sold me a wooden roller and showed me how to use it. A few days after, during my sleep I was moving my right foot for exercise and also moved my left foot to see the difference in feeling, I must have forced it, because I had trouble walking as of then.

I then registered for a 10 session shiatsu with Darryl. During the sessions Darryl talked about a doctor his pregnant wife went to see, which happened to be a friend of ours from Tai Chi Chuan classes. We called him for an appointment. He uses a lot of alternative medicine including polarity. He told me I had a lumbar and sacroiliac problem whatever that is, and referred me to Ginette, a therapist that had studied the Meltzer's method in France. The very same day we managed to have a session with her. After two sessions I was walking properly, but my toes still had a string wrapped around them, so I continued with the therapist to ease the tension I had built around my shoulders and the rest of my body. I also kept on taking my shiatsu sessions. As we kept exchanging conversations with Darryl on how important food was, he recommended us a light health restaurant that also had a selection of medical and health books. Every time we went for a small snack we would pick up a book. We learned the effect of having meat, and from then on we decided to have fish and chicken only. Eventually we picked up Aveline Kushi in macrobiotic cooking. We enjoyed every recipe and felt good about it. As we were discussing with Darryl about our improvement in nutrition items, we have been buying from there ever since.

One day after making a grocery order, by the cash we picked up an *East West Journal* that mentioned a two day Seminar-I for beginners of macrobiotics at 17 Station Street in Brookline, Massachusetts by Michio Kushi. We joined in January 1983, and also got a consultation with Michio about my feet and diabetes. The conclusion was: No more Tsicken (chicken), no more baked foods, very little fruits, and a list of do's and don'ts.

In April 1983 Seminar-II was given, again I attended and got another consultation with Michio. My diabetes was down from 405 to 170 on my life span machine. I was rather pleased. Richard my husband and I had also stopped eating Tsicken, but still had the problem of circulation.

In August of the same year at the Berkshire Summer Conference, I had a shiatsu treatment from Shizuko Yamamoto. Shizuko told us both to lose weight and to eat macrobiotically as much as possible. This proved to be difficult as our social activities in our type of business did not permit us always to have good wholesome food at home. I must say getting used to macrobiotic cooking was very easy and we enjoy it, but the fact that we did not always have access to it, made it harder and prolonged my recovery. To us, it was all common sense and very close to my mother's cooking from the old country. We kept visiting Shizuko at the Macrobiotic Center of New York almost every four to six weeks and in Montreal kept visiting the therapist and a Japanese friend, known to the Japanese society Mr. T. Kagemori, almost every week. We also took shiatsu from Shizuko and Patrick McCarty, Intensive I and II, which helped us a great deal in our home workouts.

In September 1990 after hot and cold baths I noticed some blotches on both legs on the outer sides. As I was visiting the therapist, she said, I am better to call a doctor to see this. The doctor looked at it and said, "These are skin ulcers from diabetes, for which I use zinc and sea vegetable treatments and is very expensive, but you are not advanced enough. For now use saltines for about a week, come and see me after." After I go home Richard saw me being scared thinking it was going to get worse, I decided to call Shizuko and explained what was happening. She replied "Sarah, don't be scared, you are discharging, wash your ulcers with salt and water, apply sesame oil to loosen it, then apply miso on top." I started this procedure and kept visiting Shizuko. By the middle of November 1990 it was healed, but left my skin the color of dark miso and is now gradually going away. When I am not lazy, Shizuko recommended that I rub the skin with green vegetable paste, it really does help the color to disappear. Thanks to Shizuko and her patience for helping so many people including me.

November 25, 1990, I came out of a restaurant having trouble breathing, I again called Shizuko thinking I was having a heart attack. Shizuko asked, "Are you coughing Sarah?" I said yes. "Is there milky white mucus coming out?" "Yes." "No Sarah, you are not having a heart attack, you are discharging again, take lotus tea, that will help dissolve the mucus, have a lot of round vegetables and sea vegetables." By then we were also having a lot of hato mugi (pearl barley) as hot and cold salads, soups, and so on. I found my sugar level dropped down considerably in comparison to brown rice.

I visited Shizuko again, she told me to keep losing weight, that it will help my sugar level. I replied under circumstances it is not easy, the fact that we do not always eat at home, but that definitely we are determined to make an effort.

One night Richard was going through a medical book and was telling me everything he read about congestive heart failure corresponded to my symptoms. He insisted that we meet Dr. Martha Cottrell with Shizuko's approval, for a checkup. Dr. Cottrell agreed with Richard that I was having a congestive heart failure and suggested that I see a heart specialist. My pulse was high, even higher than usual the fact that I was seeing a doctor, made me nervous. We asked her what was the normal pulse, she said, between 70 and 84, but I was 101. She insisted that I see a heart specialist the fact that we only have one heart and I should get some treatment. By that time I believed so strongly in macrobiotics, I figured I will return home and practice macrobiotics in a very strict manner. Dr. Cottrell and I agreed, that I should at least take a prescription of "Lasix" (water pills). I ended taking them as prescribed, but reluctantly, I thanked her for being so very nice and very patient with me. I will be seeing her in the future.

From then on I made sure to have good balanced meals, light exercises, walks, lots of fresh lotus, natural diuretics, and kept cutting our consumption of oil to very strict minimum, which proved to be an unbelievable breakthrough, that dropped my sugar level to between 98 and 110 within two to three days. With experiments here and there, we confirmed that oil is one of the key factors in my control of diabetes.

By the time I was due for my next visit to Shizuko, I had lost more than 20 pounds, no more swollen feet, my pulse is 81 to 87, sometimes lower, hardly coughing, but I still feel the tight strings around my toes, which I am hoping one day to reverse the situation (real soon).

When Shizuko saw me, she said, "Sarah, you look so much better, both of you have such a strong constitution, keep it up, you will do alright." But my husband Richard said, "Shizuko I cannot get used to her being so small." "That is alright," she said, her famous words of assurance "Don't Worry. Make sure both of your bodies are very compact."

I take this opportunity to thank Shizuko for her patience, her good treatments, her food recommendations, her sympathetic words of kindness, and her wonderful support. MAY GOD BLESS YOU AND KEEP YOU SHIZUKO "WE LOVE YOU." Also thanks to my lovely husband Richard, for his understanding and constant support.

4. Sophie Regenstein

On August 1, 1988 I was operated on for ovarian cancer. When I got out of the recovery room the doctor informed me that he performed a complete hysterectomy and removed a lymph gland as well. In addition I was given chemotherapy treatments for six months. To add insult to injury the doctor told me I had an 80 percent chance of having a recurrence of cancer within six months to a year. This belief was reinforced by the chemotherapist as well. After the six month period of having received chemothrapy they wanted to give me another round of treatments. The side effects from these treatments, I was told, would in all likelihood affect my heart and kidneys. Routinely, I was told I would be operated again for a reevaluation.

Luckily it was at this time that I heard about macrobiotics through a friend. I checked into it further and decided to follow a macrobiotic approach rather than taking more chemotherapy treatments and following the medical route.

The first thing I did was to sign up for a series of macrobiotic cooking classes. In addition I took shiatsu treatments from Shizuko Yamamoto who was my macrobiotic counselor. I followed her suggestions as to diet, spiritual and physical practices. In addition Shizuko recommended external body treatments which I did religiously.

If it had not been for Shizuko I think that I would not have been here today to tell my story. She has given me the strength and confidence that no other human being could have given me! I am eternally grateful. Shizuko is indeed a precious human being.

After only two years of being macrobiotic I feel better than ever. I have been told and know that I look younger and feel very energetic.

Upon being examined by my medical doctor he could not believe a macrobiotic approach could help me. He believes that God was very good to me. I know that I helped God do this by being macrobiotic.

5. Lou-Ella Merin

In May of 1990, I began a detoxification diet of vegetable and fruit juices and colonics which lasted for three weeks. I then began to reintroduce solid foods, but most were raw. I had eliminated all meat and dairy, processed foods, sugar and other sweeteners, pastas, rice cakes, spreads, and oils and other condiments. I had never acquired a taste for alcohol and had long since stopped drinking coffee. Bagels with cream cheese and lox and an ice cream with mounds of whipped cream were more my speed!

I began to have weekly shiatsu treatments with a woman who recommended that I try the macrobiotic diet as a way of cleansing and healing myself. I was reluctant to do so, despite my prior knowledge of macrobiotics and its documented positive results. Slowly, I became involved with the diet and by September I was 100 percent macrobiotic, both in my eating and philosophy. I was also doing Tai Chi Chuan almost daily, not eating for three hours before going to sleep, and sleeping longer.

The macrobiotic diet was a big commitment at first, requiring discipline. It meant eliminating most of the foods that I loved to "junk out" on, which we are all familiar with. However, my motivation has been strong: That May 1, 1990, a medical doctor discovered a mass on my right breast. A urine test showed positive regarding cancer cells in my body. I have chosen to follow an alternate mode of healing myself. Thus far, one year, I have lost eighteen pounds and have never veered from the prescribed diet. With the recommendations of Shizuko Yamamoto, I have expanded my diet to include beans, grains, seasonal vegetables, pastas, fish, and certain other foods and condiments. As for my "condition" it is still too soon to know whether all is healed within me, but I take each day with pleasure and do what I can in that day to care for myself, physically, emotionally, and spiritually.

6. Miriam Hausman

In July l985, while on vacation in Israel, I heard about Elaine Nussbaum's recovery from cancer. Upon my return to New York I called Elaine's sister Phyllis, who had been in my bunk in summer camp many years ago. I was interested in learning more about macrobiotics as a very close friend of mine had been diagnosed with cancer a year early. Phyllis suggested that I read Michio Kushi's books *The Macrobiotic Way* and *The Cancer-Prevention Diet*, and that I call the Macrobiotic Center of New York for further information. I read the books and tried some of the recipes.

In January l986 I signed up for cooking classes at the center. I started with the beginner's series followed by three intermediate series: spring, summer, and fall cooking. Although at one time I was a big junk food eater— chocolate, cake, a pint of ice cream a day—but the time I started macrobiotics I had become more "health conscious." I was off sugar and meat, and was eating lots of raw foods such as salads and fruits, and drinking lots of vegetable and fruit juices. The only dairy product I liked was ice cream, so the macrobiotic diet which does not use any dairy products appealed to me.

At the time I started eating macrobiotic food I considered myself in "relatively" good health. I now know that in fact although I had no symptoms I was very toxic. The only medical problems of which I was aware were two degenerated discs in my back and fibroids of the uterus. I think it was in 1975 when I first learned that I had fibroids; a condition that my mother and grandmother also had, perhaps a result of similar eating habits. I was told that if they remained small there was nothing to worry about. However, they continued to grow.

In September l986, after eight months of being on macrobiotics without any guidance, I went to see a macrobiotic counselor. He told me the diet I had put myself on was too narrow; I was eating the same thing every day. He suggested that I add more variety. He told me that some of my organs especially my pancreas, were cold due to past eating and that the degenerated discs in my back were due to lack of minerals caused by too many fruits and juices. He recommended eating more cooked, warming foods for my fibroids.

In November 1986, the doctor told me that the fibroids had grown so large that my uterus was the size of someone who was six months pregnant, and he recommended surgery. When I told him I was going to try to heal myself with the help of macrobiotics, he patted me on the back and told me, "Don't consider yourself a failure if it doesn't work, diet can't do anything for your problem." I walked out of his office, determined to prove him wrong and I decided to see Shizuko Yamamoto.

I went to see Shizuko for the first time at the end of November 1986. Having read

Elaine Nussbaum's book *Recovery*, I had an idea of what to expect. Shizuko examined me and told me that I had eaten too much animal protein and that all my organs (liver, kidneys, pancreas, and gallbladder) were full of fat. She recommended a fairly strict diet, which included carrot-daikon drink, very little protein, no desserts, and no baked goods. In addition I was to take hip baths for my fibroids.

I began to see Shizuko for shiatsu on a regular basis once every four or six weeks. My body began to detoxify. Some of the noticeable signs were a general tiredness, the palms of my hands and the bottoms of my feet turned yellow, my skin at times was dry and flakey, my face had a yellowish color, and my body odor Shizuko told me was that of burning fat. My fibroids, however, seemed to be getting worse. Shizuko told me not to worry that the fibroids which had been deep inside were starting to come up to the surface. Shizuko added acupuncture to my shiatsu treatment and recommended nightly taro plasters. I continued this way for about three and one half years. My basic condition continued to improve but my fibroids remained about the same. There were times, when I became a little discouraged. I kept hearing about all the people who had life-threatening illnesses and who seemed to be healing much faster than I was. The more I spoke to people, however, the more I came to realize that fibroids are one of the most difficult things to discharge. Shizuko was always encouraging and told me, "When you climb a mountain don't look to the top of the mountain and see how far you have to go, look back and see how far you have come."

I think the turning point in my condition came in April 1990. Shizuko suggested that I try fasting for a week to speed things up. At this point I was willing to try anything. So for one week, under Shizuko's guidance I fasted. For the first three days I drank ume-sho-kuzu tea three times a day, but by the fourth day I lost my taste for it so I just drank bancha tea. Twice prior to my becoming macrobiotic I had gone on a week long juice fast. This fast, however, was entirely different. While on the juice fast I felt nervous, this time although I was physically weaker I felt incredibly calm. The immediate results of my fast were that I lost eighteen pounds in one week, ten of which I gained back once I starting eating, and that I had a general feeling of calmness. Shizuko explained that one does not see the results of fasting immediately but that it takes some time for the body to react. In the year and a half since my fast my condition has definitely improved. My eyes and skin are clearer, my skin color is better, even the shape of my face has changed and my energy level has improved. My fibroids although not completely gone have been reduced to one third their size.

I consider myself fortunate to have been introduced to macrobiotics and to have been able to attend cooking classes, lectures, and dinners at the Macrobiotic Center of New York. But most of all there is no way that I could have healed myself without Shizuko's support and guidance. Healing oneself is not easy. It takes patience and discipline. The reward however is the realization that one's health is not a random event and that by accepting responsibility for one's condition, macrobiotics can be used to heal oneself.

7. Maggie Dukakis

It has only been three and a half weeks since I saw you and I feel like a new person. Every day I can feel that the pain in my back is getting less and less. I have been cooking and eating very carefully and walking five miles a day which also fills me with energy. Thanks so much.

8. Lilo Mandel

For over thirty-five years I had suffered with rheumatoid arthritis. After consulting various physicians and specialists I was always told I could not be helped; I must learn to live with it or take pain relieving pills. My usual weight was 140 pounds. I had an uneven pulse. I was on various medications: aspirin (sometimes eight a day for two weeks at a time), Darvon, and Librium.

Then I had my first appointment with Ms. Shizuko Yamamoto on May 19, 1974, and my life changed dramatically. The most important fact is: I stick to the macrobiotic diet, my weight never varies from 118 to 120 pounds. I take no medication at all, I have a steady blood pressure of 130/80 and no physical problems.

Ms. Yamamoto has saved my life with her shiatsu treatments, her advise on the macrobiotic diet, and her constant reminders on the importance of balance. Not least of all she is a concerned and encouraging healer.

I have followed this whole method faithfully for the past eighteen years and would not wish to change it ever. I feel better at age seventy-three than I did at twenty years.

9. Frances Alexander

During the period between 1979 and 1982 several doctors and many laboratory tests gave me the assurance of good health. Yet at times I got so ill, hurting from the top of my head to the bottom of my feet, my joints especially hurt. Because of my deep faith in Jesus, I knew there would be a solution yet I had not found it.

In 1982, Dianne Bitte told me about the East West Center in Eureka, California. I waited until December 9, 1983, after more tests showed me to be clinically healthy. I skeptically listened to Dianne tell me that the nightshade family of vegetables (potato, tomato, eggplant, and bell pepper) could be the cause of my hurts and aches. The time for my interview with Patrick McCarty came and what he explained gave me hope. He spoke of many things such as shiatsu, macrobiotic food preparation, energy and balance of food, and treatments. All these things are supposed to enhance life and he suggested this direction could be the solution for what was ailing my system.

This natural choice for healthy living seemed not merely rigid but impossible. Macrobiotic eating, thinking, cooking, talking, and shopping was and still is like being in a different country. It is like learning a new language. I had to overcome barriers of what I thought were former healthy eating habits.

I took shiatsu lessons from Patrick and macrobiotic cooking classes by his wife Meredith. I needed to hear this kind of information many times and still I do not have it down pat. My lifestyle of traveling hampers consistent macrobiotic living. Old habits of eating and cooking are hard to break. Yet, even under these circumstances I am a healthier person and not in constant pain as I was before. Now every muscle in my body is not under attack. Sharp stabs of pain do not start at a moment's notice. I sleep through the night now and rest peacefully. Yes, truly this is a new beginning for me at age of sixty years. Until my appointment to this life is over, I plan to be healthy on macrobiotics.

Appendix B: Procedure for Whole Health Macrobiotic Shiatsu Counseling Session

1. Talk with and question the patient.
2. Skin to skin test.
3. Abdominal palpation.
4. Look at the tongue.
5. Check the eyes.
6. Feel the pulses.
7. Examine the back (checking the Back—Yu and kidney acu-points).
8. Give shiatsu treatment (observing and noting any abnormalities).
9. Tell patient an assessment of his or her condition.
10. Explain dietary and lifestyle suggestions (exercises, breathing, and so on).

Appendix C: Further Studies in Macrobiotic Shiatsu

The study of nature will consume the investigator for a lifetime. In order to maximize your time we have developed several teaching and educational tools. With the development of an international organization, practice courses, books, and videos, we have attempted to share our many years of experience. It is our hope the following tools will help the serious student in the never-ending quest for mastery. We invite you to join us and continue on your study of life's mysteries.

International Macrobiotic Shiatsu Society

Started in December of 1985 by Shizuko Yamamoto and Patrick McCarty, the I.M.S.S. represents the combination of sound lifestyle practices and powerful shiatsu treatment. Membership in the society is available in the United States and Canada, as well as Europe. Currently there are active Macrobiotic Shiatsu Society affiliates in Belgium, Great Britain, and Germany with contacts in Sweden, Italy, Switzerland, France, Spain, and Yugoslavia. Macrobiotic Shiatsu literature has been translated into Spanish, Polish, Czechoslovakian, and Hungarian languages. Membership in the International Macrobiotic Shiatsu Society includes the society's newsletter, *Healthways,* three times each year; an invitation to the annual I.M.S.S. conference, currently each winter in the Bahamas; worldwide client referral service, and an opportunity to attend Shizuko Yamamoto's unique apprentice "Masters Program." To join and to find out the names of practitioners in your area write to: International Macrobiotic Shiatsu Society, 1122 "M" Street, Eureka, CA 95501–2442, U.S.A., Telephone 707–445–2290, FAX 707–445–2391.

Recommended Reading

McCarty, Meredith. *American Macrobiotic Cuisine.* Eureka, CA: Turning Point Publications, 1986.

————. *Fresh—from a Vegetarian Kitchen.* Eureka, CA: Turning Point Publications, 1989.

————. *Natural Bread Making.* Eureka, CA: Turning Point Publications.

McCarty, Patrick. *Beginner's Guide to Shiatsu.* Eureka, CA: Turning Point Publications, 1986.

Yamamoto, Shizuko. *Barefoot Shiatsu.* Tokyo and New York: Japan Publications, Inc., 1979.

Yamamoto, Shizuko, and Patrick McCarty. *The Shiatsu Handbook.* Eureka, CA: Turning Point Publications, 1986.

Video

Yamamoto, Shizuko. *Barefoot Shiatsu Video*. Eureka, CA: Turning Point Publications, 1991.

————. *Releasing Tension between Shoulder Blades Video*. Sugarman Productions, 1985.

Index